# STROKE SERVICES & RESEARCH

# An overview, with recommendations for future research

Editors:

*Charles Wolfe MD*

*Tony Rudd FRCP*

*Roger Beech PhD*

*United Medical & Dental Schools*

*of Guy's and St Thomas' Hospitals*

*London*

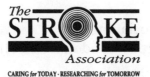

The
STR KE
Association
CARING *for* TODAY · RESEARCHING *for* TOMORROW

The Stroke Association,
CHSA House, Whitecross Street, London EC1Y 8JJ.
Tel 0171 490 7999 Fax 0171 490 2686

A catalogue record for this book is available from the British Library.

ISBN 0-901548-64-2

The Stroke Association raises funds for
Research, Prevention, Welfare, Information and Community Services.

Registered Charity No. 211015.

WL 355

© The Stroke Association 1996

Published by The Stroke Association,
CHSA House, Whitecross Street, London EC1Y 8JJ.

# FOREWORD

The Stroke Association carried out a comprehensive review of its stategy in 1996. It started by commissioning a review of the published literature on stroke services and research. The aim of the review was to identify gaps in services and knowledge about stroke, and to develop ideas for delivering practical services effectively.

The findings of this literature review provide an up-to-date overview, covering facts about stroke, services and economic evaluation. It will be of use to all those interested in developing services, carrying out services or caring for stroke patients.

I trust that this review will be read by many, to further the aim of The Stroke Association for equitable services for all aspects of stroke care by the year 2000.

*Sylvia McLauchlan, Director General of The Stroke Association.*

# Contents

Contents

# ACKNOWLEDGEMENT

We would like to thank The Stroke Association for funding this review. We are indebted to Claire O'Connor, Ana Childs and Carole Price for secretarial support, and Robert Wood for editorial assistance.

# BIBLIOGRAPHY

This review presents an overview of a range of issues and the authors have drawn on the published literature using MEDLINE searches in the relevant areas. We have also drawn heavily on local and European data from projects that we are currently undertaking as these are pertinent to any future stroke strategy.

There are certain key documents and previous reviews on stroke research and stroke services that were of particular importance and which readers will find invaluable:

- *Caplan LR. Stroke: a clinical approach. 2nd Edition. Butterworth Heinemann, 1993.*
- *Cochrane Database of Systematic Reviews. Stroke module, 1995.*
- *Ebrahim S. The clinical epidemiology of stroke, 1990.*
- *Effectiveness Bulletin. Stroke rehabilitation, 1992.*
- *King's Fund Consensus Statement on Stroke, 1988.*
- *Royal College of Physicians. Guidelines on stroke management, 1989.*
- *Wade D, 1994. Stroke needs assessment. In: Health care needs assessment Volume 1. Radcliffe Medical Press, 1994.*
- *WHO Consensus Conference on Stroke Management, 1995.*

# EXECUTIVE SUMMARY & PRINCIPLE RECOMMENDATIONS FOR RESEARCH & DEVELOPMENT OF STROKE SERVICES & RESEARCH

## Introduction

This book provides an overview of the issues spanning all aspects of stroke care. It draws on the published scientific literature, and local and European data on stroke care which are pertinent to the debate. The review has been compiled by a multidisciplinary group including medical practitioners (care of the elderly, neurology and public health medicine), a health economist, an operational researcher, therapists (physio, occupational and speech therapy), a psychologist and nurses.

The remit of the exercise was to undertake a literature review in order to identify:

• The faults or gaps, notably in the National Health Service (NHS) but more broadly in our knowledge, government policy, and individual behaviour, etc. to meet identified needs to prevent and manage stroke.

• Current ideas for correcting those faults or plugging those gaps.

• Existing evidence that the ideas are effective, thereby exposing areas where further research is necessary. Can the effective ideas be translated into practical and concrete services?

The review considers the evidence for preventive, therapeutic, rehabilitative and respite care; the current service provision for stroke and models of care for the future. Basic scientific research at the molecular and cellular level has not been reviewed but developments in these areas have implications for the development of future stroke services.

Each chapter is self-contained and is written such that readers need only read selected chapters should they wish. Consequently there is repetition, which the authors consider necessary for reinforcing key points.

The Stroke Association has achieved an enormous amount to raise the profile of stroke in the United Kingdom over the last few years. Of all the major killing and maiming diseases in this country stroke still has the least research funding and this fact needs to be reinforced to the public, government and health services.

**Levels of evidence**

In the UK there is a move towards using evidence based medicine to guide clinical practice and purchasing decisions with the establishment of the Cochrane Collaboration Centre and the Department of Evidence Based Medicine at Oxford University. The US task force on preventive health care has classified interventions on two scales with a rating both of the direction of the evidence in support of a procedure and the quality of that evidence. The strength of the recommendation ranges from good evidence to support it, to good evidence to support the rejection of the use of the procedure. The quality of the evidence ranges from grade one which includes evidence obtained from at least one properly randomised controlled trial or meta-analysis (I) through evidence obtained from well designed controlled trials without randomisation (II-1), evidence from well designed cohort or case controlled analytic studies, preferably from more than one centre or research group (II-2), evidence obtained from multiple time series with or without the intervention, from dramatic results in uncontrolled experiments (11-3), opinions of respected authorities (III) and lastly inadequate evidence owing to problems of methodology (IV).

This summary presents the areas which in the views of the editors should receive priority for funding. It is our view that the strategy of The Stroke Association should be to:

• Support research into all aspects of stroke from cell to the population.

• Promote stroke disease as an important area for funding by central government and the major research funding organisations.

• Promote the profile of stroke disease within the general population and to professionals who are involved in providing care to patients with stroke.

• Provide education and support to stroke patients, their carers and health and social service professionals.

It is important that the charity applies the same rigorous scientific and cost-effectiveness criteria to its own initiatives as well as those organisations it supports financially. No major new initiatives should be undertaken without formal evaluation.

Each chapter lists at the end priorities for research. A few of the key areas, where there are not already major projects underway are highlighted below. All projects should include economic evaluation and assess the patients' and carers' perceptions of care. We have now used the term 'evaluation' to mean a formal study with a hypothesis to be tested which is answering a question relevant to stroke. Evaluations can employ many methodologies, some of which are more appropriate than others depending on the aspect being studied and the question being asked.

It is considered that 'evaluations' will include the descriptive and analytical methodologies used by social scientists to explore such aspects as the 'black box' of rehabilitation, the views of patients, carers and professionals and quality of life. The use of case-series analysis to explore the inputs and outcomes of various forms of rehabilitation in depth is required but this would normally not substitute the need for randomised controlled trials. Case control and cohort studies are appropriate methods for the quantification of risk. Effectiveness is best assessed using randomised controlled trials and/or meta-analysis and this should be the norm for drugs, forms of rehabilitation and other health care interventions. Where a whole service requires assessment and a trial is not feasible a detailed descriptive study of the inputs to care and the outcome are required.

There have been significant changes at a Governmental level over the last decade. Stroke is now a *Health of the Nation* target, although stroke remains almost synonymous with cardiovascular disease in the minds of those developing preventive programmes in this area. The national Research and Development Programme has earmarked considerable funds for stroke research which it should be encouraged to continue over the foreseeable future and its efforts need to be co-ordinated with those of The Stroke Association.

## Summary of findings and recommendations

### *The burden of stroke*
Stroke is the third most common cause of death and the most common cause of adult disability in the UK. One man in four and one woman in five aged 45 or over can expect to have a stroke if they live to be 85. Much of the research to date has treated stroke as a single entity or at best ischaemic or haemorrhagic. Classification, for no very logical reason, has concentrated on the duration of symptoms and signs which probably has little relevance to the causation and mechanisms involved. The natural history and

long-term outcome of silent cerebral infarction, patients with multiple infarcts, small vessel disease and the other subtypes of stroke require clarification. Underpinning much of the future research must be a better understanding of the pathologies of stroke and better means of classifying them. Not only does there need to be clarification of the incidence of the subtypes of stroke but the natural history, prevalence and longer term outcomes require quantification if stroke service provision is to be based on accurate estimates of need. These estimates should be undertaken in defined populations and monitored over time. The definition of stroke type is of particular importance in the design of trials of therapy and failure to accurately define stroke type in the past may explain why few treatments so far have been shown to be effective. The major priorities for research are:

• The development of a classification of the subtypes of stroke that would be of use to researchers, clinicians and health service planners.

• The estimation of the incidence, prevalence, natural history (long-term particularly) and outcome of stroke subtype in the UK. These studies should be in contrasting locations to provide various estimates which take into account the effect of the different geographical and demographic characteristics of the population studied. Outcome should include disability, handicap and quality of life measures and be analysed alongside data on use of health and social services.

• The estimation of the prevalence and natural history of silent cerebral infarction is required and the relationship between silent infarction, multiple infarct dementia and clinical stroke established.

•The Stroke Association has a key role in lobbying the Departments of Health, Social Services and Education to raise the profile of stroke and to encourage the setting of realistic targets for improvements in the quality of care through service developments and research.

### Prevention of stroke
For too long stroke has been considered, particularly by epidemiologists, in the same breath as cardiovascular disease. Identification of separate risk factors for stroke, and especially the subtypes of stroke in different groups of the population, is fundamental to the development of a stroke prevention programme. Research should not just focus on the known risk factors but explore the role of, for example, environmental, genetic

and social factors on stroke risk. Preventive programmes should be tailored to the needs and aspirations of local populations. The development of effective methodologies to assess the requirement for, and implementation of, such strategies is a priority.

In secondary prevention the successes need further development. For example, the refinement of the criteria for carotid endarterectomy and anticoagulation with warfarin are required. The main priorities for research are:

• Cohort studies to establish the prevalence and attributable risk of risk factors in the various subtypes of stroke and in different groups of the population, particularly different ethnic and socio-economic groups.

• Studies evaluating the most effective way of implementing preventive programmes for established risk factors in district health authorities and general practices. These need to take into account attitudes and beliefs of the population to the proposed interventions.

• for The Stroke Association to play a role in maintaining the identity of stroke separate from cardiovascular disease.

### Stroke care

It is virtually impossible currently to estimate the true cost of stroke, be it to the health services, the sufferer and the family or society as a whole. Although there are estimates that 4-5% of the NHS budget are spent on stroke services it is not possible to assess the services inputs that stroke sufferers receive on a routine basis. Studies in Europe and surveys from The Stroke Association indicate that service provision is still haphazard, fragmented and often sub-optimal. Although the efficacy of many of the interventions may be unclear, there is current geographic inequality in the services that stroke patients receive. The current overall pattern of services cannot be cost-effective. Although the effectiveness of many of the potential interventions for stroke care is still to be clarified, the current variation in service provision implies that in some areas there is overprovision of ineffective services and in others underprovision of effective services. These implications demonstrate the need for developments in stroke care and for continuing research to identify which patterns of care are the most effective and cost-effective. The evaluation of the whole service rather than just its components is long overdue.

The information on the provision of services after the acute phase of stroke is paltry. Continuity of care between the primary and secondary care sectors is often lacking. There is evidence that nearly one in four residents in nursing homes are stroke sufferers. The links between the health and social services for stroke are few and far between, despite the introduction of the Community Care Act.

### Acute care

Management of an established stroke has not radically changed with the development of modern medicine and many areas of current practice are based on clinical intuition and tradition rather than research evidence. The emphasis still remains on preventing complications rather than any treatment that directly affects the pathology. The acute management of stroke to minimise cerebral damage is the subject of considerable research. The areas that particularly need addressing are aspects concerning the optimal way of delivering health care e.g. hospital or home, stroke intensive care beds or acute medical beds; the role of anticoagulation after stroke, for which there is a trial already underway, and the use of drugs to reduce oedema. The final results of some of the thrombolysis trials are awaited but so far the evidence for benefit is disappointing. Developments in pharmacology, particularly the NMDA receptor antagonists are showing promise. Interventional radiology, so effective in cardiovascular and peripheral vascular disease, may have a role in stroke and surgical intervention for cerebral haemorrhage requires further research. The future priorities for research are:

• The role of anticoagulation. The preliminary results of the International Stroke Trial have suggested that early anticoagulation at moderate doses is hazardous with regard to 14-day outcome, but that use of aspirin in the acute phase of stroke may have small benefits. Definite conclusions will not be drawn until final results are available in 1997.

• A trial of thrombolysis for stroke in evolution.

• Quantification of the extent and consequences of respiratory dysfunction after stroke and the effect of respiratory support when required to reduce potential hypoxic damage and chest infection.

### Rehabilitation

Well established rehabilitation services are available in the UK although access to them would appear to be less than optimal. These services are accepted as valuable by patients, carers and health care professionals, although often without scientific evidence. Withdrawing such services to undertake randomised controlled trials of treatment is considered by most people as unethical and it may therefore be that comparison with very different styles of service around Europe will be an alternative way of beginning to understand which forms of treatment are most beneficial to patients.

Rehabilitation has been shown to be more effective when provided in an organised way such as in a stroke unit. What is it about rehabilitation that works and would more of the effective components benefit the stroke sufferer? Is rehabilitation best provided in hospital or at home and if it is to be provided in both settings when should the transition occur? How long should therapy continue and does attention to quality early on in rehabilitation have any effect on long-term complications and levels of handicap? Is one style of physiotherapy or occupational therapy preferable to another or do different patients need different packages of care? If so how should these be defined and provided? Improvements in the clinical and radiological assessment of dysphagia and the development of percutaneous gastrostomy feeding have all occurred in recent years. These techniques need further evaluation so that clear guidelines for care can be implemented. Widespread introduction of supplemental feeding could result in improved survival of profoundly disabled people. Development of scales to predict outcome of treatment could be useful in such circumstances. Development of therapies for dysphagia to speed recovery are also required. A proportion of patients show a very prolonged pattern of recovery with improvement still evident at six or more months. Such patients are worthy of further study to elucidate the mechanism and help direct rehabilitation strategies.

The priorities for research are:

• A study to determine which components of the rehabilitation 'black box' are particularly effective for which subgroups of patients. Trials of increasing the dose of components to assess whether there is an impact on outcome are required.

• The development of clearly defined definitions and descriptions of what therapy involves.

• Randomised controlled trials of each therapy compared to no therapy, where feasible; otherwise comparing different models of care.

• A trial of prolonged rehabilitation either given continuously or intermittently to determine whether continued improvement can be achieved or deterioration prevented.

• Definition of the natural history of deficits associated with the stroke subtypes e.g. motor recovery, dysphagia.

*Psychology*

The psychological sequelae of stroke are considerable and it would appear there is an important gap in service provision in most hospitals and communities of psychology services. There is a need to train members of staff with regard to psychological aspects of stroke disease and counselling. Psychological support in the longer term is required which will necessitate the development of community services. Trials of the impact of early disorders of mood and cognition on recovery and outcome of physical function are a priority. In addition trials of pharmacological interventions such as SSRI antidepressants are needed. The interpretation of and reactions to stroke disease by patients and carers within and between different cultural groups needs to be investigated. The main priorities are:

• A study on the incidence, prevalence and natural history of cognitive, perceptual and other psychological problems following stroke, with particular attention to different ethnic and socio-economic groups.

• A longditudinal study to assess the impact of early disorders of mood and cognition on recovery and outcome of physical function.

*Nursing*

The role of the nurse and nursing techniques has received scant attention in the UK, and what has been written about has concerned the process of care rather than the effectiveness of any interventions. Nursing research in the area of stroke should be encouraged along with the evaluation of training methods in the care of stroke patients. The role of the nurse as part of the multidisciplinary team and in the rehabilitation process should be investigated. The priorities for research are:

• The provision of support for training of nurses in research methodologies applicable to stroke.

• The evaluation of methods of training nurses and the provision of information and support to carers.

• The Stroke Association has an important role in developing the concept of specialist nurse care. This may include the training of health visitors particularly in the prevention of stroke.

### *Primary health care*

The primary health care team is central to stroke prevention and the long-term management of disability and handicap. Unfortunately primary care does not appear to have taken on this role at the moment and there is a potential role in co-ordinating services for patients. Most of the research in primary care has focused on prevention but the role of the GP or practice nurse in the management of stroke patients has not been evaluated. There are particular areas that require consideration which include secondary prevention, detection of change in impairments and disability, and co-ordination of the rehabilitation of stroke patients. The priorities for research are:

• The audit of secondary prevention in primary care and the evaluation of different ways of delivering an effective secondary prevention service, with particular reference to anticoagulation.

• Evaluation of primary and secondary led care in the community for the management of long-term disability and handicap.

### *Families and carers*

With the current level of service provision for stroke that applies to most areas of the UK, the burden of support falls upon the family and carers. The evidence suggests the burden is considerable, but not well quantified. Evaluation of the need and value of providing information, emotional support and respite care is required. A formal study of the feasibility of multisectoral collaboration to provide a seamless service is long overdue. The outcome of the evaluations of The Stroke Association's Family Support Service should dictate the direction of developments in this service. The priorities for research are:

• The quantification of the need for and effectiveness of providing information and education for carers and families

• The evaluation of the effect of emotional support and respite care.

*Outcome*

There is an expectation in the health services that effective services will be provided and to assess their effectiveness, the components of quality require monitoring. Although the measurement of outcome is important, it has to be interpreted in the local context. There are currently limitations with the existing battery of measures used in stroke assessment and many have only been used in the research setting. The development of national guidelines on outcome measures for stroke that fulfil all the criteria of an effective measure are currently being discussed by a Royal College of Physicians Working Group. These measures need to be incorporated into routine practice. The relationship between the process of care and outcome requires considerable attention if planners are to be able effectively to change services to improve outcome. The development of proxy outcome measures should also be a priority as these may be more feasibly collected. The priorities for research are:

• The development of national guidelines on outcome measures for both patients and carers that fulfil all the criteria of an effective measure.

• Further development of effective patient and carer measures which sensitively estimate outcome and which can be used in routine practice.

*Health economics*

Considering the significant burden of stroke and the services required to manage stroke patients, very little attention has been placed on the health economics of the disease. This may be in part due to the lack of data on which to assess these aspects of stroke but in a health service where cost-effective options are the preferred ones for purchasing authorities, there is little evidence on which they can draw for stroke services. All future research should consider including an economic component. The cost burden of stroke both in hospital and the community requires quantification and the cost to carers should not be forgotten. In the short-term data should be collected which allow the variation between institutions in key services received by patients to be estimated. These data would allow a basis for cost comparisons and, by linkage with routine data on outcomes, a basis for identifying which patterns of overall care appear to be most effective. The priorities for research are:

• All future clinical research to have a health economic component where relevant.

• The development of health economic models for stroke that can be used to evaluate cost-effectiveness both in research and routine clinical practice.

*Models of stroke care*

There have been many documents written by individuals or groups about model stroke services which all strike the same cord. Unfortunately much of what is written is jargon, unsupported by evidence of cost-effectiveness and untried and untested. There would appear to be a current trend for purchasing authorities to undertake local needs assessments of stroke, duplicating effort around the country but putting stroke on the agenda. Perhaps what would be more effective would be for The Stroke Association, along with the professional bodies involved in stroke care, to agree models of service that could be evaluated in different locations before wider implementation. The key components to a model service are outlined in this review but many components and the service as a whole require formal evaluation. The training of health care professionals and support for carers are an integral part of such a service. Consideration should be given to the introduction of specialist medical and nurse training. A key aspect to any service should be to provide a co-ordinated service. The priorities for research are:

• The formal evaluation of a district stroke service, including an economic evaluation.

• Evaluation of the benefits of clinical co-ordination of stroke services, which should include the benefits of a clinical nurse specialist.

• Estimating the components of an effective team and the measurement of the 'chemistry' of a team.

*Conclusion*

Stroke is certainly higher on the nation's agenda than a decade ago but there is a long way to go. Research into prevention, treatment and rehabilitation must continue in parallel but evaluations of the provision of services are equally important if research findings are to be implemented effectively.

# The role of voluntary stroke organisations in service development

This chapter has so far outlined the research priorities in the field of stroke. It has stressed the need to evaluate services provided by voluntary organisations.

The organisations have a key role in lobbying politicians regarding the burden of stroke. Specifically, the areas that require discussion with Government departments include issues associated with prevention of stroke, acute stroke care and longer-term care.

In the area of prevention, the Government's policies on salt in diet, alcohol and cigarette consumption and education of the population with regard to stroke risk factors needs to be addressed.

In the area of acute care, voluntary organisations have a role in disseminating the evidence of effectiveness and trying to identify, with commissioners of health care, the inequalities in health care provision for stroke around the country. By linking with national initiatives on stroke care and professional bodies, powerful arguments can be developed to effect change at a local level. This is the prime role of such organisations rather than providing services in a haphazard way around the country to plug the gaps.

The voluntary organisations have a long history of providing support to patients, carers and families after stroke, although many of these services have not been formally evaluated. There are still inequalities in the provision of these services which require rectification. This may best be achieved by more formal collaboration with health and social services rather than the voluntary organisations working in isolation. Their role in facilitating, rather than purely providing, support services should be considered.

In collaboration with educators, professional bodies and local communities a strategy for teaching and training should be developed by the voluntary organisations. The strategy should incorporate the priorities for training and education outlined above. It is clear that health care professionals require training in stroke and families and carers require appropriate information.

## References

Report of the US Preventive Services Task Force. Guide to clinical preventive services. An assessment of the effectiveness of 169 interventions. Baltimore: Williams and Wilkins, 1989.

# CHAPTER 1

## THE BURDEN OF STROKE

Charles Wolfe

**Chapter outline**

## Introduction

This chapter will summarise the epidemiology of stroke, focusing on the gaps in current knowledge and outlining the need for effective services to reduce the identified burden of disease. There are many publications on the incidence, mortality and natural history of stroke and these will be reviewed but with a particular focus on the UK literature. The review has relied heavily on the comprehensive review of stroke for purchasing authorities by Wade (1994) which should be read for detailed estimates of the burden of stroke in a typical district health authority, although these are estimated using the limited data there is in the UK.

## Definition of stroke

For the purposes of the review the definition of stroke will be that used by the World Health Organisation: 'a syndrome of rapidly developing clinical signs of focal (or global) disturbance of cerebral function, with symptoms lasting 24 hours or longer or leading to death, with no apparent cause other than of vascular origin' (Hatona 1976). This definition includes subarachnoid haemorrhages but excludes transient ischaemic attacks (TIA), subdural haematomas, and haemorrhage or infarction caused by infection or tumour. It also excludes silent cerebral infarcts.

Asymptomatic cerebral infarction is often found in elderly people presenting with epilepsy and inpatients presenting with their first symptomatic attack (Roberts *et al.* 1988; Kase *et al.* 1989). Shinkawa *et al.* studied autopsy records in Japan and estimated that 12.9% of subjects had suffered a silent cerebral infarction and its frequency increased with age (Shinkawa *et al.* 1995). The subjects with silent infarcts were older, had higher diastolic blood pressure, and suffered atrial fibrillation more frequently than subjects in the non-infarction group. The autopsy rate in Hisayama was 82% at the time of the study and during the study period a stroke register had been functioning. Although several studies have reported the prevalence of silent stroke, most only describe the frequency of prior asymptomatic or unreported cerebral infarction on CT among patients with stroke (Ricci *et al.* 1993; Kase *et al.* 1989). Brainin *et al.* (1995) studying hospitalised stroke patients concluded that neither a history of transient ischaemic attacks, or evidence of silent infarct diagnosed at the time of the presenting major stroke in first-ever ischaemic stroke patients, exert an important influence on neurological or epidemiological outcome variables. On reviewing the evidence it would appear that epidemiological studies are likely to underestimate the total burden of cerebrovascular disease.

## Classification of stroke

There are various classifications of stroke that have been developed for varying purposes but there appears to be no classification which fulfils the criteria required by all those involved with stroke care i.e. health service managers, clinicians and researchers.

Routine NHS data are available in the Department of Health hospital episode statistics and Office of Population Censuses and Surveys (OPCS) mortality data (Department of Health 1995; OPCS 1995). These utilise International Classification of Disease (ICD) codes which are an eclectic grouping of pathological type, anatomical location and presumed cause (World Health Organisation 1977, ICD codes 430-438). They are reliant on doctors coding correctly and for health service use the subcategories are best amalgamated to describe 'stroke'. In the United States the drive to link resource use to case mix of disease has resulted in the development of Diagnostic Related Groupings which for stroke are clinically meaningless but perhaps relevant to resource allocation (Health Systems International 1986). In the United Kingdom, the Department of Health case-mix office has developed similar Health Resource Groups which use the ICD codes grouped together according to resource use and which are now starting to be used in the contracting process although their advantage over the ICD classification has not been demonstrated. The Department of Health is developing a classification of stroke based on the elements of care that are required for different categories of stroke; these 'Health Benefit Groupings' will be discussed further in the Developing District Services chapter and may represent a way forward, linking clinically relevant groupings with the resource elements of a stroke service.

It would be of importance both for treating individual patients and planning preventive services to be able to estimate the size of the underlying disease processes or risk factor(s) that led to the stroke. As the chapter on risk factors for stroke outlines, the risk attributed to individual risk factors is poorly estimated and for many individuals the disease has multiple risk factors. A useful clinically based classification has been developed by Bamford *et al.* (1991) in which prognosis is related to subtype of stroke and which has been repeated in other studies (Ricci *et al.* 1991). A pathological distinction between haemorrhage and infarction is most reliably made by CT scan within 7-14 days of the stroke (Dennis *et al.* 1987). Subclassification of infarction into thrombosis or embolism based on CT scan is not possible although an informed judgement based on further investigation can identify the possible source of emboli.

The severity of stroke is of clinical relevance for the management of individual patients and in predicting outcome in populations. There is no widely used categorisation of severity of stroke, but possibilities exist which require further investigation along with an assessment of their usefulness in planning services for individuals or groups of patients. The use of imaging techniques to assess the extent of cerebral damage and predict disability and prognosis have been described for CT (Allen 1985).

Much work has been performed to derive rules for predicting stroke outcome, such as those reviewed by Hier and Edelstein (1991). The predictors commonly studied have included impaired level of consciousness, extent of stroke, and neurological weakness, while demographic variables often have not been examined. Multivariable methods such as multiple logistic regression have been used to derive rules of prediction that efficiently combine information from the severity indicators. Gladman *et al.* (1992) validated five previously published multivariable models and estimated the predictive value to be between 50-75% which was not convincingly better than the 65% accuracy achieved by the initial level of consciousness alone. Taub *et al.* (1994), in a population based study, concluded that multivariable predictors of disability had little advantage over incontinence within 24 hours of the stroke as a predictor of one year outcome.

## Mortality

Stroke accounts for 10-12% of all deaths in industrialised countries. Some 88% of stroke deaths are in the over 65s. In 1992 there were 66,300 deaths in England and Wales from stroke, with 2,500 from subarachnoid haemorrhage (OPCS 1995). Stroke is the third most common cause of death in the United Kingdom after myocardial infarction and cancer (OPCS 1995). It was for this reason that the Government considered it an important public health issue and included it in *The Health of the Nation* targets (Department of Health 1992).

There are noticeable differences in the standardised mortality ratios (SMR) for stroke (i.e. mortality rates adjusted for age and sex differences in populations) between countries (Fratiglioni *et al.* 1983; European Community Atlas of Avoidable Deaths, 1991) and between regions of the same country. Japan has the highest cerebrovascular disease mortality rate. Finland, Scotland, Portugal, Northern Ireland, Austria and Czechoslovakia also have high rates. The USA and England and Wales have intermediate rates whereas Poland, Denmark, Sweden and Canada have low rates.

In the UK, SMRs vary considerably from 122 (Northern Region) to 83 (NW Thames) in males and 115 (Mersey) to 84 (NW Thames) in females (national SMR =100)(Public Health Common Data Set 1990). The relationship between the prevalence of risk factors and SMRs has not been investigated. Wolfe *et al.* (1993) did however demonstrate that the variation in the SMR for stroke in three health authorities of southern England was due to variations in incidence rather than case-fatality.

In terms of years of life lost as a result of stroke, in England and Wales between 1986-1990 an average of 36.6 years of life were lost per 10,000 male population and this varied from 26 in the Oxford region to 48.7 in the Northern region. In females the average was 29.5 ranging from 21.6 in South West Thames to 42.9 in East Anglia (Public Health Common Data Set 1991).

There has been a significant decrease in mortality from stroke over time and in the western world this started in the early 1900s and has accelerated in the past 30 years (Whelton and Klag 1987, Klag *et al.* 1989; Fratiglioni *et al.* 1983). In the US there has been a marked acceleration in the rate of decline in stroke mortality since 1973, consistent across all age-sex groups but an increase in the same period in Bulgaria by 42% and Poland by 59%. In an ecological analysis Whelton and Klag (1987) did not consider that the treatment of hypertension alone explained these trends but probably accounted for the acceleration in the decline seen in the US. The downturn in mortality after 1950 in the US and UK occurred prior to the widespread use of anti-hypertensive therapy, and some researchers believe that the treatment of hypertension may not be the principle reason for the decline in mortality, although it may be relevant to the accelerated decline since 1970 (Klag *et al.* 1989; Whelton and Klag 1987; Bonita and Beaglehole 1986). Others have, however, attributed this decline to the improved treatment and control of hypertension (Anonymous 1983). Are there any other plausible explanations for the decline in stroke mortality? The remarkable consistency of the change in slope in each age-race-sex group suggests some widespread environmental agent.

Wolfe and Burney (1992) challenge the assumption that mortality from stroke in England and Wales will remain constant or decline over the next few decades. A decline in stroke mortality could be brought about by changes in factors acting close to the time of death (period effect) or by risk factors determined by the generation into which a person is born (cohort effect). Age-specific death rates for stroke (1931-1985) in England and Wales were analysed to estimate the influence of these different effects. There were significant effects for age, period, and cohort on mortality from stroke with significantly different age and period effects in each sex. The effect of age was linear, with an increasing mortality with age in both sexes. Cohort analysis demonstrated a deceleration away from the previous trend in the mortality rates associated with birth cohorts born after 1980, followed by an acceleration in the trend of mortality rates in cohorts born after 1910. These relative increases in risk for cohorts born after 1910 were offset by a deceleration in mortality associated with periods from around 1951-1954. Since cohort effects are likely to be associated with a lifetime increase in risk of stroke mortality, it is difficult to predict the extent of any long-term fall in stroke incidence.

Factors operating around the time of death (period effects) may include methods of classifying and coding the cause of death (Miller and Kuller 1973) and the short-term effects of anti-hypertensive therapy (Klag *et al.* 1989; Garraway *et al.* 1983). Cohort effects include those risk factors which act early in life or which are characteristic of a given generation over a prolonged part of life. These might include smoking habits, alcohol use, diet, or the long-term effects of prolonged anti-hypertensive treatments.

# Incidences of transient ischaemic attacks (TIA), subarachnoid haemorrhage (SAH) and stroke

The incidence is defined as the number of first-in-a-lifetime strokes occurring per unit time. Most studies express an incidence rate per 1000 population.

## TIA

Although not part of this overall review, the relationship between TIAs and subsequent stroke risk must not be excluded. The incidence of TIAs is about 42 per 100,000 per year, about 80% being in the carotid territory (Dennis *et al.* 1989). The OCSP study suggests a risk of stroke of 11.6% over the first year following the first TIA, reducing thereafter to about 5% (Dennis *et al.* 1990). Forty per cent of the strokes following a TIA were in vascular territories not involved in the original TIA (Dennis *et al.* 1990). In Holland this figure reached 45% (Cillessen *et al.* 1993).

## SAH

The incidence is about 9-14 per 100,000 per year (Sandercock 1984-MD thesis). Other published estimates are as high as 33 per 100,000 per year for men and 25 per 100,000 per year in women (Sarti *et al.* 1991; Bonita and Thompson 1985).

The case-fatality rate is high, 46% within 30 days and 48% at one year (Bamford *et al.* 1990; Sarti *et al.* 1991).

## Stroke

Although there have been many population based studies of stroke most have had significant methodological flaws and Malmgren has outlined the criteria for an ideal register; only one UK study fulfilled the criteria, the Oxford Community Stroke Project (OCSP) (Malmgren *et al.* 1987; Oxford Community Stroke Project 1983; Bamford *et al.* 1988 and 1990). Although this study is the gold standard for incidence studies in the UK it commenced over 15 years ago when mortality rates were higher and the study area was predominantly in rural Oxfordshire with no ethnic minority groups. The fulfilment of all the Malmgren criteria may be ideal but much valuable information can be obtained by limiting the scope of a register. There have been two population based registers in southern England over the past few decades. Weddell and Beresford (1979) registered all stroke patients in 1971-2 who were registered with 38 local general practices in Frimley, Surrey. Patients were followed up for up to four years. A more recent register has assessed the variation in incidence of stroke in southern England but the study was restricted to those residents aged under 75, thereby studying only half of all possible strokes (Wolfe *et al.* 1993 and 1995). Data from these three studies form the basis of the epidemiology of stroke in the UK described here but all have their limitations and extrapolation of the results should be made with considerable caution.

The overall incidence of first-in-a-lifetime stroke is 2.4 per 1000 per year. The Oxford age/sex specific rates per 1000 population for first-ever strokes are shown in Table 1. These estimates are similar to other studies in the Malmgren review of the world literature and subsequent European registers including the recently published MONICA studies (Bamford *et al.* 1988; Malmgren *et al.* 1987; D'Alesandro *et al.* 1992; Thorvaldsen *et al.* 1995). The latter project has involved 16 European and two Asian populations. Age-standardised stroke incidence rates per 100,000 varied from 101 to 285 in men and from 47 to 198 in women. Stroke incidence rates were very high among the population of Finnish men studied. The incidence of stroke was, in general, higher among populations in eastern than in western Europe. It was relatively high in the Chinese population studied, particularly among women. The MONICA study has provided a unique opportunity to perform cross-sectional and longitudinal comparisons of stroke epidemiology in many populations. The present data show how large differences in stroke incidence and case-fatality rates contribute to the more than threefold differences in stroke mortality rates among populations.

In the UK, a one-year incidence study in three districts in southern England (Wolfe *et al.* 1993) demonstrated a significant difference in the incidence rates between district health authorities in those residents aged less than 65. Incidence was higher in the higher standardised mortality ratio districts and case-fatality was not significantly different (26% at three weeks). In a two-year incidence study in two of these districts (West Lambeth and Tunbridge Wells) there was a significant difference in incidence and after age and sex adjustments the inner city district had a 26% higher incidence rate than the average of the two and the rural district a 16% lower incidence rate than the average (Wolfe *et al.* 1995). The independent risk factors associated with the risk of having a stroke were increasing age, being male, living in West Lambeth and being black. It was not possible to estimate incidence rates by ethnic group over this time period as too few events had occurred. In this study the overall one year case-fatality rate was 36% among the under 75s. These studies highlighting differences in incidence rate would indicate that where the SMR for stroke is high there is a need to assess the prevalence of risk factors for stroke and develop a health promotion programme in line with *The Health of the Nation* strategy (see Chapter 2).

There are, however, considerable methodological problems to be taken into account when comparing data from different registers in different time periods with different methods of case ascertainment and follow-up. In the MONICA study there were ten centres with a low ratio of registered strokes compared with routine statistics of stroke mortality and/or with a low proportion of non-fatal out-of-hospital events of such a magnitude that clarification of such biases would be needed before these populations could be included in a comparative study. The proportion of non-fatal stroke cases diagnosed and treated out of hospital varied between 0%-16% and was 5% or less in 13 populations (Asplund *et al.* 1995).

The statistical methodology of 'capture-recapture' has been used to estimate the underestimation of cases for such chronic diseases as diabetes mellitus but it has not been researched for stroke (La Porte 1994). Data to enable such estimations to be made could be incorporated into stroke register data sets and provide a more objective assessment of the reliability of the case ascertainment.

The incidence of all acute strokes (first and recurrent) is in the region of 20-30% higher than the first in a lifetime rate (Herman *et al.* 1982; Bonita *et al.* 1984) with no recent UK data to draw upon.

### Incidences of subtypes of stroke

In most registers, particularly the older ones, the incidence by subtype has not been published. This may be in part because this subclassification had no particular relevance to clinical management but it will be important to estimate the effect of any acute stroke intervention and rehabilitation package on the various subtypes of stroke in the future.

Intracerebral haemorrhage (excluding SAH) accounts for just over 10% of all strokes, the remainder being cerebral infarction (Ricci *et al.* 1991; Bamford *et al.* 1988). Lacunar stroke syndrome constitutes about 21% of first strokes, and has a crude annual incidence of 0.33 per 1,000 (Ricci *et al.* 1991; Bamford *et al.* 1987). These stroke patients have a much lower case-fatality rate (10% at one year) and 66% are functionally independent at one year. The Bamford classification is purely clinical and may not be sufficiently reliable for some studies but is currently the best clinical classification available. It probably underestimates premorbid silent vascular disease and small vessel disease which may affect prognosis and the definition of lacunar infarction is arbitrary. Using the Bamford classification the following proportions of first strokes can be expected based on several studies (Ricci *et al.* 1991; Bamford *et al.* 1990):

*Cerebral infarction* 76%

Partial anterior circulation syndrome 56%

Lacunar syndrome 20%

Total anterior circulation syndrome 15%

Posterior circulatory syndrome 8%

Unclassified 1%

*Primary intracerebral haemorrhage* 10%

*Subarachnoid haemorrhage* 4%

*Not known* 10%

# Trends in stroke incidence and case-fatality

## *Incidence*

As described earlier, mortality rates have been declining since the 1950s but whether this reduction is due to reduced incidence or improved survival requires clarification. There have been few stroke incidence registers that have been maintained over long enough periods of time to document a change in incidence. Garraway *et al.* (1983) reported a 54% decrease in stroke incidence in Rochester, Minnesota, USA, between 1945-49 and 1975-79 but Broderick *et al.* (1988) reported a reversal in this trend with a 17% increase in incidence between 1975-79 and 1980-84. An increase in stroke incidence in younger women was also reported from a study in Soderhamn, Sweden, but the reverse was shown in a Danish study, in which an increase in incidence in men, but not women, was observed between 1972-74 and 1989-9 (Terent 1988, Jorgensen *et al.* 1992). Another Danish study, based on a randomly selected sample of an urban population who were followed up for 12 years, showed no change in incidence in men or women between 1976 and 1988 (Lindenstrom *et al.* 1992). Findings in Goteborg, Sweden, among people aged 15-65 years followed since 1971 were similar; in that study case-fatality improved during the same period (Harmsen *et al.* 1991). Bonita *et al.* (1993), reporting on trends in incidence in the 1980s in Auckland, New Zealand, estimated that there had been no overall change in rate but increases in younger women and reductions in older men.

Since stroke rates increase greatly with age and the number of elderly people is increasing, the burden of stroke on individual families, and the health services is unlikely to fall rapidly. Malmgren *et al.* (1989) estimated that between 1983 and 2023 in England and Wales there will be an absolute increase in the number of patients experiencing a first ever stroke of about 30%. There will be an increase in the number of deaths from stroke of about 40%, and there will only be an increase of 4-8% in the number of disabled long-term survivors. There can be an anticipated increase in the need for acute care and early rehabilitation services over this time period but not in longer term care.

The relationship of stroke incidence with the various demographic, biological, social and behavioural characteristics is discussed in detail in Chapter 2.

To summarise, the all-age first-in-a-lifetime risk of suffering a stroke is around 2.4 per 1,000 population per year. Stroke incidence rates rise exponentially with age (Table 1), with a 100-fold increase from the 4th decade to the 9th decade of life. Incidence rates vary significantly between countries but how much this is due to different methodologies employed in the different registers remains unclear (Malmgren *et al.* 1987). The cumulative risk of stroke - i.e. the lifetime risk of having a stroke (assuming no competing risks) - is calculated by means of life tables from age-specific incidence data. Bonita (1992) has estimated that the risk of a person 45 years of age having a stroke within 20 years is very low (about one in 30). However, almost one in four men and nearly one in five women aged 45 can expect to have a stroke if they live to their 85th year. Although the lifetime risk of having an acute stroke is higher in men than women, the converse is true for the lifetime risk of dying of a stroke. Thus about 16% of all women are likely to die of a stroke compared with 8% of men; this difference is largely attributable to the higher mean age at stroke onset in women, and to their greater life expectancy. Typically, first events account for about 75% of all acute events. The cumulative risk of recurrence over 5 years is high, ranging from about a third to almost a half of people who have a stroke.

**Table 1 AGE-SEX INCIDENCE RATES PER 1,000 PER YEAR**

| Age | Sex | SAH | TIA | Stroke |
|-----|-----|-----|-----|--------|
| 15-24 years | M | 0.039 | - | 0.02 |
| | F | 0.007 | - | 0.10 |
| | M&F | 0.023 | - | 0.06 |
| 25-34 years | M | 0.088 | - | 0.05 |
| | F | 0.053 | - | 0.12 |
| | M&F | 0.070 | - | 0.08 |
| 35-44 years | M | 0.161 | - | 0.26 |
| | F | 0.215 | - | 0.20 |
| | M&F | 0.189 | - | 0.23 |
| 0-44 | M | - | 0.02 | 0.08 |
| | F | - | 0.01 | 0.11 |
| | M&F | 0.04 | 0.01 | 0.09 |
| 45-54 years | M | - | 0.25 | 0.67 |
| | F | - | 0.26 | 0.46 |
| | M&F | 0.14 | 0.25 | 0.57 |
| 55-64 years | M | - | 1.22 | 3.47 |
| | F | - | 0.63 | 2.35 |
| | M&F | 0.16 | 0.92 | 2.91 |
| 65-74 years | M | - | 2.43 | 8.11 |
| | F | - | 0.90 | 5.84 |
| | M&F | 0.29 | 1.61 | 6.90 |
| 75-84 years | M | - | 3.01 | 15.87 |
| | F | - | 2.29 | 13.39 |
| | M&F | 0.39 | 2.57 | 14.34 |
| 85+ years | M | - | 0.70 | 18.42 |
| | F | - | 2.87 | 20.36 |
| | M&F | - | 2.38 | 19.87 |
| All | M | 0.105 | 0.39 | 1.50 |
| | F | 0.183 | 0.31 | 1.71 |
| | M&F | 0.144 | 0.35 | 1.60 |
| | UK population M&F | | ? | 0.42 |

From Wade DT 1994

## Case-fatality

Case-fatality measures the proportion of people who die within a specified period after the stroke; comparisons are based on the first-ever stroke in a lifetime since recurrent strokes have a higher case-fatality. One-month case-fatality rates are dependent on the age structure and health status of the populations studied and vary from 17-49% amongst men in the MONICA studies and 18-57% in women (Thorvaldsen *et al.* 1995) with an average of about 24% from the literature. In the UK the OCSP 28-day case-fatality was 19% overall, that for cerebral infarction being 10%, primary intracerebral haemorrhage 50%, and subarachnoid haemorrhage 46% (Bamford *et al.* 1990). About half the deaths within the first month are due to the direct neurological sequelae of the stroke (Bamford *et al.* 1990). After 30 days non-stroke cardiovascular disease becomes increasingly important and is the most common cause of death after the first year (Dennis *et al.* 1993). The one-year case-fatality rate in the OCSP study was 31% but with marked differences between subtypes: cerebral infarction 23%, primary intracerebral haemorrhage 62%, and subarachnoid haemorrhage 48%. The most important prognostic factors for survival are unfortunately not currently amenable to health service intervention (retention of consciousness, younger age, no history of stroke, urinary incontinence) (Bonita *et al.* 1988; Wolfe *et al.* 1993).

In the OCSP study the five-year survival rate was 55%, which compares with 52% (male), 60% (female) in the Framingham study, USA, 46% in Rochester, 28% in Moscow and 39% in Ikawa (Dennis *et al.* 1993; Sacco *et al.* 1982; Dyken *et al.* 1983; Scmidt *et al.* 1988; Kojima *et al.* 1990). Predictably, older patients have a worse absolute survival but, relative to the general population, stroke also increased the relative risk of dying in younger patients. In patients who survive the first month after a stroke, cardiovascular disease is the most common cause of death in the following 11 months (Dennis *et al.* 1993).

Data on trends in case-fatality rates based on epidemiological studies are scarce. A reduction of 50% in the 30-day case-fatality following stroke from 33 to 17% was observed in the Rochester study during the periods 1945-49 and 1980-84 (Garraway *et al.* 1983). Since some of the improvements in case-fatality occurred during the time when incidence was declining, increased detection of milder cases is unlikely to be the only reason for the observed changes. In the Soderhamn study, three-year survival improved by 15.4% and 5.5% for men and women respectively between the two study periods, 1975-78 and 1983-87; there was no difference in 30-day survival. Most of the long-term improvement occurred between two and six months after the stroke and was attributed to fewer fatal complications rather than a reduced risk of recurrent stroke (Terent 1989). In New Zealand the overall 28-day case-fatality declined from 27.1% to 21.9% in men and from 37.6% to 25.8% in women from 1981-1991, but the decline was not statistically significant in any age or sex group (Bonita *et al.* 1993).

## Prevalence of stroke

The prevalence is the number of stroke sufferers in the population. There have been very few prevalence surveys of stroke, the prevalence rates being estimated using the incidence and survival data from stroke registers. A cross sectional survey is the best method for determining the prevalence of a chronic condition such as a stroke. O'Mahony *et al.* (1995) validated a simple self-completed questionnaire to screen for cases of stroke in the community which they suggest could form the basis for subsequent studies of prevalence and health needs. Ten per cent of respondents reported a history of stroke and the question "have you ever had a stroke?" had a sensitivity of 95% and a specificity of 96%. It will be important to undertake surveys of prevalence using such methodologies as knowledge of the prevalence of stroke is necessary for determining the burden on patients, social services, health care providers and purchasers. This methodology would have the advantage of providing an estimate in a relatively short period of time although the detail of the health and social service inputs would not be as detailed as could be collected prospectively by a register.

There have been estimates of the prevalence of stroke, such as in Australia where it was estimated there are 5-8 stroke sufferers per 1000 population over the age of 25 years (Chrystie 1981). It was estimated that about 50% of prevalent survivors could use public transport unaided. Aho *et al.* (1986) estimated the prevalence of stroke in a Finnish population in the 1970s (Table 2 from Wade 1994). The overall prevalence rate was 6.4 per 1,000 (men 7.9, women 4.8). Of the 87% assessed for disability 24% had no significant disability, 33% only slight disability, 28% moderate disability, and 16% more severe disability. Overall, about 44% had difficulties with walking. A study in

Copenhagen estimated the prevalence to be 5.18 per 1,000 persons (Table 2) (Sorensen *et al.* 1982). Hillman *et al.* (1995) have reported preliminary findings of a survey in Nottinghamshire of stroke survivors living in the community. They used a postal questionnaire methodology and estimated a total prevalence rate of 46.8 (95% confidence intervals 42.5-51.6) per 10,000 population.

Table 2  PREVALENCE RATES OF STROKE FROM TWO STUDIES (Wade 1994)

| Age band | Sex | Rate per 1,000,000 | Age band | Sex | Rate per 100,000 |
|---|---|---|---|---|---|
| 20-39 | M | 98 | 20-44 | M | 160 |
|  | F | 88 |  | F | 110 |
|  | M&F | 93 |  | M&F | 140 |
| 40-49 | M | 417 | 45-54 | M | 750 |
|  | F | 235 |  | F | 250 |
|  | M&F | 322 |  | M&F | 500 |
| 50-59 | M | 745 | 55-64 | M | 2,290 |
|  | F | 716 |  | F | 1,480 |
|  | M&F | 728 |  | M&F | 1,870 |
| 60-69 | M | 1,648 | 65-74 | M | 3,860 |
|  | F | 845 |  | F | 1,490 |
|  | M&F | 1,170 |  | M&F | 2,490 |
| 70+ | M | 4,595 | 75+ | M | 2,750 |
|  | F | 1,628 |  | F | 3,510 |
|  | M&F | 3,157 |  | M&F | 3,240 |

# Impairment, disability and handicap

*The World Health Organisation definitions are used (WHO 1980).*

Impairment refers to abnormalities arising at the level of the organism. Impairments are usually the external manifestations of the pathology: the symptom and signs. Impairments are 'objective' and cover a wide range of states which carry no personal meaning to the patient: hemianopia, sensory loss, muscle weakness, spacticity, pain etc. Some medical and surgical treatments aim to reduce these impairments and these are outlined in Table 3.

About 40% of patients will have a reduced level of consciousness in the first 24 hours, with half being unconscious; about 80% will have a hemiparesis (Herman *et al.* 1982).

**Table 3 ACUTE (0-7 DAYS), THREE WEEK & SIX MONTH IMPAIRMENT/DISABILITY RATES (Wade 1994)**

| Phenomenon | | Acute | 3 Week | 6 Month |
|---|---|---|---|---|
| Impairments | Initial loss/depression of consciousness | 5% | - | - |
| | Not oriented (or unable to talk) | 55% | 36% | 27% |
| | Marked communication problems (aphasia) | 52% | 29% | 15% |
| | Motor loss (partial or complete) | 80% | 70% | 53% |
| Disabilities | Incontinent of faeces | 31% | 13% | 7% |
| | Incontinent of urine | 44% | 24% | 11% |
| | Needs help grooming (teeth, face, hair) | 56% | 27% | 13% |
| | Needs help with toilet/commode | 68% | 39% | 20% |
| | Needs help with feeding | 68% | 38% | 33% |
| | Needs help moving from bed to chair | 70% | 42% | 19% |
| | Unable to walk independently indoors | 73% | 40% | 15% |
| | Needs help dressing | 79% | 51% | 31% |
| | Needs help bathing | 86% | 65% | 49% |
| | Very severely dependent | 38% | 13% | 4% |
| | Severely dependent | 20% | 13% | 5% |
| | Moderately dependent | 15% | 15% | 12% |
| | Mildly dependent | 12% | 28% | 32% |
| | Physically independent | 12% | 31% | 47% |

**Note:** The 'acute' figures are of limited accuracy as many patients were not assessed within the first week; many of these were very ill and probably very dependent. Consequently the figures relating to acute disability are minimum estimates. These data relate only to survivors.

Disability refers to changes in the interactions between the patient and the environment. It is the behavioural consequences, which manifest within the patient's environment, or the personally meaningful functions or activities which are no longer executed, or are altered. Altered behaviours stretch from continence and turning over in bed to dressing and bathing and gardening, interacting with other people and specific work skills. In practical terms, especially in relation to health and social services, disability manifests itself as an increasing dependence upon people and/or environmental adaptations.

Most studies describe disability levels at three months and rarely longer term, although British studies have been good in this regard. In the 1970s Weddell and Beresford (1979) assessed a population in Frimley, Surrey, and estimated at three months that, of survivors, 81% were able to transfer, 12% drive a car, 75% walk out of doors and 20% to use public transport. These data are useful in defining abilities to perform specific activities but it is not possible to compare findings with later studies which have used the Barthel and Rankin scales of disability.

Some representative data of disability for the acute phase and six months are shown in Table 4 and taken from Wade (1994) using mainly UK data (Wade *et al.* 1989; Wade *et al.* 1985 a and b; Wade *et al.* 1987; Wade *et al.* 1986). The OCSP study has estimated the disability levels at one year. 65%(95% confidence intervals (CI) 61-69) of survivors were functionally independent, which varied by subtype: cerebral infarction 65%(95% CI 60-70%), intracerebral haemorrhage 68%(95% CI 50-86), and subarachnoid haemorrhage 76%(95% CI 56-96). Due to the small numbers involved these estimates are not robust. Martin *et al.* (1989) estimated that stroke was the most common cause of adult disability in the UK. The longer term outcome of stroke is considered in Chapter 13.

**Table 4 SOME FIGURES PER 100,000 POPULATION (PER YEAR WHERE RELEVANT) (Wade 1994)**

| | | |
|---|---|---|
| General - SAH, TIAs, stroke - diagnosed | Cases SAH per year | 14 |
| | New cases TIA per year | 42 |
| | - carotid territory TIAs | 34 |
| | First strokes per year | 200 |
| | All acute strokes per year | 240 |
| | Stroke survivors alive in community | 600 |
| | Presenting for diagnosis | Unknown |
| Impairment/disability- presentation (i.e. need acute care), all stroke | With reduced consciousness | 84 |
| | Severely dependent | 140 |
| | Incontinent of urine | 106 |
| | Disoriented/unable to communicate | 132 |
| | Unable to get out of bed unaided | 168 |
| Impairment/disability-at three weeks (i.e. need rehabilitation), all stroke | Needs help dressing | 86 |
| | Needs help walking | 67 |
| | Needs help with toilet | 66 |
| | Communication problems | 49 |
| Impairment/disability - at six months (i.e. needing long-term support) | Needs help bathing | 71 |
| | Needs help walking | 22 |
| | Needs help dressing | 45 |
| | Difficulty communicating (aphasia) | 22 |
| | Confused/demented (or severe aphasia) | 39 |
| | Severely disabled (Barthel <10/20) | 13 |
| Services - at six months | Needs long-term institutional care | 23 |
| | Possibly needs speech therapy | 24 |

**Note:** This assumes:
- all stroke, first and recurrent (2.4 per 1,000 per year)
- 30% die by three weeks
- 40% die by six months
- minimal contribution from SAH to care and rehabilitation needs

Handicap is the most difficult level to define and measure and is the change in social position which arises from illness; it also refers to the social, societal and personal consequences of the disease. It is the roles and expectations which are performed less readily if at all.

The outcome measures which have been used and advocated for stroke patients are described in the chapter on outcome in stroke. Levels of impairment have been well described in both hospital series and some epidemiological studies (Table 3). In the OCSP and other stroke registers the Barthel activity of daily living disability scale and the modified Rankin scale, purporting to measure handicap, have been used (Mahoney *et al.* 1965; Collins *et al.* 1968; Rankin 1957; van Swieten *et al.* 1988), probably inappropriately.

# Executive summary and priorities for research

This chapter summarises the epidemiology of stroke, and consequently the need for stroke services. Although much has been written on the epidemiology of stroke there are few good, current data available in the United Kingdom on which to plan service developments. Using the World Health Organisation definition of stroke it would appear that epidemiological studies are likely to underestimate the total burden of stroke, silent cerebral infarction not being included.

Routine mortality data are available but the coding by ICD subtype of stroke is virtually non-existent and the quality of these data in an ageing population is questionable. Recent NHS classifications used to determine groups of stroke patients rely on the inadequate ICD coded data and have no proven advantage and are not adequate for clinicians, researchers or health service managers.

Ten to 12 per cent of deaths in the UK are due to stroke and 88% of stroke deaths occur in the over 65s. Although there has been a decline in stroke mortality this century the reasons remain largely unexplained indicating the lack of knowledge there is on the risk factors for stroke.

The overall incidence of stroke is about 2.4 per 1000 population per year but these data are over 10 years old and estimated in a predominantly rural community. One in four men and one in five women aged 45 can expect to have a stroke if they live to 85. The incidence of the subtypes of stroke is poorly estimated. The variations in incidence between different geographical areas and groups of society are not known. It is this lack of precision in the estimation of the need for preventive and acute stroke services that hampers stroke service development. Robust estimates of incidence are required especially as over the next 30 years it has been crudely estimated that there will be a 30% increase in stroke incidence as a result of an ageing population.

The overall case-fatality rate is 24% at one month, 31% at one year and 55% at five years. The natural history by subtype is not well defined. More importantly estimates of the prevalence of stroke are based on incidence data and, again, robust estimates are essential if health and social services are to plan effective, equitable services for stroke sufferers and their families.

One year post-stroke, 35% of survivors are not functionally independent but studies have inadequately described the resultant handicap. The longer-term outcome of stroke is discussed in Chapter 13 but studies are few and not large enough to provide adequate estimates of the need for long-term support.

The following suggested areas of research could redress the current situation with regard to the epidemiological and clinical estimates of the burden of stroke. They are in order of priority:

1. The development of a classification of the subtypes of stroke that would be of use to researchers, clinicians and health service planners.

2. The estimation of the incidence, prevalence, natural history (long-term particularly) and outcome of stroke subtypes in the UK. These studies should be in contrasting locations to provide various estimates which take into account the effect of the different geographical and demographic characteristics of the populations studied. Outcome should include disability, handicap and quality of life measures and be analysed alongside data on use of health and social services.

3. The estimation of the prevalence and natural history of silent cerebral infarction and investigation of the relationship between silent infarction, multi-infarct dementia and clinical stroke.

4. The investigation of differences in the prevalence of risk factors for stroke in different geographical locations and groups of society.

5. Permanent monitoring of trends in cerebrovascular disease (mortality, incidence, prevalence) and its determinants for defined populations.

6. Investigation to achieve an understanding of the epidemiology of stroke in different ethnic groups.

7. The development of a stroke severity scale that could be used by researchers, clinicians and health care planners.

8. The development of tools of prediction that are sensitive enough for clinical use.

# References

Aho K, Reunanen A, Aromma A, Knekt P, Maatela J. Prevalence of stroke in Finland. Stroke 1986; 17: 681-6.

Allen CMC. The accurate diagnosis and prognosis of acute stroke. Correlation of clinical features with computed tomographic appearance and functional outcome. MD Thesis, University of Cambridge, 1985.

Anonymous: Why has stroke mortality declined? (Editorial). Lancet 1983; 1: 1195-6.

Asplund K, Bonita R, Kuulasmaa K et al. Multinational comparisons of stroke epidemiology. Stroke 1995; 26: 355-60.

Bamford J, Sandercock P, Dennis M et al. A prospective study of acute cerebrovascular disease in the community: the Oxfordshire Community Stroke Project. 1. Methodology, demography and incident cases of first-ever stroke. J Neurol Neurosurg Psychiatry 1988; 51: 1373-80.

Bamford J, Sandercock P, Dennis M, Warlow C. Classification and natural history of clinically identifiable subtypes of cerebral infarction. Lancet 1991; 337: 1521-6.

Bamford J, Sandercock P, Jones L, Warlow C. The natural history of lacunar infarction: The Oxfordshire Community Stroke Project. Stroke 1987; 18: 545-51.

Bamford J, Sandercock, Dennis M, Warlow C. A prospective study of acute cerebrovascular disease in the community: The Oxfordshire Community Stroke Project. 2. Incidence, case fatality rates and overall outcome at one year of cerebral infarction, primary intracerebral and subarachnoid haemorrhage. J Neurol Neurosurg Psychiatry 1990; 53: 16-22.

Bonita R. Epidemiology of stroke. Lancet 1992; 339: 342-4.

Bonita R, Beaglehole R. Does treatment of hypertension explain the decline in mortality from stroke? BMJ 1986; 293: 191-2.

Bonita R, Beaglehole R, North JDK. Event, incidence and case fatality rates of cerebrovascular disease in Auckland, New Zealand. Am J Epidemiol 1984; 120: 236-43.

Bonita R, Broad JB, Beaglehole R. Changes in stroke incidence and case-fatality in Auckland, New Zealand, 1981-91. Lancet 1993; 342: 1470-3.

Bonita R, Ford M, Stewart AW. Predicting survival after stroke: a three-year follow-up. Stroke 1988; 19: 669-73.

Bonita R, Thompson S. Subarachnoid haemorrhage: epidemiology, diagnosis, management and outcome. Stroke 1985; 16: 591-4.

Brainin M, McShane LM, Steiner M, Dachenhaursen A, Seiser A. Silent brain infarcts and transient ischaemic attacks. A three year study of first-ever ischaemic stroke patients: the Klosterneuburg Stroke Data Bank. Stroke 1995; 26: 1348-52.

Broderick JP, Phillips SJ, Whisnant JP, O'Fallon WM. Stroke incidence in Rochester Minnesota, 1945-84. The end of the decline in stroke? Neurology 1988; 38(Suppl) 146.

Cillessen JPM, Kappelle LJ, van Swieten JC, Algra A, van Gijn J. Does cerebral infarction after a previous warning occur in the same vascular territory? Stroke 1993; 24: 351-4.

Christie D. Prevalence of stroke and its sequelae. Med J Aust 1981; ii: 182-4.

Collins C, Wade DT, Davis S, Horne V. The Barthel ADL Index: a reliability study. Int Disab Stud 1988; 10: 61-3.

D'Alessandro G, Giovanni M, Roveyaz L et al. Incidence and prognosis of stroke in the Valle d'Aosta, Italy. Stroke 1992; 23: 1712-15.

Dennis MS, Bamford JM, Molyneux AJ, Warlow CP. Rapid resolution of signs of primary intracerebral haemorrhage in computed tomograms of the brain. BMJ 1987; 295: 379-81.

Dennis MS, Bamford JM, Sandercock PAG, Warlow CP. Incidence of transient ischaemic attacks in Oxfordshire, England. Stroke 1989; 20: 333-9.

Dennis MS, Bamford JM, Sandercock PAG, Warlow CP. Prognosis of transient ischaemic attacks in the Oxfordshire Community Stroke Project. Stroke 1990; 21: 848-53.

Dennis MS, Burn JPS, Sandercock AG et al. Long-term survival after first-ever stroke: The Oxfordshire Community Stroke Project. Stroke 1993; 24: 796-800.

Department of Health. Hospital Episode Statistics. Volumes 1 and 2. England. Financial year 1993-94. Leeds: Department of Health, 1995.

Department of Health. The Health of the Nation: a strategy for health in England. (Cm 1989) London: HMSO, 1992.

Dyken ML. Natural history of ischaemic stroke in cerebrovascular disease. In: Harrison MJG, Dyken ML (eds): Butterworth International Medical Reviews: Neurology, edition 3, London, Butterworth 1983, pp 139-170.

European Community Atlas of Avoidable Deaths. 2nd Edition. Project Director WW Holland. Oxford University Press. Oxford 1991.

Fratiglioni L, Massay E, Shoenberg D, Shoenberg B. Mortality from cerebrovascular disease. Neuroepidemiol 1983; 2: 281-311.

Garraway W. Whisnant J, Drury I. The continuing decline in the incidence of stroke. Mayo Clin Proc 1983; 58: 520-3.

Garraway WM, Whisnant JP, Drury I. The changing pattern of survival following stroke. Stroke 1983; 14: 699-703.

Gladman JRF, Harwood DMJ, Barer DH. Predicting the outcome of acute stroke: prospective evaluation of five multivariate models and comparison with simple methods. J Neurol Neurosurg Psychiatry 1992; 55: 347-51.

Harmsen P, Tsipogianni A, Wilhelmsen L. Stroke incidence rates were unchanged, while fatality rates declined, during 1971-1987 in Goteborg, Sweden. Stroke 1991; 23: 1410-5.

Hatona S. Experience from a multicenter stroke register: a preliminary report. Bull WHO 1976; 54: 541-53.

Health Systems International. Diagnostics Related Groups, 3rd revision: definitions manual. New Haven, Connecticut: Health Systems International, 1986.

Herman B, Leyten ACM, Van Luijk JH, Frenken CWGM, Op de Coul AAW, Schulte BPM. Epidemiology of stroke in Tilburg, The Netherlands. The population-based stroke incidence register: 2. Incidence, initial clinical picture and medial care, and three-week case fatality. Stroke 1982; 13: 629-34.

Hier DB, Edelstein G. Deriving clinical prediction rules from stroke outcome research. Stroke 1991; 22: 1431-6.

Hillman M, Geddes JML, Tennant A, Chamberlain MA. Benefits and services; Stroke survivors living in the community. Stroke Association Annual Scientific Conference. London 1995.

Jorgensen HS, Plesner AM, Hubbe P, Larsen K. Marked increase of stroke incidence in men between 1972 and 1990. Frederiksberg, Denmark. Stroke 1992; 23: 1701-4.

Kase CS, Wolf PA, Chodosh EH, Zacher HB, Kelly-Hayes M, Kannel WB, D'Agostino PB, Scampini L. Prevalence of silent stroke in patients presenting with initial stroke: the Framingham Study. Stroke 1989; 20: 850-2.

Klag MJ, Whelton PK, Seidler AJ. Decline in US stroke mortality. Demographic trends and antihypertensive treatment. Stroke 1989; 20: 14-21.

Kojima S, Omura T, Wakamatsu W, Kishi M, Yamazaki T, Iida M, Komachi Y: Prognosis and disability of stroke patients after 5 years in Akita, Japan. Stroke 1990; 21: 72-7.

La Porte RE. Assessing the human condition: Capture-recapture techniques. BMJ 1994; 308: 5-6.

Lindenstrom E, Boysen G, Nyboe J, Appleyard M. Stroke incidence in Copenhagen, 1976-1988. Stroke 1992; 23: 28-32.

Mahoney FI, Barthel DW. Functional evaluation. The Barthel Index. Maryland State Med J 1965; 14: 61-5.

Malmgren R, Bamford J, Warlow C, Sandercock P, Slattery J. Projecting the number of patients with first ever strokes and patients newly handicapped by stroke in England and Wales. BMJ 1989; 298: 656-60.

Malmgren R, Bamford J, Warlow C, Sandercock P. Geographical and secular trends in stroke incidence. Lancet 1987; ii: 1196-200.

Martin J, White A, Meltzer H. Office of population censuses and surveys. Disabled adults: services, transport and employment (report 4, Disability in Greater Britain). London: HMSO, 1989.

Miller GD, Kuller LH. Trends in mortality from stroke in Baltimore, Maryland: 1940-1941 through 1968-1969. Am J Epidemiol 1973; 98: 233-42.

O'Mahony PG, Dobson R, Rodgers H, James OFW, Thomson RG. Validation of a population screening questionnaire to assess prevalence of stroke. Stroke 1995; 26: 1334-7.

Office of Population Censuses Surveys. Series DH 2 no.19. Mortality statistics causes. England and Wales 1992. London: HMSO, 1995.

Oxford Community Stroke Project. Incidence of stroke in Oxfordshire: first year's experience of a community stroke register. BMJ 1983; 287: 713-7.

Public Health Common Data Set 1958-9. Office of Population Censuses and Surveys. Department of Health 1990.

Rankin J. Cerebral vascular accidents in patients over 65. 2. Prognosis. Scot Med J 1957; 2: 200-15.

Report of the US preventive Services Task Force. Guide to clinical preventive services. An assessment of the effectiveness of 169 interventions. Baltimore: Williams and Wilkins, 1989.

Ricci S, Celani MG, La Rosa F et al. SEPIVAC: a community-based study of stroke incidence in Umbria, Italy. J. Neurol, Neurosurg Psychiatry 1991; 54: 695-8.

Ricci S, Celani MG, La Rosa F, Righetti E, Duca E, Caputo N. Silent brain infarctions in patients with first ever stroke: a community based study in Umbria, Italy. Stroke 1993; 24: 647-651.

Roberts RC, Shorvon SD, Cox TCS, Gilliat RW. Clinically unsuspected cerebral infarction revealed by computed tomography scanning in late onset epilepsy. Epilepsia 1988; 29: 190-4.

Sacco RL, Wolf PA, Kannel WB, McNamara PM. Survival and recurrence following stroke: The Framingham Study. Stroke 1982; 13: 290-6.

Sandercock PAG. The Oxfordshire Community Stroke Project and its application to stroke prevention. The University of Oxford, MD Thesis, 1984.

Sarti C, Tuomilehto J, Salomaa V et al. Epidemiology of subarachnoid haemorrhage in Finland from 1983 to 1985. Stroke 1991; 22: 848-53.

Scmidt EV, Smirnov VE, Ryabova VS. Results of the seven-year prospective study of stroke patients. Stroke 1988; 19: 942-9.

Shinkawa A, Ueda K, Kiyohara Y et al. Silent cerebral infarction in a community-based autopsy series in Japan. The Hisayama Study. Stroke 1995; 26: 380-5.

Sorensen PS, Boysen G, Jensen G, Schnohr P. Prevalence of stroke in a district of Copenhagen: The Copenhagen City Heart Study. Acta Neurol Scand 1982; 66: 68-81.

Taub NA, Wolfe CDA, Richardson E, Burney PGJ. Predicting the disability of first-time stroke sufferers at 1 year. Stroke 1994; 25: 352-7.

Terent A. Survival after stroke and transient ischaemic attacks during the 1970s and 1980s. Stroke 1989; 20: 1320-6.

Terent A. Increasing incidence of stroke among Swedish women. Stroke 1988; 19: 598-603.

Thorvaldsen P, Asplund K, Kuutasmaa K, Rajaknagas AM, Schroll M, for WHO MONICA Project. Stroke 1995; 26: 361-7.

Van Swieten JC, Koudstaal PJ, Visser MC, Schouten HJA, Van Gijn J. Interobserver agreement for the assessment of handicap in stroke patients. Stroke 1988; 19: 604-7.

Wade D. Stroke (acute cerebrovascular disease) in Health Care Needs Assessments vol 1. Ed Stevens A, Raftery J. Radcliffe Medical Press, Oxford 1994.

Wade DT, Langton-Hewer R. Functional abilities after stroke: measurement, natural history and prognosis. J Neurol, Neurosurg Psychiatry 1987; 50: 177-82.

Wade DT, Langton-Hewer R. Outcome after an acute stroke: urinary incontinence and loss of consciousness compared in 532 patients. Q J Med 1985b; 221: 347-52.

Wade DT, Langton-Hewer R, Skilbeck CE, Bainton D, Burns-Cox C. Controlled trial of home care service for acute stroke patients. Lancet 1985a; 1: 323-6.

Wade DT, Parker V, Langton-Hewer R. Memory disturbance after stroke; frequency and associated losses. Int Rehab Med 1986; 8: 60-4.

Wade DT, Skilbeck CE, Langton-Hewer R. Selected cognitive losses after stroke. Frequency, recovery and prognostic importance. Int Disability Stud 1989; 11: 34-9.

Weddell JM, Beresford AA, Planning for stroke patients. A four-year descriptive study of home and hospital care. Department of Health and Social Security. HMSO 1979.

Whelton PJ and Klag MJ. Recent trends in the epidemiology of stroke: what accounts for the stroke decline in Western nations? Curr Opin Cardiol 1987; 2: 741-7.

Wolfe CDA, Burney PGJ. Is stroke mortality on the decline in England? Am J Epidemiol 1992; 136: 558-65.

Wolfe CDA, Taub NA, Bryan S, Beech R, Warburton F, Burney PGJ. Variations in the incidence, management and outcome of stroke in residents under the age of 75 in two health districts of Southern England. J Pub Health Med 1995; 17: 411-8.

Wolfe CDA, Taub NA, Woodrow J, Richardson E, Warburton FG, Burney PGJ. Does the incidence, or case fatality of stroke vary in southern England? J Epidemiol Community Health 1993; 47: 139-143.

World Health Organisation. International classification of disease, 9th revision, volume 1. London: HMSO, 1977.

World Health Organisation. The international classifications of impairments, disabilities and handicaps. WHO, Geneva, 1980.

# CHAPTER 2

# THE EFFECTIVENESS OF MEASURES AIMED AT REDUCING THE INCIDENCE OF STROKE

*Charles Wolfe, Nada Stojcevic, Judy Stewart*

**Chapter outline**

## Introduction

As the mortality and disability that result from stroke are considerable (Chapter 1), strategies for prevention in communities should form the basis of public health policy. In the United Kingdom care of stroke patient consumes approximately 4% of the National Health Service (NHS) budget. However, effective medical and surgical treatments for most types of stroke are a long way off. The effectiveness of many of the components of rehabilitation are also uncertain.

Many of the risk factors identified for stroke have been those also associated with coronary heart disease, having been identified in observational studies mainly considering coronary heart disease outcome, such as the Multiple Risk Factor and Intervention Trial (MRFIT 1990) and Framingham studies (Wolf *et al.* 1986). There are risk factors which are specific to stroke and generally the attributable risk fraction of these have not been accurately estimated. Most studies have only considered the risk factors for total stroke or for ischaemic strokes and relative risks are weighted towards describing the risk factors for thrombotic events, which do, however, constitute 76% of strokes.

The risk factors identified through cohort and case control studies will be outlined along with the evidence from randomised controlled trials and community intervention projects of the effectiveness of risk factor reduction on stroke incidence and mortality. Public health physicians can use the evidence from these studies to devise risk factor reduction strategies for stroke which will be in keeping with targets for stroke outlined in *The Health of the Nation* (Department of Health 1992). Strategies should also be developed in primary care to deal with high risk individuals and through initiatives involving multisectoral collaboration to encourage healthier life styles for the whole population.

When planning services to reduce the incidence of stroke and mortality from stroke it is necessary to be cognisant of those factors not currently amenable to reduction by health service interventions and that continuing research is required to further elucidate the causes of the different types of stroke.

# The changing epidemiology of stroke in relation to risk factors

In Chapter 1 the geographical variations in stroke mortality were described. Research is required to elucidate how much of this is due to variation in the prevalence of risk factors for stroke in the different areas. The fall in mortality from stroke, although encouraging, remains largely unexplained and recent incidence data do not suggest that the decline is continuing.

# Classification of types of risk factors

When considering risk factors for stroke it is important to distinguish between factors which are amenable to reduction and those which are not. In the former group the evidence on how to effectively reduce their prevalence will be presented. The broad categories under which risk can be considered are outlined:

**1. Inherited biological traits. (Table 1)**

These include age, sex and genetic predisposition.

**2. Social characteristics. (Table 2)**

These include ethnic background with cultural effects and socio-economic status. These traits overlap with behavioural and biological factors.

**3. Environmental factors.**

Factors such as temperature and other climatic variables which may affect seasonal and geographical variations in stroke incidence and mortality.

**4. Physiological characteristics. (Table 3)**

These include blood pressure, serum factors such as cholesterol and glucose and obesity.

**5. Behavioural characteristics. (Table 4)**

These include smoking, alcohol intake, dietary factors and the use of the oral contraceptive and hormone replacement therapy.

## 1. Inherited biological traits

*Age:*

Both in the US and UK the risk of stroke doubles with each successive decade over the age of 55 (Robins and Baum 1981; Oxfordshire Community Stroke Project (OCSP), 1983). In the UK population projections predict an increasingly aged population, at increased risk of stroke. Malmgren and colleagues (1989) estimate, however, that this will result in a net increase of only 4% of moderately or severely handicapped individuals. The incidence rates increase from 0.2/1000 population per year aged 45-54 to 10/1000 in people aged over 85 (OCSP 1983).

*Sex:*

The Framingham study demonstrated an overall 30% increased incidence in men compared with women, which was slightly higher in those aged under 65 (Wolf *et al.* 1986). In the Oxfordshire Community Stroke Project in the UK, the odds of a male sustaining a first stroke were 26% greater than that of a female (Bamford *et al.* 1988).

Fetal and infant influences: Some groups have attributed the inequalities in health seen in Great Britain to fetal and infant influences (Barker 1991). There is controversy over the early origins of cardiovascular disease (Robinson 1992). Traditionally, factors related to lifestyle have been blamed and operate mainly in adult life but attention has now focused on factors in fetal life. Barker and his colleagues, using longitudinal data of 50 year olds whose birth records were available, suggest that fetal growth, and growth and nutrition in infancy, importantly affect risk factors for cardiovascular disease in later life (Barker *et al.* 1990). Stroke is also linked to earlier maternal and neonatal mortality (Barker and Osmond 1987). The risk factors thought to be influenced by early life include plasma concentrations of cholesterol, apolipoprotein B, fibrinogen, blood pressure, body fat distribution and impaired glucose tolerance (Barker *et al.* 1992). The authors suggest that factors influencing infant mortality along with factors associated with later affluence account for the pattern of stroke incidence. Critics suggest these ecological studies fail to take fully into account the continuing social disadvantages in these areas (Elford *et al.* 1991 and 1992). The effect of migration as described by the British Regional Heart Study suggested, contrary to the findings of Osmond *et al.* (1990), that where men live is more important than where they were born in determining blood pressure (Elford *et al.* 1990) and mortality from ischaemic heart disease (Elford *et al.* 1989). The data used by Barker *et al.* is from selected populations with variable follow-up periods and the validity of the routinely collected data cannot be assessed.

A study from Israel failed to show the relationship between birthweight and blood pressure at the age of 17 previously found in several population groups at different ages by Barker and his colleagues (Barker *et al.* 1989, 1991; Law *et al.* 1991; Seidman *et al.* 1991). However the British Regional Heart Study also reported that the pattern of systolic blood pressure differences in children was similar to that observed in the study of middle aged men and concluded that the geographical differences in blood pressure observed in British men may have its origins in early life (Whincup *et al.* 1988). If this shift in paradigm for the origins of cardiovascular and cerebrovascular disease is correct, research and treatment of intrauterine pathologies may be an alternative strategy to the activities of risk factor reduction in middle life. However, more detailed studies of these influences on cardiovascular and stroke risk factors in childhood and early adulthood are required.

Migration studies of Japanese men living in Japan, Hawaii and California have shown the 'paradoxical' occurrence of high rates of stroke and low rates of coronary heart disease observed in Asian populations. Reed (1990) infers that the high risk of stroke is not due to atherosclerosis in the major cerebral arteries. Rather, it is more likely due to lesions in the small intracerebral arteries and appears to be related to low levels of serum cholesterol, high alcohol intake, and some aspects of a traditional oriental diet.

*Family history:*
A family history of stroke in any first degree relative was an independent predictor of stroke in women only of a middle-class Caucasian cohort, with a relative risk of 2.3 after controlling for age, cholesterol, blood pressure, cigarette smoking and diabetes (Khaw and Barrett-Connor 1986). Welin and colleagues (1987), in a Swedish cohort study of middle-aged men, demonstrated that men with mothers who had died of a stroke had a three-fold increased risk of stroke and the population attributable risk was estimated to be 0.19. Studies of the occurrence of stroke among twins indicate that stroke deaths are up to 20 times more common than expected in both monozygotic and dizygotic twins which implies that a shared family environment is an extremely strong risk factor for stroke (De Faire *et al.* 1975).

Bromberg *et al.* (1995) estimated that subarachnoid haemorrhage (SAH) occurs almost seven times more often in first-degree relatives than in second-degree relatives and this is the first report to distinguish between the type of relative and risk. This means that the lifetime risk of subarachnoid haemorrhage is between 2% and 5% in first-degree relatives. Therefore, screening for unruptured aneurysms should at least be considered in first-degree relatives of patients with subarachnoid haemorrhage.

The genetic basis for stroke is not known although sporadic reports are now emerging describing the prevalence of various genes in stroke patients. Without adequate data on control subjects these data are difficult to interpret. This emerging field of molecular biology is considered to be an important issue for the future but is not dealt with further in this review.

Table 1  INHERITED BIOLOGICAL TRAITS

| Factor | Relative Risk |
| --- | --- |
| Male | 1.3 |
| Age (55-64 vs. 75+) | 5 |
| Family history | 2.3 |
| - SAH | 7 |

## 2. Social characteristics

*Socio-economic status (SEC):*
In the United Kingdom Acheson and Sanderson (1978) estimated a relative risk of 1.6 in the lowest (SEC V) compared with the highest (SEC 1) group. There is also a tendency for the SMR for stroke to be higher in northern regions of the UK and inner-city districts where the highest proportion of SEC IV and V reside (European Community Atlas of Avoidable Deaths 1991). This may reflect numerous factors such as social deprivation, environmental and geographical differences and dietary differences. The British Regional Heart Study found no significant difference in stroke risk between socio-economic groups after adjustment for other risk factors (Shaper *et al.* 1991).

### Ethnic group:

In the United States mortality data consistently show higher death rates from stroke amongst black communities, probably partly because of a higher prevalence of ischaemic heart disease and hypertension in these communities (Comstock 1957; Otten *et al*. 1990; Fray and Douglas 1993; Deubner *et al*. 1975; Gaines *et al*. 1995). In the US Kittner *et al*. (1990) documented a relative risk of stroke incidence of 1.4 for black females and 1.1 for black males after adjustment for age, hypertension and diabetes mellitus. The possibility that a specific type of stroke accounts for racial differences has been suggested (Heyman *et al*. 1971). Even amongst black communities, there is an association between darker skin colour and hypertension in lower socio-economic groups (Klag *et al*. 1991). Wang *et al*. (1991) advocate that sickle cell patients who have had a stroke must receive long-term transfusions indefinitely to reduce the risk of recurrence although this recommendation is not based on trial evidence.

Balarajan (1991) demonstrated significantly differing mortality rates between ethnic groups in England and Wales. In general, ethnic groups that experienced lower mortality rates from ischaemic heart disease in the 1970s showed the greatest improvement over the following decade. For ischaemic heart disease the highest rates were observed in those of Indian origin. Those born in the Caribbean, United States, old Commonwealth and Western Europe had the lowest rates. For stroke the highest rates were in Afro-Caribbeans followed by Africans, Indians and Irish and showed a decline of 28% from 1970-2 to 1979-83. There were, however, classification problems in this analysis and no adjustment was made for social class or other factors. These data only relate to country of origin and not ethnic group and therefore do not take into account the second generation ethnic groups. The highest mortality rates for stroke are in Indian men (53% above the national average) and Indian women (25% above the national average). These data reinforce the need to establish the prevalence of the more conventional risk factors for stroke in large representative samples of these communities. A 76% excess of deaths in Caribbean men has been reported by Cruickshank *et al* (1980). These observed differences in mortality have never been satisfactorily explained (Cruickshank *et al*. 1980; Marmot *et al*. 1984).

In Britain, the Northwick Park Heart Study examined the blood pressure of factory workers in north-west London and found that black workers had higher blood pressure than white workers on the day-shift, but no difference in blood pressure between night-shift workers. They also found that blacks had 55% lower plasma renin than whites (Meade *et al.* 1978). Sever *et al.* (1979) investigated 115 factory workers and found that blood pressure was higher in blacks than whites and rose with age in both groups. Cruickshank reported a 76% excess of deaths from stroke and cardiovascular disease in Caribbean men and these high rates are in accordance with the high levels of blood pressure in these subjects, particularly in younger age groups (Cruickshank 1980, 1985, 1991). A study by Chaturvedi *et al.* (1993) found median systolic blood pressure in Afro-Caribbean men to be 6mmHg higher than in European men and 17mmHg higher in Afro-Caribbean women than in European women. Haines *et al.* (1987), however, did not find a significant difference between blood pressure levels in white and black subjects attending a London inner-city general practice, but more blacks than whites were being treated for hypertension. Some authors have argued that there is no difference in the mean blood pressure between the different ethnic groups studied, but that rather more blacks than whites may have a blood pressure above a given cut-off value for hypertension. The effect of different ethnic group observers on blood pressure measurement needs to be considered when assessing these results.

Whether or not differences in blood pressure between different ethnic groups are genuine, hypertension alone cannot account for the high stroke rates in black populations. A further important consideration is the difference in the prevalence of diabetes mellitus between ethnic groups. Higher mortality and hospital admission rates have been found in Afro-Caribbeans than for other ethnic groups (Shanket and Cruickshank 1993; Cruickshank *et al.* 1980). Miller *et al.* (1988) surveyed 209 men (81% of all registered in a general practice) and found that hyperglycaemia was present in 29% of Afro-Carribbeans compared with 9% of Europeans. To investigate the underlying mechanism for these ethnic differences, Cruickshank *et al.* (1991) measured plasma C-peptide and insulin concentrations after an overnight fast and during an oral glucose tolerance test in subjects aged between 45 and 74. They failed to find differences in insulin secretion, but there were variations in the C-peptide response relative to the insulin response and the authors speculated that this may be due to an impaired hepatic processing of insulin in Afro-Caribbeans. Gaines *et al.* (1995), reviewing the literature on black/white differences in stroke risk factors, conclude that apart from hypertension, smoking, diabetes and obesity are also more prevalent in blacks.

There are probably other relevant factors predisposing to stroke in these groups which include sickle cell disease, cholesterol levels, dietary factors such as increased sodium content, incidence of phospholipid antibodies and specific genetic differences.

In the USA, Howard *et al.* (1995) estimated that socio-economic status accounted for less than 25% of the excess male deaths from stroke amongst blacks aged 45-64 and in women it did not significantly reduce the estimated excess black stroke mortality.

**Table 2  SOCIAL CHARACTERISTICS**

| Factor | | Relative risk |
|---|---|---|
| SEC | 1 | 1.00 |
| | V | 1.6 |
| Ethnic group black | M | 1.1 |
| | F | 1.4 |

## 3. Environmental factors

Seasonal variation in stroke mortality has been reported by many groups (Haberman *et al.* 1981; Knox 1981; Christie 1981; Barer *et al.* 1984) which may be due to an effect on survival or a direct effect on incidence. Many of the studies are based on small numbers and have poor documentation of the stroke. These reports indicate a preponderance of strokes occurring during the winter or colder months in both hemispheres. In hot arid climates, the converse pattern emerges, with a risk of stroke of 2.76-times greater on hot days with temperatures above 30C, than cold ones. This trend was reported in the Negev Desert, Israel, based on 895 patients (Beringer *et al.* 1989). These apparently conflicting reports may be explained by Ohno's studies (1969), which found that climatic effects tend to increase as one moves away from the "comfort zone" with increased cases of stroke being reported when the temperature was greater than 30C or less than -10C.

Wroe *et al.* (1992) reported that in Oxford, England, all types of stroke are most likely to occur after waking in the morning, although other hospital-based and retrospective studies, have suggested that stroke is more common at night (Marshall 1977, Caplan *et al.* 1983).

The possible mechanisms for these observations may relate to the effects of temperature on blood pressure and clotting mechanisms and further research is required on the environment in which the stroke occurred in relation to blood pressure and haemostatic factors.

## 4. Physiological characteristics

*Hypertension: Observational and ecological data:*
Approximately 4 million people in the UK have raised diastolic blood pressures between 100-120mmHg. Observational studies have all demonstrated hypertension to be the single most important risk factor for stroke and one which has been shown to be eminently reducible by antihypertensive treatment in the randomised controlled trial setting. The attributable risk factor has, however, varied from 0.6 in the Framingham study (Whisnant 1984) to 0.75 in the Whitehall study (Reid *et al.* 1976; Reid *et al.* 1990; Reid 1994), Also in the bi-racial community of Evans County, US, the attributable risk was only 0.46-0.56 (Heyman 1971). In the British Regional Heart Study the relationship between blood pressure and stroke seemed to be predicted by systolic blood pressure alone (Shaper *et al.* 1991).

Secular trends in hypertension and its cardiovascular sequelae are of great public health importance. The decline in both stroke and coronary heart disease mortality predates effective antihypertensive therapy and the reasons remain unclear as to the contribution of antihypertensive therapy to this decline (Kannel and Wolf 1992, see Chapter 1).

Casper *et al.* (1992), in an ecological analysis, could find no evidence to support the hypothesis that increased antihypertensive pharmacotherapy has been the primary determinant of recent declines in stroke mortality in the US. However, they consider that the implications of the results from their study neither address nor challenge the efficacy of antihypertensive drugs to reduce the risk of stroke among individuals under conditions of clinical and community trials. McGovern *et al.* (1992) have also reported findings of only a small effect of antihypertensive medication on the stroke mortality decline, because antihypertensive treatment explains only part of the average population blood pressure decline. Other explanations for the population decline in blood pressure may be associated with physical activity (Jacobs *et al.* 1991), body weight, smoking and cholesterol (McGovern *et al.* 1992). Bonita and Beaglehole (1986) have estimated that the treatment of hypertension accounted for only 10% of the decline in stroke mortality seen in New Zealand between 1973-1982. A later analysis suggested that at least three quarters of the decline in stroke mortality in the US in the period 1970-80 was due to factors other than antihypertensive treatment (Bonita and Beaglehole 1989).

*Intervention data - trials:*

It has been clear for many years that antihypertensive therapy reduces the incidence of stroke in moderate and severe hypertension (diastolic phase IV >115mmHg). However, 70% of hypertensives are in the stratum 90-104mmHg in which 60% of the excess mortality from hypertension lies (Hypertension Detection Follow-up Program HDFP 1979). In the Medical Research Council trial (MRC 1985) and European working party on high blood pressure in the elderly (Amery *et al.* 1985) there were similar reductions (45% and 52%) in stroke rate but the reduction in fatal strokes was not significant in either study and in the MRC trial it was estimated that 1 stroke was averted for every 850 patient years of treatment in patients under the age of 65. In the HDFP study a 35% reduction in stroke mortality in favour of the special intervention group was observed after 8.3 years of follow-up (HDFP 1988) and was considered not solely to be the effect of drugs but the whole antihypertensive programme. Hydrochlorthiazide and amiloride have been shown to reduce the risk of stroke, coronary events, and all cardiovascular events in older hypertensive adults (aged 65-74) (MRC 1992). This reduction in stroke events was mainly in non-smokers taking diuretics.

In the Framingham observational studies, USA, diastolic blood pressure in the over 65s in both sexes did not exert a significant effect on stroke mortality. A rise in systolic and diastolic blood pressures occurs with increasing age (Kannel and Gordon 1978) and it has been considered unsafe to await the appearance of target-organ involvement in elderly hypertensives before treating them. The systolic hypertension in the elderly program (SHEP 1991) showed that in persons aged 60 years and over with isolated systolic hypertension, antihypertensive stepped-care drug treatment with low-dose chlorthalidone as step 1 medication, reduced the incidence of total stroke by 36%, with a five-year absolute benefit of 30 events per 1000 participants.

*Meta-analysis:*

Macmahon and colleagues (1990) undertook a meta-analysis of nine major prospective observational studies in subjects aged 25-84, but with 98% male subjects. After correction for 'regression dilution' bias, prolonged differences in usual diastolic blood pressure of 5, 7.5 and 10 mmHg were respectively associated with at least 34%, 46% and 56% fewer stroke events and for the large majority of individuals whether conventionally 'hypertensive' or 'normotensive', a lower blood pressure should eventually confer a lower risk of vascular disease. This effect was seen throughout the blood pressure range and there was no evidence of any 'threshold' below which levels of diastolic blood pressure were not associated with lower risk of stroke. Therefore for populations where strokes are common a substantially lower diastolic blood pressure should eventually confer a substantially lower relative risk of vascular disease. The absolute benefits of a lower blood pressure would be greatest for large countries with high stroke rates, such as China. They concluded that there is still a need for better understanding of the dietary and other determinants of population blood pressure levels.

Collins *et al.* (1990) analysed 14 randomised trials of antihypertensive drugs. Long-term differences seen in observational studies of 5-6 mmHg in usual diastolic blood pressure were associated with about 35-40% fewer stroke events. Stroke was reduced in trials by 42% (SD6) suggesting that virtually all the epidemiologically expected stroke reduction appears rapidly. For stroke the overview provides direct and highly significant evidence that both fatal and non-fatal strokes are prevented within just a few years of lowering blood pressure, even if the diastolic blood pressure is below 110mmHg at the start of treatment. There were proportionally similar sized reductions among those with mild, moderate and severe hypertension (Collins *et al.* 1990). This suggests that as part of a primary care programme, patients with borderline blood pressures of 140-160 systolic and 90-100 diastolic should also be included for consideration of approaches to reduce blood pressure.

*Concerns over trial data:*

Grimley-Evans (1987) emphasised that caution was needed in the extrapolation of USA data to the UK. He demonstrated, in a follow-up study in Newcastle, that hypertension in people aged 65 and over, especially systolic blood pressure was only associated with stroke in men and not in women. In the population studied there seemed little scope for the primary prevention of stroke in elderly women by detecting and treating hypertension. There has also been concern in Britain over the undesirable side effects of antihypertensive treatment, especially in the elderly (Anonymous 1977; Jackson *et al.* 1976).

The best method of detecting hypertension is by case-detection (D'Souza *et al.* 1976) but in general practice the detection rate, treatment and follow-up is poor (Kurji *et al.* 1985; Weinstein and Stason 1976; Heller and Rose 1977). This is why extrapolation from trials to clinical practice should be treated with caution. Morgan and Watkins (1988) studied lay beliefs and responses to antithypertensive therapy and found that whereas the level of adherence to the prescribed medication was high among white patients, less than half of the West Indians were classified as compliers. This reflected their particular beliefs and concerns, and was often associated with the use of herbal remedies, an expression of a continuation of traditional cultural patterns. The prevalence of hypertension and stroke is greater amongst black communities who share the following characteristics which predispose to stroke: lower potassium intake, increased obesity, salt sensitivity and low renin hypertension (Klag *et al.* 1991).

Other strategies for reducing hypertension have been described. Elliot and colleagues (1987) in the Caerphilly Heart Study found no relationship between dietary intakes as measured by seven-day weighed dietary record and blood pressure. This group also could not confirm the relationship between potassium and blood pressure described by Khaw and Barrett-Connor (1986). Yamori *et al.* (1984) showed a blood pressure lowering effect of dietary protein.

Both weight loss (Reisen *et al.* 1978) and sustained abstention from alcohol (Saunders *et al.* 1987) are associated with a lowering of blood pressure. The effect of weight loss has however been shown not to be sustained (Haynes *et al.* 1984).

Community-based stroke registers indicate a prevalence of hypertension in patients with stroke of 52-70% which has important implications for secondary prevention (Sandercock *et al.* 1989).

*Cardiac disease:*
After age, sex and hypertension, cardiac disease is said to be the most important risk factor for stroke. In the hypertensive population of Framingham, the ratio of myocardial

infarction to stroke was two in men and one in women, whereas it was six in men and three in women who were not hypertensive (Wolf 1986). The study also showed in men that in the presence of coronary heart disease the relative risk of stroke was 2.5, in the presence of congestive heart failure it was 2.5, and in the presence of left ventricular hypertrophy (LVH) it was 4.4. This risk was more pronounced in females (3.2, 4.3 and 7.9 respectively). The Evans County Study (Heyman 1971) found similar but weaker evidence for this. Conversely, Welin and colleagues (1987) in multivariate analysis, did not find coronary heart disease or left ventricular hypertrophy to be significant factors.

### Left ventricular hypertrophy (LVH):

 Ten per cent of persons aged 30-62 can expect to have ECG changes of LVH within ten years (Kannel 1983). ECG patterns of LVH do to some degree reflect the anatomical hypertrophy, as evidenced at autopsy. LVH may be evident prior to overt hypertension which is contrary to conventional theories, neurohumoral control being important in the development of both LVH and hypertension. ECG changes may be influenced by several non-cardiac factors and do not allow accurate quantification of alterations of left ventricular mass. More precise measurements of LV thickness and mass are possible with echocardiography, which has been shown to be cost-effective in the detection of LVH in hypertensive patients. The sensitivity of the ECG to detect LVH is between 15-57% and echocardiography up to 98% (Devereux *et al.* 1987).  LVH on ECG indicated a high risk of stroke in the Framingham study (relative risk 7.5 in men and 8.6 in women). To some extent this is a reflection of the severity and duration of the associated hypertension, but the residual effect of ECG LVH is substantial (4-8 fold) after adjustment for a co-existent increase in blood pressure (Kannel *et al.* 1983).

### Atrial fibrillation (AF):

AF affects 2% of the population ( 0.5% at 50-59 to 8.8% at 80-89) and the Framingham Study has estimated that AF accounts for between seven and 31% of all strokes in patients under the age of 60 and increases the risk of stroke by a factor of five (1.5% in the fifth decade to 23.5% in eighth decade) (Wolf *et al.* 1978, 1991). Up to 20% of those with AF who suffer a first stroke have a further episode within one year (Sherman *et al.* 1986). In addition, atrial fibrillation is associated with a greater early mortality in patients admitted to hospital with acute stroke (Lowe *et al.* 1983) and a greater risk of recurrent stroke (Sage and Van Uitert 1983) although these associations were not found in the Framingham Study (Wolf *et al.* 1983). Kopecky *et al.* (1987) suggested lone atrial fibrillation in patients under 60 as diagnosis was not associated with increased risk of stroke but the cohort study did not include subjects with cardiovascular disease, hypertension or diabetes at the onset. People with AF without underlying rheumatic heart disease are five to six times more likely to have a first stroke or TIA compared with a control population of matched age and blood pressure (Wolf *et al.* 1978); in those with AF and rheumatic heart disease the risk is 17 times greater than in controls. Gustafsson *et al.* (1992), in an ecological analysis in Sweden, suggested that treatment with anticoagulants or aspirin is cost-effective provided that the risk of serious haemorrhage complications is kept low (savings of £2 million per million inhabitants/year).

*Trial evidence:*

Non-rheumatic AF increases the risk of stroke and five randomised controlled trials of the use of warfarin in the primary prevention of stroke have shown consistent reductions in the region of two thirds with moderate anticoagulation long-term (Stroke Prevention in Atrial Fibrillation Study Group Investigators 1991; Peterson *et al.* 1989a; Boston Area Anticoagulant Trial for Atrial Fibrillation Investigators 1990; Connolly *et al.* 1991; Ezckowitz *et al.* 1992; Albers *et al.* 1991; Kistler *et al.* 1993). Warfarin reduces the incidence of ischaemic stroke or embolus from 4.5% to 1.4% per year (31 events per 1000 treated). Only two of these trials also reported a beneficial effect of aspirin in patients with AF (Stroke Prevention in Atrial Fibrillation Investigators 1991, Peterson *et al*, 1989b). The Stroke Prevention in Atrial Fibrillation trial reported that primary events or death were reduced by 58%(p=0.01) by warfarin and 42% by aspirin (p=0.02). The risk of significant bleeding was 1.5%, 1.4% and 1.6% per year in patients assigned to warfarin, aspirin and placebo respectively. In this trial, very stringent exclusion criteria were applied for eligibility for the warfarin group and monitoring was extremely thorough, which is reflected in the low risk of bleeding. In the non-trial setting, where criteria are not always met, the benefits will be reduced.

In the SPAF II study (1994) although warfarin seemed more effective than aspirin for the prevention of ischaemic strokes, this agent was associated with more haemorrhagic strokes, which are generally more disabling than ischaemic strokes. In patients less than 75 years of age, without a history of hypertension, heart failure or previous thromboembolism, the absolute risk of ischaemic stroke or embolism with aspirin was

0.5% per year. Previously warfarin has been recommended unless there were contraindications for anticoagulation. In the light of the SPAF II results treatment with aspirin can now be recommended for many patients because of its efficacy, safety, cost and ease of administration. Warfarin is indicated for high-risk individuals such as those who have had a previous TIA or stroke.

Although those over 75 have the highest risk of a stroke from atrial fibrillation, they are at higher risk of bleeding with anticoagulants. These trials need to be replicated in the primary care setting if management is to be based in primary care. Further trials of the benefits and risks of various combinations of doses of aspirin and warfarin are also required.

The European Atrial Fibrillation Trial Study Group (1993) concluded that anticoagulation is effective in reducing the risk of recurrent vascular events in patients with non-rheumatic atrial fibrillation with a recent TIA or minor ischaemic stroke. In absolute terms 90 vascular events (mainly stroke) are prevented if 1000 patients are treated with anticoagulants for one year. Aspirin prevents 40 such deaths. The same group have analysed the optimal intensity of anticoagulation (EAFT 1995).

The Copenhagen Atrial Fibrillation Aspirin Study (1989) showed a 12% reduction in serious vascular events (stroke, myocardial infarction or vascular deaths) and the Antiplatelet Trialists Collaboration overview of 25 trials (1994) reported a 25% reduction across all types of vascular death with aspirin therapy. Most of the trials to date evaluating the benefit of aspirin in these patients have produced results which fail to reach statistical significance and larger trials are required to determine the benefit. The SPAF II study has continued to randomise patients between aspirin and warfarin and the results will inform this debate (Stroke Prevention in Atrial Fibrillation Investigators 1994).

Community stroke registers have estimated the prevalence in first-time stroke patients of cardiac emboli to be between 8-20% and ischaemic heart disease between 13-38% (Sandercock *et al.* 1989). The scope for secondary prevention is therefore considerable.

*Previous transient ischaemic attack (TIA):*
Whisnant (1984) estimated the attributable risk of a previous TIA to be 10% and estimates of a 13-fold increased risk of stroke for subjects who have had a TIA have been observed in the first year after a TIA and a seven-fold risk for the seven years thereafter

(Harrison 1983). Eighty per cent of TIAs originate from emboli in the region of the carotid artery. Approximately 20% of patients with first-time stroke have had one or more preceding TIAs.

### Carotid artery stenosis:

Clinical evaluation and duplex carotid ultrasound are required to assess patients with previous TIAs for possible carotid endarterectomy. To detect carotid stenosis of greater than 75% it is most cost-effective to screen all patients with ultrasound and thereby reduce the requirement for angiography and the risk of stroke (Hankey and Warlow 1990). Duplex ultrasound can detect occlusion of the internal carotid artery with a sensitivity of 80-96% and specificity of 95% but requires skill, is costly and not widely available, certainly in the UK. The use of duplex ultrasound alone in the investigation of carotid stenosis should reduce the associated mortality and morbidity of angiography and would allow all investigations to be performed on an outpatient basis but requires further evaluation.

Several large trials have reported interim or final results assessing the benefits of carotid endarterectomy and to determine the level of perioperative risk at which the procedure becomes acceptable: the European Carotid Surgery Trial (ECST 1991), the North American Symptomatic Carotid Endarterectomy Trial (1991) and the Veterans Affair Cooperative Studies Program (Mayberg *et al.* 1991) all published in 1991 with similar findings. The former two trials recruited patients with a history of a minor ischaemic event and severe stenosis of the origin of the ipsilateral internal carotid artery (70-99%). The risk of stroke or death within 30 days of surgery was 7.5% in ECST and 5.8% in NASCET. If the patient survived stroke-free, the risk of stroke in the ipsilateral territory over the next few years, assessed by life table analysis, was 2.8% for surgical patients and 16.8%, for controls at three years in the ECST study and 9% for surgical patients and 20% for controls in the NASCET study. The beneficial effect of surgery is such that between five and ten patients must be operated on to prevent one from having a stroke. Only half the strokes prevented are disabling. If all those patients with severe carotid artery stenosis who had had a TIA underwent surgery the overall reduction in the total incidence of stroke would be between 0.2%-0.5% but there would be a resultant five-fold increase in carotid surgery (Dennis and Warlow 1991; Lambert 1995).

The ECST trial included patients with mild carotid stenosis of less than 30% for whom surgery had no benefit. Less clear-cut is the value of carotid endarterectomy in the moderate stenosis group (30-69%). Both ECST and NASCET are still randomising patients in this group and their results are awaited with interest. The trials indicate that if the procedure is to be carried out it should be within a few weeks by a surgical team whose operative risks are at least as good as those in trials. It was thought at the time of the trials that the endarterectomy rates would increase five fold and decline in the US. It is unclear whether most UK districts have the facilities or expertise to cope with the potential demand.

Endarterectomy is not indicated for most, possibly all, patients with moderate symptomatic carotid stenosis (ECST 1996).

Another controversial area is the value of carotid endarterectomy in asymptomatic patients. The Carotid Artery Stenosis with Asymptomatic Narrowing: Operation Versus Aspirin Study (CASANOVA) recruited patients with stenosis of between 50 and 90%. There was no difference in the number of major vascular events between the two groups (CASANOVA study group 1991).

This suggests that the patients with moderate asymptomatic stenosis should not receive surgery, but the value of surgery in asymptomatic patients with greater than 90% stenosis remains unknown.

The lack of conclusive evidence for endarterectomy in asymptomatic disease led to the establishment of two multicentre trials, the Asymptomatic Carotid Arterosclerotic Study (ACAS) and in its European counterpart the Asymptomatic Carotid Surgery Trial (ACST). Recent ACAS data suggests that if stenosis is greater than 60% endarterectomy is beneficial with a relative risk reduction of 55% but absolute risk reduction of 5.9% (Barnett *et al.* 1993). The problem with the study is that 9% of the study group did not receive the allocated treatment and median follow-up time was short (Irvine *et al.* 1995).

*The role of carotid endarterectomy in the following areas requires clarification:*

1) Moderate stenosis
2) Asymptomatic stenosis
3) Predicting which factors increase the risk of stroke from carotid endarterectomy.
4) The effect of plaque morphology on the risk of stroke rather than just the measurement of stenosis.

### Secondary prevention after TIA or ischaemic stroke:

The Antiplatelet Trialists Collaboration performed a meta-analysis of trials assessing the benefit of aspirin therapy in secondary prevention of stroke and estimated that long-term anticoagulant therapy reduces the risk of stroke and other major vascular events by about 25% (Antiplatelet Trialists Collaboration 1988). This benefit has been shown clearly for doses of aspirin of 300mg to 1300mg/day but it remains unclear whether low-dose aspirin would be effective for certain high-risk groups.

There have been two recent clinical trials suggesting the benefit of lower doses of aspirin. The Dutch TIA trial (1991) compared 30mg of aspirin with 300mg, and in the former group, stroke, myocardial infarction or vascular death occurred in 14.7% versus 15.2% in the 300mg group. However, there were too few events for the difference to reach statistical significance. The second trial, the Swedish Aspirin Low-dose Trial (1991), was the first to show a clear beneficial effect of aspirin with daily doses of less than 300mg. This group compared the effect of 75mg aspirin with placebo and showed a significant 17% risk reduction in the treatment group compared with placebo.

The UK-TIA Study Group (1991) results also suggested similar beneficial effects for different aspirin doses above 300mg, but that side effects are probably dose-dependent. The beneficial effect of aspirin appears to be similar in people with hypertension and diabetes, in all age groups and in both sexes.

Ticlopidine is another antiplatelet agent which has been shown to be effective as a secondary preventative agent with similar if not greater efficacy than aspirin, but which is associated with significantly more side effects. It is recommended for those who are unable to tolerate aspirin. Interestingly, its mechanism of action is different from aspirin and there is some evidence that combined aspirin and ticlopidine therapy has a greater beneficial effect than each individually, but with a considerably increased bleeding risk (Uchiyama *et al.* 1989; Albers 1992; Grotta *et al.* 1992).

With regard to secondary prevention after TIA, it is important to note that only 12% of strokes are preceded by TIA and only about half of these are reported to a doctor. Therefore if secondary prevention is introduced at this stage, this could prevent no more than 5% of all strokes.

The Antiplatelet Trialists Collaboration (1994a) undertook an overview of randomised trials of prolonged antiplatelet therapy. They concluded that there is, as yet, no clear evidence on the balance of risks and benefits of antiplatelet therapy in primary prevention among low-risk subjects. Among a much wider range of patients at high risk of occlusive vascular disease than is currently treated routinely (e.g. unstable angina, suspected acute myocardial infarction, stroke, TIA and other high-risk groups such as those with stable angina or peripheral vascular disease), some years of antiplatelet therapy with aspirin 75-325mg/day or some other antiplatelet regimes offers worthwhile protection against myocardial infarction, stroke and death.

The same group (Antiplatelet Trialists Collaboration 1994b) indicates that antiplatelet therapy, chiefly aspirin alone or aspirin plus dipyridamole, greatly reduces the risk of vascular occlusion in a wide range of patients at high risk of this complication, but when treatment should be started and for how long requires further study.

Compliance and safety with warfarin are less likely to be assured when warfarin is prescribed in general practice than in the selected trials (Lowe 1992).

### Recurrent stroke:
Burn *et al.* (1994) estimated the chance of at least one recurrence in the OCSP was 30% (95%CI 20-39%) by five years, about nine times the risk in the general population. The risk was highest in the first year, 13% (10-16%) and 4% thereafter. Smoking was a prognostic variable associated with recurrence that was significant at the time of stroke. In other European countries the MONICA Project has reported a median recurrence rate of 20% (Thorvaldsen *et al.* 1995).

### Obesity:
Many studies fail to distinguish obesity from its associated feature, hypertension and it is not clear how much of an independent effect obesity has on the incidence of stroke. The Framingham study provides some evidence for obesity as an independent factor (Wolf *et al.* 1986), however, much of the effect of obesity is mediated through other risk factors. Larsson (1984) showed clearly that an increased waist/hip ratio was associated with stroke but was not an independent long-term predictor. In univariate analysis comparing subjects with a waist/hip ratio at the 95th centile or greater with those in the lowest quintile an 11.5 risk ratio was demonstrated by Welin *et al.* (1987) and an attributable risk fraction of 0.21 for a high waist/hip ratio, and 0.21 for large waist circumference. In multivariate analysis Welin found abdominal obesity to be an independent variable, but not body mass index.

*Diabetes mellitus:*

The Framingham study documented a relative risk of stroke of 2.6 in men and 3.1 in women with diabetes and an attributable risk of about 10% (Wolf *et al.* 1983). More recently Stegmayr and Asplund (1995), using population-based registry data, estimated the risk at 4.1 in men and 5.8 in women. They estimated that the attributable risk was 18% in men and 22% in women and 50 strokes are annually directly attributable to diabetes per 100,000 population, although how the authors controlled for other factors such as hypertension and atrial fibrillation is unclear. Treatment had no effect on risk but if diabetes was poorly controlled the risk doubled. In a cohort study Welin and colleagues (1987) found no such association. Barrett-Connor (1988) using multivariate analysis of data from a cohort in California adjusted for age, systolic blood pressure, cholesterol, obesity and smoking habits, demonstrated a relative risk of 1.8 in men and 2.2 in women. In Finland Salonen *et al.* (1982) concluded that diabetes confirmed a four-fold excess risk of stroke, as did Abbott in Hawaii (1986) but Roelmholdt (1983) considered that hypertension entirely explains the excess risk of stroke in diabetic patients.

Diabetes has been reported as a significant independent risk factor for ischaemic stroke by other groups (Ellekjaer *et al.* 1992; Marmot and Poulter 1992). Diabetic patients with proteinuria or ischaemic electrocardiogram abnormalities are at highest risk of new cerebrovascular disease (Kiers *et al.* 1992).

*Infection:*

Syrjanen and colleagues (1988), in a case control study, estimated that febrile infection in the previous month to a stroke in patients aged under 50 inferred a relative risk of nine (CI 2.2 to 80). The most common infection was respiratory (80%), with a relative risk of 14.5 (CI 1.9-112.3) estimated in conditional logistic regression analysis for matched pairs. The study used community controls. A case control study, again using community controls, by Grau *et al.* (1995) indicated that recent infection, primarily of bacterial origin, may be a risk factor for cerebrovascular ischaemia in older as well as younger patients.

*Homocysteinuria:*

Premature arteriosclerosis and thromboembolic events are well known complications of homozygous homocysteinuria due to cystathionine syntheses deficiency which damages vascular endothelial cells. Heterozygosity for homocysteinuria can be assessed after methionine loading and is said to occur in one in 70 of the population and predisposes to premature occlusive arterial disease, including cerebral disease (Boers *et al.* 1985). Perry at al. (1995) reported in the British Regional Heart Study that total homocysteine levels are a strong independent risk factor for stroke with a graded increase in the relative risk of stroke in the second, third and fourth quartiles of the total homocysteine distribution (odds ratio 1.3 to 2.8). Nygard *et al.* (1995), in a survey of a community in western Norway, demonstrated that elevated plasma total homocysteine levels were associated with major components of the cardiovascular risk profile, i.e. male sex, old age, smoking, high blood pressure, elevated cholesterol and lack of exercise. High doses of vitamin B6 treatment could theoretically reduce the risk of thromboembolic disease in these heterozygote subjects, and a trial of vitamins for primary or secondary prevention is being considered by Professor Ebrahim at the Royal Free Hospital, London.

### Sickle cell disease:
Serjeant (1985) estimated that a patient with sickle cell disease has an approximately 10-fold increased risk of stroke compared with the general population. The risk is greatest for homozygous HbSS individuals, but heterozygote carriers also carry significant risk.

### Fibrinogen:
Elevation of the fibrinogen level increases blood viscosity, which may further enhance the risk of thrombus formation. Wilhelmsen (1984) showed a significant relationship with stroke when the systolic blood pressure was above 200 mmHg and fibrinogen 5-6 g/L, when a 12% incidence of stroke was seen compared with 0 if the systolic was between 100-120 mmHg and fibrinogen 1-3g/L. The Framingham study (Wolf *et al.* 1986) showed a significant independent relationship of fibrinogen with stroke but the coefficient was not significant. Welin (1987) estimated the population attributable risk to be 0.18 and in multivariate analysis fibrinogen was shown to be an independent risk factor. Qizilbash (1990), in a case control study adjusting for other variables, estimated the odds ratio for ischaemic stroke to be 1.78 (0.91-3.18) for fibrinogen greater than 3.6g/L.

### Clotting factors:
In the Northwick Park Study, Meade and colleagues (1986) demonstrated elevated factor VII levels to be the strongest predictor of myocardial infarction five years before

the event, followed by elevated cholesterol and fibrinogen levels. Patients with hyperlipoproteinaemia associated with raised serum triglyceride with or without high cholesterol, have increased activity of factors VII and VIIp1 which are both associated with increased risk of coronary heart disease (Norday *et al.* 1990). Uchiyama *et al.* (1983) studying patients with cerebrovascular disease suggested that a systematic increase of hyperaggregable platelets and of plasma activators of platelets exist in thrombotic cerebrovascular disease and may be related to pathogenesis. The induced and spontaneous platelet aggregation and proportion of megathrombocytes could be reduced with 600mg aspirin treatment daily.

There has also been recent attention to antiphospholipid antibodies such as anticardiolipin antibody and lupus anticoagulant. These may be found in association with a variety of systemic diseases, but most commonly in systemic lupus erythematosis. In some instances they are an isolated finding with no clinical correlates of connective tissue disease (Hess 1992). These antibodies are associated with increased risk of thrombotic episodes both in venous and arterial vessels. In a study of 100 consecutive patients hospitalised with first-ever strokes, Chakravarty (1991) found that 21% were positive for anticardiolipin antibody compared with 0 in 100 age matched controls. In the patient group which was positive for anticardiolipin antibody, the three-month case-fatality was 62% compared with 21.5% in the antibody negative group. In addition, the proportion of patients with significant disability after stroke (Barthel score 0-9) was significantly higher in the antibody group. The authors suggested that the presence of anticardiolipin antibodies may represent an independent prognostic marker for mortality and outcome from stroke. Studies have been on selected groups and long-term follow-up of patients is required to assess whether the presence of antibodies is an epi phenomenon.

### Haematocrit:
Increased blood pressure and cigarette smoking increase the haematocrit and account for most of the association with stroke. The Framingham study showed a significant independent correlation in the under 65s only (Wolf 1986). Welin (1987) was not able to demonstrate an association. Yiyohara (1986) found a low haematocrit was important as an independent risk factor in women.

## Table 3 PHYSIOLOGICAL CHARACTERISTICS

| Factor | Relative risk | Attributable risk |
| --- | --- | --- |
| Hypertension | 7 | 0.46-0.75 |
| Cardiac disease | 3 | 0.11 |
| LVH | 4.4 | |
| AF | 3-7 | 0.015 (age 50-59) |
| | | 0.24 (age 80-89) |
| Previous TIA | 5-13 | 0.1 |
| Diabetes mellitus | 4.1 M | 0.18 |
| | 5.8 F | 0.22 |
| Epilepsy | 4 | |
| Snoring | 3 | |
| Infection | 9 | |
| Homocysteinuria | 10 | |
| Sickle cell disease | 10 | |
| Fibrinogen >3.6 g/1 | 1.8 | |

## 5. Behavioural characteristics

*Physical activity:*

Herman *et al.* (1982), in a case control study, indicated that those undertaking little physical activity had a 2.5-fold increased risk of stroke compared with heavy activity but there was no adjustment for other risk factors. Another case control study examined the effect of lifelong exercise on stroke risk and found that a history of vigorous exercise during the ages 15-25 years appeared to protect against stroke with an age and sex adjusted odds ratio of 0.33 (Shinton and Sagar 1993). In the British Regional Heart Study physical activity was inversely associated with risk of stroke independent of coronary risk factors, heavy drinking, and pre-existing ischaemic heart disease or stroke (relative risk 1 for inactivity, 0.6 moderate activity, and 0.3 vigorous activity) (Wannamethee and Shaper 1992). Also in the Framingham study, at the 14-year follow-up point there was a similar inverse relation between physical activity and risk of stroke (Kannel and Sorlie 1979) but this was not significant after adjustment for age, and the classification of physical activity was broad. The Allied Dunbar National Fitness Survey (1992) found that approximately 25% of the population do not take any exercise. With a relative risk of 2.5, the attributable risk of inactivity could be as high as 60%.

### *Lipids:*

The story is far less clear or consistent than for coronary heart disease. In the Framingham study there was a negative association of low density lipoprotein (LDL) cholesterol with stroke, especially in women over 65 after other risk factors had been accounted for. There was no clear cut relationships with triglycerides and no protective effect of high density lipoprotein (HDL) (Wolf *et al.* 1983, 1986). Multivariate regression coefficients, used to assess the impact of the factors on stroke incidence in males and females for LDL, were 0.18 and 0.42 respectively. The Evans County study (Heyman 1971) did not find any such association. It may be that subjects with raised lipids die of a myocardial infarct before they reach the age for stroke. Other studies have suggested that increased concentrations of total cholesterol (Heyman *et al.* 1971; Ueda *et al.* 1980) and or triglycerides (Gertler *et al.* 1975; Taggart and Stout 1979) are related to risk for stroke.

In observational studies there have been reports of an inverse relationship between serum cholesterol and mortality from intracerebral and subarachnoid haemorrhage, particularly for cholesterol levels below 4.4 mmol/L (Yano *et al.* 1989; Multiple Risk Factor Intervention Trial Research Group 1982; Dolecek and Grandits 1991) which was only seen for men in the lowest quintile of serum cholesterol. It was considered that perhaps low cholesterol levels were a marker of poor nutrition which enhances the vulnerability of small cerebral arteries and that this factor has only a very low population attributable risk as the association is only with very low levels of cholesterol. The separation of cerebral infarction into subtypes based on mechanism may help clarify lipid-related risk factors in cerebrovascular disease.

In more recent investigations only a low concentration of HDL cholesterol has been consistently implicated as an indicator of risk for brain infarction (Taggart and Stout 1979). Adams *et al.* (1989) observed no differences in the concentrations of total cholesterol, triglycerides, LDL cholesterol, very low density lipoprotein cholesterol, or apoproteins A1 and B. Patients with lacunar infarction, however, had higher concentrations of HDL cholesterol than patients with cortical stroke which suggests that previously demonstrated differences in HDL cholesterol concentrations between patients with ischaemic stroke and control subjects without stroke may apply to patients with cortical but not lacunar infarction. HDL cholesterol was also found to be lower in whites than in blacks among survivors of cortical and lacunar stroke. Salonen *et al.* (1982) estimated that in men a raised blood triglycerides level (>6.5 mmol/L) conferred a relative risk of stroke of 2.4.

Median concentrations of serum lipoprotein (a) were twice as high in blacks compared with whites in a cross-sectional survey of 25-64 year olds in the Seychelles and Switzerland (Bovet *et al.* 1994). Lindenstrom *et al.* (1994) indicated in the Copenhagen City Heart Study that total cholesterol was only positively associated with risk of non-haemorrhagic stroke when levels were greater than 8mmol/L (upper 5% of the distribution in the study population). Plasma triglyceride concentration was significantly and positively associated with risk of non-haemorrhagic events. The relative risk corresponding to an increase of 1 mmol/L was 1.12 (95% CI 1.07-1.16). There was a negative, log linear association between HDL and risk of non-haemorrhagic events (0.53(0.34-0.83)). They concluded that the association between very high cholesterol and stroke does not itself justify advice for the normal population. Trials of dietary modification should focus on triglyceride and HDL cholesterol and evaluate the risk of the subtypes of stroke.

In a meta-analysis on ten prospective studies Qizilbash *et al.* (1990, 1993) described a pooled relative risk of 2.9 (CI 1.43-5.87) for people with a total cholesterol of greater than 5.7 mmol/L compared with lower levels. In Caucasians, the population attributable risk of stroke due to a cholesterol level of greater than 5.7 mmol/L has been calculated at 0.2. In a case control study the same group found fibrinogen and lipids to be important risk factors for ischaemic stroke. Adjusted for other variables the odds ratio of ischaemic events were 1.73 (0.9-3.29) for total cholesterol >6 mmol/L; 1.34 (0.69-2.61) for LDL >3.5 mmol/L; and 0.32 (0.15-0.69) for HDL >1.2 mmol/L (Qizilbash 1991).

Overviews of the effect of cholesterol-lowering trials have focused on coronary heart disease and conclusions on the effect on stroke mortality and morbidity remain unclear (Peto *et al.* 1985).

Law *et al.* (1994) in a meta-analysis of cohort studies based on half a million men and 18,000 ischaemic heart disease events, estimate that a long-term reduction in serum cholesterol concentration of 0.6mmol/L (10%), which can be achieved by moderate dietary change, lowers the risk of ischaemic heart disease by 50% at age 40, falling to 20% at age 70. The randomised trials, based on 45,000 men and 4,000 ischaemic heart disease events show that the full effect of the reduction in risk is achieved by five years. This risk affects only those people with a very low concentration and even in these will be outweighed by the benefits from the low risk of ischaemic heart disease.

At the six year follow-up point in the Multiple Risk Factor Intervention Trial Research Group (MRFIT) study, Iso and colleagues (1989) demonstrated that a reduced serum cholesterol level was associated with a three fold increased risk of intracranial haemorrhage after controlling for age, smoking, diastolic blood pressure, and race or ethnic group. The group stressed that the excess risk was almost exclusively among men with high blood pressure and that intracranial haemorrhage accounted for only 2.9% of all deaths from cerebrovascular disease. There was an overwhelming positive association between high serum cholesterol and death from non-haemorrhagic stroke and total cardiovascular disease. Similar findings of the inverse relationship of serum cholesterol to intracranial haemorrhage have been observed in prospective studies of Japanese-American men (Tanaka *et al* . 1982)

*Cigarette Smoking:*
In a case control study, Bonita *et al.* (1986) demonstrated a three-fold increase in risk of stroke in smokers compared with current non-smokers. This association remained significant after adjustment for hypertension. Those who smoked and were hypertensive had an increased risk of stroke of almost 20-fold compared with those who had neither factor. Overall 37% of events in this study from a community-based register were attributed to smoking and 37% to hypertension.

In the British Regional Heart Study the combination of a raised systolic blood pressure and cigarette smoking resulted in a more than 10-fold increase in the risk of stroke compared with that of normotensive men who were not cigarette smokers (Shaper *et al* . 1991).

In the Nurses Health Study cohort (Colditz *et al.* 1988) a dose response effect of the number of cigarettes smoked and stroke was observed with those who smoked 1-14 cigarettes per day having an age-adjusted relative risk of 2.2 (1.5-3.3) compared with those that never smoked, whereas those who smoked 25 or more had a relative risk of 3.7 (2.7-5.1). Adjustment for known risk factors for stroke did not appreciably alter the association. Ex-smokers had reduced risk compared to current smokers (Abbott *et al.* 1986; Wolf *et al.* 1988; Colditz *et al.* 1988). In the US the prevalence of ex-smokers had increased from 1965 to 1980 and it is conceivable that smoking cessation could have accounted for some of the large decline in stroke mortality that began in 1973 (Klag *et al.* 1989).

Various degrees of association of smoking with stroke have been documented but many studies have a small number of cases. In Framingham, only in males under the age of 65 could an association be found which was not statistically significant but at the 16-year point, smokers were found to have a three-fold increased risk (Wolf *et al.* 1988). Abbott *et al.* (1987), in the Honolulu Heart Program, stated that smoking in men was an independent risk factor with a two to three-fold increased risk after controlling for age, diastolic blood pressure, coronary heart disease, and other major risk factors. If patients continued to smoke during follow-up this risk increased to four to six-fold compared to non-smokers. If patients gave up smoking, the risk was halved. Colditz *et al.* (1988) estimated a relative risk of two for females who smoked 1-14 cigarettes a day, and 3.7 for those that smoked five or more a day and in regression analysis these associations did not appreciably change.

A meta-analysis of the relation between cigarette smoking and stroke provided strong evidence of an excess risk of stroke among smokers with an overall relative risk of 1.5 (1.4-1.6) (Shinton and Beevers 1989).

*Alcohol:*
Alcohol is a risk factor for hypertension and studies have shown a positive association between alcohol consumption and stroke which may be linked with hypertension rather than alcohol acting independently (Camargo 1989). There is evidence that chronic and heavy drinking (>60g ethanol/day) are associated with increased risk of all types of stroke (Camargo 1989). The role of low or moderate alcohol intake remains unclear.

Evidence from case control and cohort studies provides some conflicting evidence of an association. All studies have been hampered by lack of a gold standard for estimating alcohol intake, the lack of differentiation of binge from chronic and regular alcohol intake, and the evidence is mainly from moderate alcohol intake. Controls have often been selected in such a way that bias has been introduced into the study (Camargo 1989). The evidence, until recently, has been based on total stroke rather than subtypes. Overall, the evidence from case control studies demonstrates that moderate drinkers appear to have an equal or modestly elevated risk of total stroke compared with non-drinkers. There is some evidence of a J-shaped association between level of alcohol intake and total stroke in White populations with reduced risk for those reporting light drinking (Camargo *et al.* 1989). All studies specifically addressing ischaemic stroke risk found no association with alcohol use (Abu-Zeid *et al.* 1977; Gorelick *et al.* 1989; Stemmermann *et al.* 1984). A non-linear association cannot be ruled out in two of these studies (Abu-Zeid *et al.* 1977; Stemmermann *et al.* 1984) but was not present in the third in a predominantly black population (Gorelick *et al.* 1989). For haemorrhagic stroke, a non-significant positive linear association was found between customary alcohol consumption and the relative risk of stroke in 2 nested case control studies but a high relative risk was estimated in a 3rd (Stemmermann *et al.* 1984; Sacco *et al* . 1984; Petitti *et al* . 1979).

Kiyohara *et al.* (1995), in the Hisayama study, found that amongst hypertensive individuals, heavy drinking (greater than 34g of ethanol per day) significantly increased the risk of cerebral haemorrhage. However, light alcohol consumption (less than 34g per day) significantly reduced the risk of cerebral infarction.

Evidence from over 19 prospective cohort studies provides no strong evidence of any association for total stroke except for an apparently modest increase in risk in the highest level of alcohol intake. When the data are segregated according to the two broad categories of stroke type, consistent patterns emerge. For haemorrhagic stroke, there is strong evidence for an association, with typically about a three-fold excess risk for higher levels of alcohol consumption. In contrast, there is equally strong evidence against any material adverse association with ischaemic stroke (Camargo 1989; Stampfer *et al.* 1988; Kono *et al.* 1986; Klatsky *et al.* 1990; Okada *et al.* 1976).

*Sodium/Salt:*

Reduced salt intake over the last century has been put forward as an explanation for the reduced prevalence of high blood pressure (Cummins 1983). The Intersalt study (1988) showed a significant relationship between blood pressure and urinary sodium within centres and between the slope of blood pressure and sodium with age across populations. Overall this study confirmed only a weak relationship between salt intake and blood pressure, but there were few data points with low or high sodium intake. Law and colleagues (1991) did show that the evidence on the relationship between salt and hypertension is consistent and that the association between salt and blood pressure is substantial. A reduction of 50 mmol (3g) sodium per day in subjects over 50 years lowers blood pressure by about 5 mmHg on average and 7-8 mmHg in hypertensive subjects. This salt restriction was considered adequate to reduce the incidence of stroke by 22% and ischaemic heart disease by 16%. If national policy mandated manufacturers to reduce sodium content in products then a near 40% reduction in stroke events would be achieved which is equivalent in the UK to preventing 6,500 deaths and much disability each year. In an Australian randomised controlled trial of salt restriction (<80 mmol/day) (Australian NH and MRC Dietary Salt Study 1989) blood pressure fell by 6.1 mmHg systolic and 3.7 mmHg diastolic on a low sodium diet compared with 0.6 and 0.9 mmHg on a normal diet. MacGregor and colleagues (1989) observed a progressive fall in blood pressure as salt intake was reduced and noted that in many patients with mild essential hypertension, blood pressure was controlled without the need for drugs. All 20 patients controlled their salt restriction for one year and in 16 blood pressure remained well controlled but how typical these subjects were was not discussed.

*Potassium:*

In the Intersalt study (1988) potassium was negatively associated with blood pressure. Khaw *et al.* (1987) estimated the relative risk of stroke in a Californian cohort in those whose potassium intake was in the lowest tertile compared to the top two tertiles to be 2.6 in men and 4.6 in women. In multivariate analysis a 10mmol increase (one serving of fresh fruit and vegetable) in daily potassium intake was associated with a 40% reduction in risk of stroke-associated mortality which was independent of other dietary variables and known cardiovascular risk factors. Tobias *et al.* (1985) suggested that high potassium diets protect against stroke events even though blood pressure was not affected. Siari and colleagues (1987) did show that a moderate (48 mmol potassium) oral supplement was associated with a reduction of blood pressure in mild hypertensives but the observation period was only 15 weeks.

The relationship between dietary sodium, saturated fat, potassium, alcohol consumption and stroke mortality was examined by Sasaki *et al*. (1995). The highest correlation was found between urinary excretion levels of sodium and stroke mortality. Saturated fatty acids and alcohol also correlated positively with stroke mortality and urinary excretion of potassium correlated negatively.

### The oral contraceptive:
Reports of a four-fold increase in haemorrhagic stroke in over 35s, particularly those that smoke have been documented (Vessey *et al*. 1984). The relative risk of ischaemic stroke is about three and the absolute risk is estimated at one in 10,000 oral contraceptive users.

### Hormone replacement therapy:
Meade and Berra (1992) reviewed ten cohort studies and estimated a 15% reduction in stroke deaths in women on hormone replacement therapy (HRT), although there was considerable variation between centres.

### Vitamin C:
Acheson and Williams (1983) in an ecological analysis demonstrated a possible protective effect of Vitamin C in fresh fruit and vegetables on stroke occurrence.

### Polyunsaturated fatty acids:
Results from the MRFIT study support the hypothesis that long chain fatty acids, found primarily in fish oils, protect against cardiovascular disease but no stroke-specific results have been presented. (Dolecek and Grandits 1991).

**Table 4 BEHAVIOURAL TRAITS**

| Factor | | Relative Risk | Attributable Risk |
|---|---|---|---|
| Obesity | | 1.8 | |
| Increased waist/hip ratio | | 1.5 | |
| Physical inactivity | | 2.5 | |
| Total cholesterol > 5.7 mmol/L | | 2.9 | |
| Alcohol (acute intoxication) | | 5 | |
| Smoking | | 1.5 | 0.37 |
| Potassium | M | 2.6 | |
| | F | 4.6 | |
| HRT | | 0.53 | |

# Population based intervention trials

Strategies to reduce stroke incidence or recurrence can be directed either to those at high risk for a particular factor or to the whole population. Both approaches are probably required to reduce the incidence of stroke but the optimum strategy is still to be determined. The high risk approach may involve population screening or opportunistic case finding and the selective treatment of the few individuals at highest risk. An alternative, complementary, strategy is to try to produce a small reduction in the risk factor in every individual in the community by some form of intervention.

There have been several major intervention trials at a community level, largely set up to determine the effectiveness of risk factor reduction strategies on cardiovascular (CHD) mortality but with cerebrovascular mortality also being recorded. The majority of the evidence is also based on males.

The Stanford Five-City Project (Farquhar *et al.* 1990) was a multiple risk factor reduction project of 14 years' duration with a comprehensive, integrated programme of community organisation and health education. Two treatment and two non-treatment cities were tested for change in knowledge of risk factors, blood pressure, cholesterol, smoking, body weight and resting pulse in a five-year programme which included: social learning theory, communication-behaviour change model, community organisation principles and social marketing methods (of which there were 26 hours of exposure to multichannel and multifactual education). After 30 to 34 months there were significant net reductions in community averages favouring intervention which occurred in plasma cholesterol (2%), blood pressure (4%), resting pulse (3%) and smoking rate (13%). There was a reduction in composite mortality scores (15%) and coronary heart disease scores (16%).

The task force on arteriosclerosis convened by the National Heart and Lung Institution in the USA recommended that a Multiple Risk Factor Intervention Trial (MRFIT) be set up in individuals at high risk of CHD (aged 35-57) due to combinations of elevated lipids, hypertension and cigarette smoking, to determine whether an intervention programme would result in a significant reduction in CHD mortality, non-fatal myocardial infarct, cerebrovascular mortality and mortality from all causes over a period initially of six years. In total 361,662 men were screened (1974-76) and those at the upper end of the risk scale for CHD were randomly allocated to either a special intervention group or the usual source of care. The interventions occurred over the period 1976-1982 and 12,866 men aged 35-57 at increased risk of coronary heart disease were randomised to receive either stepped care or ordinary care. Stepped care included hypertension control, counselling for cigarette smokers and dietary advice for lowering cholesterol. There were uniform protocols with the aims of reducing natural fat to less than 10% of the diet and cholesterol to less than 300 mg per day. Cigarette smokers were switched to low tar cigarettes and nicotine intake modified by various strategies such as behaviour modification, aversion and hypnosis along with group sessions. The subjects received continuous education in the community along with four to five risk factor education programmes per year e.g.: lower cholesterol, salt, cigarettes, check blood pressure and treat hypertension, and increase physical activity. The mass media and schools were also involved and educational exposure comprised 26 hours in five years. Follow up was at 17, 39 and 60 months and cross sectional surveys were undertaken at 25, 51 and 73 months.

At seven years there was no significant reduction in CHD mortality in the stepped care group because of a possible unfavourable response in certain, but not all, subjects to antihypertensive treatment (MRFIT 1982). If a subject was in the upper 15% of risk score for cigarettes, cholesterol and blood pressure based on the Framingham risk score then a reduction of 10% was observed. At 10.5 years a 13% reduction in fatal stroke in the special intervention group was observed (MRFIT 1990). When considering follow-up of subjects, blacks and smokers were more likely to discontinue their participation between screening exams (Neaton *et al.* 1987). The effect that healthier lifestyle practices had on control subjects is not known but may have detected the possible effect in the intervention arm.

In North Karelia, Finland (Puska *et al.* 1983) a whole community package to represent 'real life' tested the feasibility of such intervention programmes by using existing services and other resources. In the ten years 1972-82 in 30-59 year olds the following significant reduction in risk factors levels for coronary heart disease were observed:

| F | M | |
|---|---|---|
| 14% | 28% | reduction in smoking |
| 1% | 3% | reduction in cholesterol |
| 5% | 3% | reduction in systolic blood pressure |
| 2% | 1% | reduction in diastolic blood pressure |

The study reports that the reduction in mortality from CHD among the male population in North Karelia was significantly greater than in the rest of the country which may possibly be attributed to the decline in the factor levels.

Male subjects followed up 10 years after a five-year intervention trial of 1222 business men in Finland reported more non-fatal myocardial infarctions and cardiac deaths in the intervention group (Strandberg *et al.* 1991; Miettinen *et al.* 1985) and the authors could find no convincing explanation for their findings. The higher rates of death associated with violence in the intervention group is consistent with reports of several cholesterol lowering trials (Smith and Pekkanen 1992; Muldoon *et al.* 1990). Although this is the first report of increased mortality from coronary heart disease after multifactorial intervention, previous reports have suggested that mortality from CHD does not necessarily fall with intervention to reduce multiple risk factors. After ten years in the Gothenburg trial and 10.5 years in the MRFIT trial there were no significant falls in the coronary deaths (Wilhelmsen *et al.* 1986; MRFIT 1990). Similarly the World Health Organisation factors study of multiple intervention for risk factors for CHD showed no significant reductions in deaths from coronary heart disease after six years of intervention (WHO European Collaborative Group 1986).

Vartiainen and colleagues (1995) estimated the extent to which the changes in the main CVD risk factors (blood pressure, smoking and serum cholesterol concentration) could explain the observed changes in mortality from stroke in North Karelia during the past 20 years. They found that two-thirds of the fall in mortality from stroke in men, and half in women, could be explained by changes in the three above CVD risk factors.

General health checks by nurses in England are ineffective in helping smokers to stop smoking, but they help patients to modify their diet and total cholesterol concentration (Imperial Cancer Research Fund OXCHECK Study Group 1994). The public health importance of this dietary change depends on whether it is sustained. The British Family Heart Study is a randomised controlled trial in general practices in 13 towns in Britain to measure the impact of a programme of cardiovascular screening and lifestyle intervention led by nurses (Family Heart Study Group 1994). As most general practices in the UK are not using such an intensive programme the changes in coronary risk factors achieved by the voluntary health promotion package for primary care are likely to be even smaller. It appears that this style of approach to the population through primary care alone is not going to produce large reductions in the risk of cardiovascular disease. Instead more effective legislation needs to be in place to control the use of tobacco and promote the consumption of healthy food.

Coppola *et al.* (1995) assessed a method for detecting men aged 40-59 at high risk of stroke in primary care. Using logistic regression factors such as age, systolic blood pressure, current cigarette consumption and evidence of angina, they were able to detect over 80% of all strokes. Such methodologies could be exploited by health promotion initiatives to target high-risk groups.

## Lay attitudes and beliefs about risk factors for stroke

A knowledge of the role and prevalence of risk factors for stroke is necessary before any attempts can be made to reduce them. However, in order to develop a health promotion strategy for primary and secondary prevention of stroke, an important consideration is the patient's own attitudes; their perception of personal risk perceived as controllable or hereditary and therefore fixed, and their desire to modify their controllable risk behaviour.

Very little work has been done in this field with regard to stroke, patients' perceptions or the social image and meaning of stroke in society. A study of patient perception of cardiovascular risk by Silagy *et al.* (1993) showed that the health risks of smoking and lack of exercise were recognised by most people. Attitudes towards diet were more complex. Being overweight was the main predictor of an individual's perception of diet as harmful to health. Interestingly there were major sex differences in attitude towards the role of diet in that obese women were more likely to believe that their diet was harmful than obese men. Motivation to reduce risk factors was high for smoking but low for exercise.

There are also important differences in attitudes and lifestyle between ethnic groups reflecting cultural differences in lifestyle and social habits. Cigarette smoking and alcohol consumption appear to be higher in white than black men (Meade *et al.* 1978) and may form an integral part of social activities in this population which may therefore be resistant to change. The control of weight is influenced by attitudes to body size held by different cultural groups and by the practical problems associated with changes in diet in a family context. Differences in attitudes towards Western medical practice between different cultural groups is an important factor determining compliance with recommended drug therapies for primary and secondary stroke prevention. At UMDS we are currently undertaking a prevalence study of stroke risk factors in African, Afro-Caribbean and white subjects and their attitudes to reducing these factors.

When developing a programme of stroke prevention, not only does the potential benefit in stroke reduction by individual risk factor modification need to be considered, but also the patient's own perception of personal and social costs of behavioural change.

Pharoah and Sanderson (1995) estimated in Cambridge, England, that with current general practice health promotion programmes for CHD and stroke, there would be a 17% reduction in stroke deaths in the 10 years after screening. The assumptions were those of the OXCHECK results in which only modest changes in risk factor profiles in the intervention group were seen and results of randomised controlled trials for smoking and antihypertensive interventions which are known not to be extrapolated to the population setting.

# Executive summary and principle recommendations for research

As the mortality and disability that result from stroke are considerable, strategies for prevention should form the basis of pubic health policy.

Generally studies have focused on coronary heart disease and not stroke and the risk factors for the subtypes of stroke and for females are poorly estimated.

This review considers risk factors from five perspectives: inherited biological traits, social characteristics, environmental factors, biological characteristics and behavioural characteristics. All may influence the risk of stroke but their relative importance has still to be established.

The risk of stroke rises exponentially with age and stroke is more common in males. With an ageing population, reducing risk factors and preventing recurrent strokes in the elderly is an important primary health care issue which is encompassed to some extent in *The Health of the Nation* strategy.

The new paradigms that suggest that fetal and early life experiences influence the risk of stroke have attracted much attention but require further study as they would suggest that the current health promotion strategies geared solely towards middle-aged and elderly people are inappropriate and that consideration needs to be given to interventions earlier in life or during pregnancy.

As with most disease processes, the effect of socio-economic and other demographic characteristics, such as ethnic group, on stroke risk are considerable although the proportion of total risk that they account for has not been estimated. Particularly in inner cities, the specific risk factors associated with stroke in ethnic groups require elucidation, as cultural attitudes to prevention may differ in these groups. This would need to be taken into consideration when developing health promotion strategies.

There have been reports of variations in the risk of stroke in different geographical and climatic settings but the effect of environmental factors on the risk of stroke is not known.

Of the physiological factors, hypertension is considered the most important and the one which, in the trial setting, can most effectively be treated. However, in ecological studies, the effect of antihypertensive treatment on the risk of stroke over the past four decades has been shown not to be as dramatic as the trial data would suggest. The presence of cardiac disease is another major risk factor for stroke and there are effective preventive strategies that can be employed to reduce this risk. The treatment of non-rheumatic atrial fibrillation with warfarin effectively reduces the risk of stroke but evidence of efficacy in primary care is required. Treatment with aspirin is also effective. Aspirin is less effective than warfarin but may provide a useful alternative in particular groups of patients.

In patients who have had a transient ischaemic attack or previous stroke, carotid endarterectomy has been shown to be effective for severe carotid artery stenosis but there are still questions to be answered on the appropriate selection of patients, the most sensitive methods of diagnosis of carotid stenosis and whether surgery is effective in lesser degrees of stenosis or asymptomatic people.

There are effective secondary preventive interventions that can be effectively utilised. Aspirin can reduce the risk of major vascular events by up to 25% and even low-dose aspirin has a significant protective effect. Antiplatelet therapy, particularly aspirin alone or in combination with dipyridamole, has not been shown to be effective in low-risk subjects but in a much wider group of patients at high risk of vascular disease it offers worthwhile protection against stroke.

Other physiological factors increase the risk of stroke but there is not good evidence that health service interventions are able to reduce the risk, particularly at a population level. These factors include obesity, diabetes mellitus, infection, homocysteinuria, sickle cell disease, elevated fibrinogen and clotting factor levels.

Considering behavioural characteristics, the effect of the various subfractions of cholesterol remains unclear although it would appear that raised total cholesterol levels increase the risk of stroke three-fold. Cigarette smoking, particularly when associated with hypertension, is a major risk factor for stroke. The effect of alcohol on stroke risk is complex and the evidence is only strong for binge and heavy drinking. It has been estimated, using ecological analysis, that if national policy mandated manufacturers to reduce sodium content in products then a near 40% reduction in stroke events would be achieved but whether this is feasible or acceptable remains to be seen.

Population-based prevention programme evaluations have not been conducted in the United Kingdom and extrapolation from data in the United States and Scandinavia is problematic, the British having different cultural and social attributes. There have been few studies involving the female population particularly since the advent of low-dose oestrogen oral contraceptives and hormone replacement therapy. In Scandinavia, it has been suggested that two-thirds of the fall in mortality from stroke in men, and half in women, could be explained by changes in blood pressure, smoking and serum cholesterol. In the United Kingdom health checks appear to be ineffective at reducing the major risk factors for stroke.

*The priority areas for research and service development are considered below:*

1. Cohort studies are required to establish the prevalence and attributable risk of risk factors in the various subtypes of stroke and in different groups of the population, particularly the different ethnic and socio-economic groups.

2. Studies evaluating the most effective way of implementing preventive programmes for established risk factors in district health authorities and general practices are required which need to take into account attitudes and beliefs of the population to the proposed interventions.

3. The influences of environmental, including climatic, factors on stroke risk need to be established, as do other less well defined factors such as homocysteine.

4. There is a need to refine the criteria for carotid endarterectomy and to find methods of assessing risk of stroke other than purely the degree of stenosis.

5. A trial is required of balloon angioplasty compared to carotid endarterectomy for secondary prevention.

# References

Abbott RD, Donahue P, MacMahon S. Diabetes and the risk of stroke: The Honolulu Heart Program. JAMA 1987; 257; 949-52.

Abbott RD, Yin Yin MA, Reed DM, Yano K. Risk of stroke in male cigarette smokers. N Eng J Med 1986; 315: 715-20.

Abu-Zeid HA, Choi NW, Maini KK, Hsu P, Nelson NA. Relative role of factors associated with cerebral infarction and cerebral haemorrhage: A matched pair case control study. Stroke 1977; 8: 106-12.

Acheson RM, Sanderson C. Strokes: social class and geography. Population Trends 1978; 13-7.

Acheson RM, William DRR. Does consumption of fruit and vegetables protect against stroke? Lancet 1983; i: 1191-3.

Adams RJ, Carroll RM, Nichols FT, McNair N, Feldman DS, Feldman EB, Thompson WO. Plasma lipoproteins in cortical versus lacunar infarction. Stroke 1989; 20: 448-52.

Albers GW. Role of ticlopidine for prevention of stroke. Stroke 1992; 23: 912-6.

Albers GW, Sherman DG, Gress DR, Paulseth JE, Petersen P. Stroke prevention in nonvalvular atrial fibrillation: a review of prospective randomised trials. Ann Neurol 1991; 30: 511-18.

Allied Dunbar National Fitness Survey. London: Sports Council and Health Education Authority, 1992.

Amery A, Broxho P, Clement D *et al.* Mortality and morbidity results from the European Working Party on High Blood Pressure in the Elderly Trial. Lancet 1985; i: 1349-54.

Anonymous: Trials and tribulations of a symptom-free hypertensive physician receiving the best of care. Lancet 1977; ii: 291-2.

Antiplatelet Trialists Collaboration. Secondary prevention of vascular events by prolonged antiplatelet therapy. BMJ 1988; 296: 320-31.

Antiplatelet Trialists Collaboration (a). Collaborative overview of randomised trials of antiplatelet therapy - 1: Prevention of death, myocardial infarction, and stroke by prolonged antiplatelet therapy in various categories of patients. BMJ 1994a; 308: 81-106.

Antiplatelet Trialists Collaboration (b). Collaborative overview of randomised trials of antiplatelet therapy - II: Maintenance of vascular graft or arterial potency by antiplatelet therapy. BMJ 1994b; 308: 159-66.

Australian National Health and Medical Research Council Dietary Salt Study Management Committee. Fall in blood pressure with modest reduction in dietary salt intake in mild hypertension. Lancet 1989; : 399-402.

Balarajan R. Ethnic differences in mortality from ischaemic heart disease and cerebrovascular disease in England and Wales. BMJ 1991; 302: 560-4.

Bamford J, Sandercock P, Dennis M, Burn J, Warlow C. A prospective study of acute cerebrovascular disease in the community: The Oxfordshire Community Stroke Project - 1981-86. 2. Incidence, case fatality rates and overall outcome at one year of cerebral infarction, primary intracerebral and subarachnoid haemorrhage. J Neurol Neurosurg Psychiatry 1990; 53: 16-22.

Bamford J, Sandercock P, Dennis M, Warlow C *et al.* A prospective study of acute cerebrovascular disease in the community: the Oxfordshire Community Stroke Project 1981-86. I. Methodology, demography and incident cases of first ever stroke. J Neurol Neurosurg Psychiatry 1988; 51: 1373-80.

Barer D, Ebrahim S, Smith C. Factors influencing day to day incidence of stroke in Nottingham. BMJ 1984; 289: 662.

Barker DJP. The foetal and infant origins of inequalities in health in Britain. J Public Health Med 1991; 13: 64-8.Barker DJP, Bull AR, Osmond C, Simmonds SJ. Fetal and placental size and risk of hypertension in adult life. BMJ 1990; 301: 259-62.

Barker DJP, Meade TW, Fall CHD, Lee A, Osmond C, Phipps K, *et al.* Relation of fetal and infant growth to plasma fibrinogen and factor VII concentration in adult life. BMJ 1992; 304: 148-52.

Barker DJP, Osmond C. Death rates from stroke in England and Wales predicted from past maternal mortality. BMJ 1987; 295: 83-6.

Barker DJP, Osmond C, Golding J, Kuh D, Wadsworth MEJ. Growth in utero, blood pressure in childhood and adult life, and mortality from cardiovascular disease. BMJ 1989; 298: 564-7.

Barnett HJ, Haines SJ. Carotid endarterectomy for asymptomatic carotid stenosis (editorial comment). N England J Med 1993; 328: 276.

Barrett-Connor E, Khaw K. Diabetes mellitus: An independent risk factor for stroke. Am J Epidemiol 1988; 128: 116-23.

Berginer VM, Goldsmith J, Batz U, Vardi H, Shipiro Y. Clustering of strokes in association with meteorological factors in the Negev Desert of Israel. Stroke 1989; 20: 65-9.

Boers GHJ, Smals AGH, Trijbels FJM, Fowler B. *et al.* Heterozygosity for homocystinuria in premature peripheral and cerebral occlusive arterial disease. N Engl J Med 1985; 313: 709-15.

Bonita R, Beaglehole R. Does treatment of hypertension explain the decline in mortality from stroke? BMJ 1986; 293: 191-2.

Bonita R, Beaglehole R. Increased treatment of hypertension does not explain the decline in stroke mortality in the United States, 1970-1980. Hypertens 1989; 13(Suppl. 1): 1-69-1-73.

Bonita R, Scagg R, Stewart A, Jackson R, Beaglehole R. Cigarette smoking and risk of premature stroke in men and women. BMJ 1986; 293, 6-8.

Boston Area Anticoagulation Trial for Atrial Fibrillation Investigators. The effect of low-dose warfarin on the risk of stroke in patients with non-rheumatic atrial fibrillation. N Engl J Med 1990; 323: 1505-11.

Bovet P, Rickenbach M, Wietlishbach V, Riesen W, Shambye C, Darioli R, Burnard B. Comparison of serum lipoprotein(a) distribution and its correlates among Black and White populations. Int J Epidemiol 1994; 23: 20-7.

Bromberg JEC, Rinkel GJE, Algra A, Greebe P, van Duyn CM, Hasan D, Limburg M, ter Berg HWM, Wijdicks EFM, van Gijn J. Subarachnoid haemorrhage in first and second degree relatives of patients with subarachnoid haemorrhage. BMJ 1995; 311: 288-9.

Burn J, Dennis M, Bamford J, Sandercock P, Wade D, Warlow C. Long-term risk of recurrent stroke after a first-ever stroke. Stroke 1994; 25: 333-7.

Camargo CA. Moderate alcohol consumption and stroke. The epidemiological evidence. Stroke 1989; 20: 1611-26.

Caplan LR, Hier DB, D'Cruz I. Cerebral embolism in the Michael Reese Stroke Registry. Stroke 1983; 14: 530-6.

CASANOVA Study Group. Carotid surgery versus medical therapy in asymptomatic carotid stenosis. Stroke 1991; 22: 1229-35.

Casper M, Wing S, Strogatz D, Davis CE, Tyroler HA. Antihypertensive treatment and US trends in stroke mortality, 1962 to 1980. Am J Public Health 1992; 82: 1600-06.

Chakravarty KK, Byron MA, Webley M, Durkin CJ, al-Hillawi AH, Bodley R, Wozniak J. Antibodies to cardiolipin in stroke: association with mortality and functional recovery in patients without systemic lupus erythematosus. Quarterly J Med 1991; 79: 397-405.

Chaturvedi N, McKeigue PM, Marmot MG. Resting and ambulatory blood pressure differences in Afro-Caribbeans and Europeans. Hypertension 1993; 22(1): 90-6.

Christie D. Stroke in Melbourne, Australia: an epidemiological study. Stroke 1981; 12: 467-9.

Colditz GA, Bonita R *et al.* Cigarette smoking and risk of stroke in middle-aged women. N Eng J Med 1988; 318: 937-41.

Collins R, Peto R., MacMahon S, Herbert P, Fiebach N *et al.* Blood pressure, stroke and coronary heart disease part 2. Short-term reductions in blood pressure: overviews of randomised drug trials in their epidemiological context. Lancet 1990; 335: 827-38.

Comstock GW. An epidemiologic study of blood pressure levels in a bi-racial community in the southern United States. Am J Hygiene 1957; 65: 271.

Connolly SJ, Laupacis A, Gent M, Roberts RS, Cairns JA, Joyner C. Canadian atrial fibrillation anticoagulation (CAFA) study. J Am Coll Cardiol 1991; 18: 349-55.

Copenhagen AFASAK Study. Placebo-controlled randomised trial of warfarin and aspirin for prevention of thromboembolic complications in chronic atrial fibrillation. Lancet 1989; 1: 175-9.

Coppola WGT, Whincup PH, Papacosta O *et al.* Scoring system to identify men at high risk of stroke: a strategy for general practice. Br J Gen Prac 1995; 45: 185-9.

Cruickshank JK, Akinkugbe OO, Nicholson GD. Heart disease in Blacks of Africa and the Caribbean. Cardiovascular Clinics 1991; 21(3): 377-91.

Cruickshank FB, Beevers D, Osbourne V, Haynes R, Corlett J, Selby S. Heart attack, stroke, diabetes and hypertension in West Indians, Asians and Whites in Birmingham, England. BMJ 1980; 281: 1108.

Cruickshank JK, Cooper J, Burnett M, Macduff J, Drubra U. Ethnic differences in fasting plasma C-peptide and insulin in relation to glucose tolerance and blood pressure. Lancet 1991; 338: 842-7.

Cruickshank JK, Jackson SH, Beevers DG, Bannan LT. Similarity of blood pressure in Blacks, Whites and Asians in England: The Birmingham factory study. J Hypertens 1985; 3(4): 365-71.

Cummins RO. Recent changes in salt use and stroke mortality in England and Wales. Any help for the salt hypertension debate? J Epidemiol Community Health 1983; 37: 25-8.

D'Souza M, Swan AV, Shannon DJ. A long-term controlled trial of screening for hypertension in general practice. Lancet 1976; i: 1228-31.

De Faire U, Friberg L, Lundman T. Concordance for mortality with special reference to ischaemic heart disease and cerebrovascular disease. Preventive Med 1975; 4: 509-17.

Dennis M, Warlow C. Strategies for stroke. BMJ 1991; 303: 636-8.

Dennis MS, Burn JB, Sandercock PAG, Bamford JM, Wade DT, Warlow CP. Long-term survival after first-ever stroke: The Oxfordshire Community Stroke Project. Stroke 1993; 24: 796-800.

Deubner DC, Tyroler HA. Attributable risk, population attributable risk and population attributable fraction of death associated with hypertension in a biracial population. Circulation 1975; 52: 901-8.

Department of Health. Health of the Nation: a strategy for health in England (Cm 1986); London HMSO 1992.

Devereux RB, Casale PN, Wallerson DC, Kligfield P, Hammond IW, Liebson PR, Campo E, Alonso DR, Laragh JH. Cost-effectiveness of echocardiography and electrocardiography for detection of left ventricular hypertrophy in patients with systemic hypertension . Hypertens 1987; 9: II-69-II-76.

Dolecek TA, Grandits G. Dietary polyunsaturated fatty acids and mortality in the Multiple Risk Factor Intervention Trial (MRFIT). World Rev Nutr Diet 1991; 66: 205-16.

Dutch Transient Ischaemic Attack Trial Study Group. A comparison of two doses of aspirin (30mg versus 283mg a day) in patients after a transient ischaemic attack or minor ischaemic stroke. N Eng J Med 1991; 325: 1261-6.

Elford J, Phillips AN, Thomson AG, Shaper AG. Migration and geographic variations in blood pressure in Britain. BMJ 1990; 300: 291-5.

Elford J, Phillips AN, Thomson AG, Shaper AG. Migration and geographic variations in ischaemic heart disease in Great Britain. Lancet 1989; i: 343-6.

Elford J, Shaper AG, Whincup P. Early life experience and cardiovascular disease - ecological studies. J Epidemiol Community Health 1992; 46: 1-8.

Elford J, Whincup P, Shaper AG. Early life experience and adult cardiovascular disease - longitudinal and case control studies. Int J Epidemiol 1991; 20: 833-44.

Ellekjaer E F, Wuller T B, Sverre J M, Holmen J. Life style factors and risk of cerebral infarction. Stroke 1992; 23:829-34.

Elliott P, Fehily AM, Sweetnam PM, Yarnell JWG. Diet, alcohol, body mass and social factors in relation to blood pressure: the Caerphilly Heart Study. J Epidemiol Community Health 1987; 4: 37-43.

European Atrial Fibrillation Trial Study Group. Optimal oral anticoagulant therapy in patients with non-rheumatic atrial fibrillation and recent cerebral ischaemia. N Eng J Med 1995; 333:5-10.

European Atrial Fibrillation Trial Study Group. Secondary prevention in non-rheumatic atrial fibrillation after transient ischaemic attack or minor stroke. Lancet 1993; 342: 1255-62.

European Carotid Surgery Trialists Collaborative Group. MRC European Carotid Surgery Trial: interim results for symptomatic patients with severe (70-99%) or with mild (0-29%) carotid stenosis. Lancet 1991; 337: 1235-43.

European Carotid Surgery Trialists Collaborative Group. Endarterectomy for moderate symptomatic carotid stenosis: interim results from the MRC European Carotid Surgery Trial. Lancet 1996; 347:591-3.

European Community Atlas of Avoidable Deaths. 2nd Edition. Project Director WW Holland. Oxford University Press. Oxford 1991.

Ezckowitz MD, Bridgers SL, James KE, Carliner WH, Colling CL, Gornick CC, et al. Warfarin in the prevention of stroke associated with nonrheumatic atrial fibrillation. N Engl J Med 1992; 327: 1406-12.

Family Heart Study Group. Randomised control trial evaluating cardiovacular screening and intervention in general practice: principal results of British family heart study. BMJ 1994; 308: 313-20.

Farquhar JW, Fortmann SP, Flora JA, Taylor CB et al. Effects of community wide education on cardiovascular disease risk factors. The Stanford Five-City Project. JAMA 1990; 264: 359-65.

Fray J, Douglas J. Pathophysiology of hypertension in Blacks. Oxford University Press, 1993.

Gaines SK, Burke G for the SECORDS Investigation. Ethnic differences in stroke: Black-White differences in the United States population. Neuroepidemiology 1995; 14: 209-39.

Gertler HM, Leetma HE, Koutrouby RJ. The assessment of insulin, glucose and lipids in ischaemic thrombotic cerebrovascular disease. Stroke 1975; 6: 77-84.

Gore JG, Dalen JE. Cardiovascular disease. JAMA 1990; 263: 2629-31.

Gorelick PB, Rodin MB, Langenberg P, Hier DB, Costigan J. Weekly alcohol consumption, cigarette smoking and the risk of ischaemic stroke. Results of a case control study at three urban medical centers in Chicago, Illinois. Neurology 1989; 39: 339-43.

Grau AJ, Buggle F, Heindl S *et al.* Recent infection as a risk factor for cerebrovascular ischaemia. Stroke 1995; 26: 373-9.

Grimley-Evans J. Blood pressure and stroke in an elderly English population. J. Epidemiol Community Health 1987; 4: 275-82.

Grotta JC, Norris JW, Kamm B. Prevention of stroke with ticlopidine: who benefits most? Neurol 1992; 42: 111-5.

Gustafsson C, Asplund K, Britton M, Norrving B, Olsson B, Marke LA. Cost-effectiveness of primary stroke prevention in atrial fibrillation: Swedish national perspective. BMJ 1992; 305: 1457-60.

Haberman S, Capildeo R, Rose FC. The seasonal variation is mortality from cerebrovascular disease. J Neurological Science 1981; 52: 25-36.

Haines AP, Booroff A, Goldenberg E, Morgan P, Singh M. Blood pressure, smoking, obesity and alcohol consumption in Black and White patients in general practice. J Hypertension 1987; 1(1): 39-46.

Hankey GJ, Warlow CP. Symptomatic carotid ischaemic events: Safest and most cost-effective way of selecting patients for angiography, before carotid endarterectomy. BMJ 1990; 30: 1485-91.

Harrison MJ. The haematocrit and cerebrovascular accidents. Presse Medicale - Paris 1983; 12: 3095-7.

Haynes RB, Harper AC, Cosiley SR. Failure of weight reduction to reduce mildly elevated blood pressure: A randomized trial. J Hypertension 1984; 2: 535-9.

Heller RF, Rose GA. Current management of hypertension in general practice. BMJ 1977; 1: 1442-4.

Herman B, Leyton ACM, Van Luijk JH *et al.* An evaluation of risk factors for stroke in a Dutch community. Stroke 1982; 13: 334-9.

Hess D. Stroke associated with antiphospholipid antibodies. Stroke 1992; 23: 23-4.

Heyman A, Karp HR, Heyden S, Bartel A, Cassel JC, Tyroler HA *et al.* Cerebrovascular disease in the bi-racial population of Evans County, Georgia. Stroke 1971; 2: 509-18.

Heyman A, Nefzger MD, Estes EH: Serum cholesterol level in cerebral infarction. Arch Neurol 1971; 5: 264-268.

Howard G, Russell GB, Anderson R, Evans GW, Morgan T, Howard VJ, Burke GL. Role of social class in excess black stroke mortality. Stroke 1995; 26: 1759-63.

Hypertension Detection and Follow-up Program. JAMA 1988; 259: 2113-22.

Hypertension Detection and Follow-up Program: 1. Reduction in mortality of persons with high blood pressure, including mild hypertension. JAMA 1979; 242: 2562-71

Imperial Cancer Research Fund OXCHECK Study Group. Effectiveness of health checks conducted by nurses in primary care: results of the OXCHECK Study after one year. BMJ 1994; 308: 308-12.

Intersalt. An international study of electrolyle excretion and blood pressure. Results for 24 hour urinary sodium and potassium excretion. BMJ 1988; 297: 319-28.

Irvine CD, Baird RN, Lamont PM. Endarterectomy for asymptomtic carotid artery stenosis. BMJ 1995; 311: 1121-32.

Iso H, Jacobs DR, Wentworth D, Neaton JD, Cohen JD. For the MRFIT Research Group. Serum cholesterol levels and six years mortality from stroke in 350,977 men screened for the Multiple Risk Factor Intervention Trial. N Engl J Med 1989; 320: 904-10.

Jackson G, Pierscianowski TA, Mahon W, Condon J. Inappropriate antihypertensive therapy in the elderly. Lancet 1976; ii: 1317-8.

Jacobs DR, Hahn LP, Folsom AR, Hannan PJ, Sprafka JM, Burke GL. Time trends in leisure-time physical activity in the Upper Midwest 1957-1987: University of Minnesota studies. Epidemiology 1991; 2: 8-15.

Kannel WB. Prevalence and natural history of electrocardiographic left ventricular hypertrophy. Am J Pub Health 1983; 75: 4-11.

Kannel WB, Gordon T. Evaluation of cardiovascular risk in the elderly: The Framingham Study. Bull N.Y. Acad Med 1978; 54(6): 573-91.

Kannel WB, Sorlie PD. Some health benefits of physical activity: The Framingham study. Arch Intern Med 1979; 139: 857-61.

Kannel WB, Wolf PA. Inferences from secular trend analysis of hypertension control. Am J Pub Health 1992; 82: 1593-5.

Khaw K, Barrett-Connor E. Dietary potassium and stroke-associated mortality. N Engl J Med 1987; 316: 235-40.

Khaw K, Barrett-Connor E. Family history of stroke as an independent predictor of ischaemic heart disease in men and stroke in women. Am J Epidemiol 1986; 123: 59-66.

Kiers L, Davis SM, Larkins R, Hopper J, Tress B, Rossiter SC, Carlin J, Ratnaike S. Stroke topography and outcome in relation to hyperglycaemia and diabetes. J Neourol Neurosurgy Psychiatry 1992; 55: 263-70.

Kistler JP, Singer DE, Millenson MM, Bauer RA, Sheehan MA, Maraventano SW, Oertel LB. Effect of low-intensity warfarin anticoagulation on the level of activity of the hemostatic system of patients with atrial fibrillation. The Boston Area Anticoagulation Trial for Atrial Fibrillation Investigators (BAATAF). Stroke 1993; 24: 1360-5.

Kittner SJ, White LR, Losonczy KG, Wolf PA, Hebel JR. Black-White differences in stroke incidence in a national sample. The contribution of hypertension and diabetes mellitus. JAMA 1990; 264: 1267-70.

Kiyohara Y, Koto I, Iwomoto H *et al.* The impact of alcohol and hypertension on stroke incidence in a general Japanese population. The Hisayama Study. Stroke 1995; 26: 368-72.

Klag MJ, Welton PK, Seidler AJ. Decline in US stroke mortality. Demographic trends and antihypertensive treatment. Stroke 1989; 20: 14-21.

Klag MJ, Whelton PK, Coresh J, Grim CE, Kuller LH. The association of skin colour with blood pressure in US Blacks with low socio-economic status. JAMA 1991; 265: 599-602.

Klatsky AL, Armstrong MA, Friedman GD. Risk of cardiovascular mortality in alcohol drinkers, ex-drinkers and non-drinkers. Am J Cardiol 1990; 66: 1237-42.

Knox EG. Meteorological associations of cerebrovascular disease mortality in England and Wales. J Epid Comm Health 1981; 35: 220-3.

Kono S, Ikeda M, Tokudome S, Nishizumi M, Kuratsune M. Alcohol and mortality: A cohort study of male Japanese physicians. Int J Epidemiol 1986; 15: 527-32.

Kopecky SL, Gersh BJ, McGoon MD *et al.* The natural history of lone atrial fibrillation. N Engl J Med 1987; 317: 669-74.

Kurji KH, Haines AP. Detection and management of hypertension in general practice in North West London. BMJ 1985; 288: 903-6.

Lambert M. Should carotid endarterectomy be purchased? Purchasers need a broader perspective. BMJ 1995; 310: 317-8.

Larsson B, Svardsudd Ketal. Abdominal adipose tissue distribution, obesity and risk of cardiovascular and death. BMJ 1984; 288: 1401-4.

Law CM, Barker DJP, Osmond C, Bull AR, Osmond C. Maternal and fetal influences on blood pressure. Arch Dis Child 1991; 66: 1291-5.

Law CM, Frost C, Wald N. By how much does dietary salt reduction lower blood pressure? I. Analysis of observational data among populations. BMJ 1991; 302: 811-5.

Law M, Frost C, Wald N. III. Analysis on data from trials of salt reductions. BMJ 1991; 302: 819-24.

Law MR, Thompson SG, Wald NJ. Assessing possible hazards of reducing serum cholesterol. BMJ 1994b; 308: 373-9.

Law MR, Wald NJ, Thompson SG. By how much and how quickly does reduction in serum cholesterol concentration lower risk of ischaemic heart disease. BMJ 1994a; 308: 367-72.

Lindenstrom E, Boysen E, Nyboe J. Influence of total cholesterol, high density lipoprotein cholesterol, and triglyceride on risk of cerebrovascular disease: The Copenhagen City Heart Study. BMJ 1994; 309: 11-5.

Lowe GDO. Antithrombotic treatment and atrial fibrillation. BMJ 1992; 305: 1445-6.

Lowe GDO, Jaap AJ, Forbes CD. Relation of atrial fibrillation and high haematocrit to mortality in acute stroke. Lancet 1983; i: 784-6.

MacGregor GA, Markandu ND, Sagnella GA, Singer DRJ, Cappuccio FP. Double-blind study of three sodium intakes and long-term effects of sodium restriction in essential hypertension. Lancet 1989; ii: 1244-7.

MacMahon SW, Peto R, Cutler J, Collins R, Sorlie P *et al.* Blood pressure, stroke and coronary heart disease. Part 1, prolonged differences in blood pressure: prospective observational studies corrected for the regression bias. Lancet 1990: 335: 765-74.

Malmgren R, Bamford J, Warlow C, Sandercock P, Slattery J. Projecting the number of patients with first ever strokes and patients newly handicapped by stroke in England and Wales. BMJ 1989; 298: 656-60.

Marmot MG, Adelstein AM, Bulusu L. Lessons from the study of immigrant mortality. Lancet 1984; I: 1455-8.

Marmot MG, Poulter NR. Primary prevention of stroke. Lancet 1992; 339: 344-7.

Marshall J. Diurnal variation in occurrence of strokes. Stroke 1977; 8: 230-1.

Mayberg MR, Wilson SE, Yatsu F, Weiss DG, Messina L, Hershey LA, Colling C, Eskridge J, Deykin D, Winn HR. Carotid endarterectomy and prevention of cerebral ischaemia in symptomatic carotid stenosis. Veterans Affairs Cooperative Studies Program 309 Trialist Group. JAMA 1991; 266: 3289-94.

McGovern P, Burke GL, Sprafka JM, Xue S, Folsom AR, Blackburn H. Trends in mortality, morbidity and risk factor levels for stroke from 1960 to 1990: the Minnesota Heart Survey. JAMA 1992; 268: 753-9.

Meade TW, Berra A. Hormone replacement therapy and cardiovascular disease. Br Med Bull 1992; 48: 276-308.

Meade TW, Brozovic M, Chakrabarti R, Haines AP, North WR, Stirling Y. Ethnic group comparisons of variables associated with ischaemic heart disease. British Heart Journal 1978; 40: 789-95.

Meade TW, Mellows S, Brozovic M. Haemostatic function and ischaemic heart disease: principle results of the Northwick Park Study. Lancet 1986; : 533-7.

Medical Research Council Working Party. Medical Research Council trial of treatment of hypertension in older patients: Principal results. BMJ 1992; 304: 405-12.

Medical Research Council Working Party. MRC trial of treatment of mild hypertension: Principle results. BMJ 1985; 291: 97-104.

Miettinen TA, Huttunen JK, Naukkarinen VA, Strandberg T, Mattila S, Kumlin T, et al. multifactorial primary prevention of cardiovascular disease in middle-aged men. JAMA 1985; 254: 2097-102.

Miller GJ, Kotecha S, Wilkinson WH et al. Dietary and other characteristics relevant for coronary heart disease in men of Indian, West Indian, and European descent in London. Atherosclerosis 1988; 70: 63-72.

Morgan M, Watkins CJ. Managing hypertension: Beliefs and responses to medication among cultural groups. Sociology of health and illness 1988; 10(4): 561-78.

Muldoon MF, Manuck SB, Matthews KA. Lowering cholesterol concentrations and mortality; a quantitative review of primary prevention trials. BMJ 1990; 301: 309-14.

Multiple Risk Factor Intervention Trial Research Group. Mortality after 10 1/2 years for hypertensive participants in the multiple risk factors intervention trial. Circulation 1990; 82: 1616-28.

Multiple Risk Factor Intervention Trial Research Group. Multiple risk factor intervention trial. Risk factors changes and mortality results. JAMA 1982; 248: 1465-78.

Neaton JD, Grimm RH, Cutler JA. Recruitment of participants for the multiple risk factor intervention trial (MRFIT). Controlled Clin Trials 1987; 8 (4 Suppl) 415-535.

Norday A, Illingworth DR et al. Increased activity of factor VII and factor VII-phospholipid complex measured using a normotest system in subjects with hyperlipidaemia. Haemostasis 1990; 20: 65-72.

North American Symptomatic Carotid Endarterectomy Trial Collaborators, Beneficial effect of carotid endarterectomy in symptomatic patients with high-grade carotid stenosis. N Eng J Med 1991; 325: 445-53.

Nygard O, Vollset SE, Refsum H et al. Total plasma homocysteine and cardiovascular risk profile. The Hordaland Homocysteine Study. JAMA 1995; 274: 1526-1533.

Ohno Y. Biometeorological studies on cerebrovascular disease, part I (Effects of meteorological factors on death from cerebrovascular accident), Japan Circ J 1969; 33: 1285-1314.

Okada H, Horibe H, Ohno Y, Hayakawa N, Aori N. A prospective study of cerebrovascular disease in Japanese rural communities, Akabani and Asahi. Part I: Evaluation of risk factors in the occurrence of cerebral haemorrhage and thrombosis. Stroke 1976; 7: 599-607.

Osmond C, Barker DJP, Slattery JM. Risk of death from cardiovascular disease and chronic bronchitis determined by place of birth in England and Wales. J Epidemiol Community Health 1990; 44: 139-41.

Otten MW, Teutch SM, Williams DF, Mark JS. The effect of known risk factors on the excess mortality of Black adults in the United States. JAMA 1990; 263: 845-50.

Oxfordshire Community Stroke Project. Incidence of stroke in Oxfordshire: first year's experience of a community stroke register. BMJ 1983; 287: 713-17.

Perry IJ, Refsum H, Morris RW, Ebrahim SB, Ueland PH, Shaper AG. Prospective study of serum total homocysteine concentration and risk of stroke in middle-aged British men. Lancet 1995; 346: 1395-8.

Petersen P, Boysen G, Godtfredsen J, Andersen ED, Andersen B. Placebo-controlled, randomised trial of warfarin and aspirin for prevention of thromboembolic complications in chronic atrial fibrillation: The Copenhagen AFASAK Study. Lancet 1989b; 1: 175-9.

Petersen P, Boysen G, Godtfredsen J, Andersen ED, Andersen B. Warfarin to prevent thromboembolism in chronic atrial fibrillation. Lancet 1989a; 1: 670

Petitti DB, Wingerd J, Pellegrin F, Ramcharan S. Risk of vascular disease in women: smoking, oral contraceptives, non-contraceptive estrogens and other factors. JAMA 1979; 242: 1150-54.

Peto R, Yusef S, Collins R. Cholesterol lowering trial results in their epidemiological context (abstract). Circulation 1985; 72(Suppl III): 111-451.

Pharoah PDP, Sanderson SP. Health promotion in primary care: modelling the impact of intervention on coronary heart disease and stroke. J Public Health Med 1995; 17: 150-6.

Puska P, Salonen JT, Nissinen A, Tuomilehto J et al. Change in risk factors for coronary heart disease during 10 years of a community intervention programme (North Karelia Project). BMJ 1983; 287: 1840-44.

Qizilbash N, Jones L, Warlow C, Mann J. Fibrinogen and lipid concentrations as risk factors for transient ischaemic attacks and minor strokes. BMJ 1991; 303: 605-9.

Qizilbash N, Jones L, Warlow C, Mann J. Fibrinogen and lipid concentrations as risk factors for transient ischaemic attacks and minor ischaemic strokes. BMJ 1993; 303: 605-9.

Qizilbash N, Warlow CP, Mann J. Fibrinogen and lipids as risk factors for ischaemic stroke. A case control study (abstract). J Neurol 1990; 237: 143.

Reed DM. The paradox of high risk of stroke in populations with low risk of coronary heart disease. Am J Epidemiol 1990; 131: 579-88.

Reid DD, Hamilton PJS, McCarthey P, Rose G. Smoking and other risk factors for coronary heart disease in British civil servants. Lancet 1990; 131: 579-88.

Reid DD, Hamilton PJS, McCarthey P, Rose G. Smoking and other risk factors for coronary heart disease in British civil servants. Lancet 1976; ii: 979-84.

Reid JL. Hypertension and the brain. Br Med Bull 1994; 50: 371-80.

Reisin E, Abel R, Modan M, Silverberg DS, Eliahou HE, Modan B. Effect of weight loss without salt restriction on the reduction of blood pressure in overweight hypertensive patients. N Eng J Med 1978; 298: 1-6.

Robins M, Baum H. Incidence. Stroke 1981; vol 12 Suppl. 1 pp 1-45.

Robinson RJ. Is the child father of the man? BMJ 1992; 304: 789-90.

Roelmholdt MB, Palumbo PJ, Wistlant JP et al. Transient ischaemic attack and stroke in a community based cohort. Mayo Clin Proc 1983; 58: 56-8.

Sacco RL, Wolf PA, Bharucha NA, Meeks SL, Kannel WB, Charette LJ, McNamara PM, Palmer EP, D'Agostino R. Subarachnoid and intracerebral haemorrhage: Natural history, prognosis, and precursive factors in the Framingham Study. Neurology 1984; 34: 847-54.

Sage JI, Van Uitert RL. Risk of recurrent stroke in patients with atrial fibrillation and non-valvular heart disease. Stroke 1983; 14: 537-40.

Salonen JT, Puska P, Tuomilehto J et al. Relation of blood pressure, serum lipids, and smoking to the risk of cerebral stroke. A longitudinal study in Eastern Finland. Stroke 1982; 13: 327-33.

SALT Collaborative Group. Swedish Aspirin Low-Dose Trial (SALT) of 75mg aspirin as secondary prophylaxis after cerebrovascular ischaemic events. Lancet 1991; 338: 1345-9.

Sandercock PAG, Warow CP, Jones LN, Starkey IR. Predisposing factors for cerebral infarction: The Oxfordshire Community Stroke Project. BMJ 1989; 298: 75-80.

Sasaki S, Zhang XH, Kesteloot H. Dietary sodium, potassium, saturated fat, alcohol and stroke mortality. Stroke 1995; 26: 783-9.

Saunders JB. Alcohol. An important cause of hypertension. BMJ 1987; 294: 1054-6.

Seidman DS, Laor A, Gale R, Stevenson DK, Mashiach S, Danon YL. Birth weight, current body weight, and blood pressure in late adolescence. BMJ 1991; 302: 1235-7.

Serjeant GR. Sickle cell disease. Oxford: Oxford University Press 1985.

Sever PS, Peart WS, Davies IB. Ethnic differences in blood pressure with observations on noradrenaline and renin. A hospital hypertensive population. Clinical Experimental Hypertension 1979; 1: 745-60.

Shanket N, Cruickshank JK. Coronary artery disease: impact upon Black and ethnic minority people. In: Access to health care for people from Black and ethnic minorities. ed. Hopkins A. and Bahl V. London: Royal College of Physicians, 1993.

Shaper AG, Phillips AN, Pocock SJ, Walker M, Macfarlane PW. Risk factors for stroke in middle aged British men. BMJ 1991; 302: 1111-5.

SHEP Cooperative Research Group. Prevention of stroke by antihypertensive drug treatment in older persons with isolated systolic hypertension. Final results of the systolic hypertension in the elderly program (SHEP). JAMA 1991; 265: 3255-64.

Sherman DG, Hart RG, Easton D. The secondary prevention of stroke in patients with atrial fibrillation. Arch Neurol 1986; 43: 65-70.

Shinton R, Beevers G. Meta-analysis of relation between cigarette smoking and stroke. BMJ 1989; 298: 789-94.

Shinton R, Sagar G. Life long exercise and stroke. BMJ 1993; 307: 231-34.

Siari A, Strazzullo P, Russo L, et al. Controlled trial of longterm oral potassium supplements in patients with mild hypertension. BMJ 1987; 294: 1453-6.

Silagy C, Muir J, Coulter A, Thorogood M, Roe L. Cardiovascular risk and attitudes to life style: what do patients think? BMJ 1993; 306: 1657-1660.

Sixty-plus Reinfarction Study Research Group: Risk of long-term oral anticoagulant therapy in elderly patients after myocardial infaction. Lancet 1982; i: 64-8.

Stampfer MJ et al. a prospective study of moderate alcohol consumption and the risk of coronary disease and stroke in women. N Engl J Med 1988; 319: 267-73.

Stegmayr B, Asplund K. Diabetes as a risk factor for stroke. Apopulation perspective. Diabetologia 1995; 38: 1061-8.

Stemmermann GN, Hayashi T, Resch JA, Chung CS, Reed DM, Rhoads GG. Risk factors related to ischaemic and hemorrhagic cerebrovascular disease at autopsy: The Honolulu Heart Study. Stroke 1984; 15: 23-8.

Strandberg TE, Salomaa VV, Naukarinen VA, Vanhanen HT, Sarna SJ, Miettinen TA. Long-term mortality after 5-year multifactoral primary prevention of cardiovascular disease in middle-aged men. JAMA 1991; 266: 1225-9.

Stroke Prevention in Atrial Fibrillation Investigators. Warfarin versus aspirin for prevention of thromboembolism in atrial fibrillation. Stroke prevention in Atrial Fibrillation II study. Lancet 1994; 343: 687-91.

Stroke Prevention in Atrial Fibrillation Study. Final results. Circulation 1991; 84: 527-39.

Syrjanen J, Valtonen VV, Iivanainen M, Kaste M, Huttunen JK. Preceeding infection as an important risk factor for ischaemic brain infarction in young and middle aged patients. BMJ 1988; 296: 1156-60.

Taggart H, Stout RW. Reduced high density lipoprotein in stroke: Relationship with elevated triglyceride and hypertension. Eur J Clin Invest 1979; 9: 219-221.

Tanaka H, Ueda Y, Hayashi M et al. Risk factors for cerebral haemorrhage and cerebral infarction in a Japanese rural community. Stroke 1982; 13: 62-73.

Thorvaldsen P, Asplund K, Kuutasmaa K, Rajaknagas A-M, Schroll M, for WHO MONICA Project. Stroke incidence, case fatality, and mortality in the WHO MONICA project. Stroke 1995; 26: 361-7.

Tobias L, Lange J, Ulm K, Wold L, Iwai J. Potassium reduces cerebral haemorrhage and death rate in hypertensive rates, even when blood pressure is not lowered. Hypertens 1985; 7: suppl 1: 1-110-4.

Uchiyama S, Takeuchi H, Osawa M. et al. Platelet function in thrombotic cerebrovascular disorders. Stroke 1983; 14: 511-7.

Ueda K, Howard G, Toole TF. Transient ischaemic attacks (TIA's) and cerebral infarction (CI): A comparison of predisposing factors. J Chronic Dis 1980; 33: 13-9.

UK-TIA Study Group. The United Kingdom transient ischaemic attack (UK-TIA) aspirin trial final results. J Neurol Neurosurg Psychiatry 1991; 54: 1044-54.

Vartiainen E, Sarti C, Tuomilehto J, Kuulasmaa K. Do changes in cardiovascular risk factors explain changes in mortality from stroke in England? BMJ 1995; 310: 901-4.

Vessey MP, Lawless M, Yeates S. Oral contraception and stroke: findings in a large prospective study. BMJ 1984; 289: 530-1.

Wang WC, Kovnar EH, Tonkin IL, Mulhern RK, Langston JW, Day SW, Shell MJ, Wilimas JA. High risk of recurrent stroke after discontinuance of five to twelve years of transfusion therapy in patients with sickle cell disease. J Pediatr 1991; 118: 377-82.

Wannamethee AG, Shaper AG. Physical activity and stroke in British middle-aged men. BMJ 1992; 304: 597-601.

Weinstein MC, Stason WB. Hypertension: a policy perspective. Cambridge Mass, Harvard Univ Press 1976.

Welin L, Svardsudd K, Wilhelmson L, Larssson B, Tibblin G. Analysis of risk factors for stroke in a cohort of men born in 1913. N Eng J Med 1987; 317: 521-6.

Whincup P, Cook D, Shaper A, Macfarlane D, Walker M. Blood pressure in British children: Association with adult blood pressure and cardiovascular mortality. Lancet 1988; 1: 890-3.

Whisnant JP. The decline of stroke. Stroke 1984; 15: 160-8.

Wilhelmsen L, Berglund G, Elmfeldt D, Tibblis G, Wedel K, Pennert A *et al.* The multifactorial primary prevention trial in Goteborg, Sweden. Eur Heart J 1986; 7: 279-88.

Wilhelmsen L, Svardsudd K, Korsan-Bengtsen E, Larsson B, Welin L, Tibblin G. Fibrinogen as a risk factor for stroke and myocadial infarction. N Eng J Med 1984; 311: 501-5.

Wolf P, Kannel WB, Verter J. Current status of risk factors for stroke. Neurol Clin 1983; 1: 317-43.

Wolf PA, Abbott RD, Kannell WB. Atrial fibrillation as an independent risk factor for stroke: the Framingham study. Stroke 1991; 22: 983-8.

Wolf PA, D'Agostino RB, Kannel WB, Bonita R, Belanger AJ. Cigarette smoking as a risk factor for stroke. JAMA 1988; 259: 1025-9.

Wolf PA, Dawber TR, Thomas HE, Kannell WB. Epidemiologic assessment of chronic atrial fibrillation and risk of stroke. The Framingham study. Neurology 1978; 28: 973-7.

Wolf PA, Kannel WB, Cupples LA, D'Agostino. Update on epidemiology of stroke in Stroke: epidemiological, therapeutic and socio-economic aspects. Ed. F Clifford Rose. Royal Society of Medicine Services Limited. International Congress and Symposium Series no. 99. 1986; p 3-9.

World Health Organisation European Collaborative Group. European collaborative trial of multifactorial prevention of coronary heart disease: final report on the 6-year results. Lancet 1986; i: 869-72.

Wroe SJ, Sandercock PJ, Bamford J, Dennis M, Slattery J, Warlow C. Diurnal variation in incidence of stroke: Oxfordshire Community Stroke Project. BMJ 1992; 304: 155-7.

Yamori Y, Horie R, Nara Y *et al.* Dietary prevention of hypertension in animal models and its applicability to human. Ann Clin Res 1984; 16 (suppl 43): 28-31.

Yano K, Reed DM, Kagan A. Coronary heart disease, hypertension and stroke among Japanese-American men in Hawaii: the Honalulu Heart Program. Hawaii Medical Journal 1985; 44: 297-300.

Yano K, Reed DM, Maclean CJ. Serum cholesterol and haemorrhagic stroke in the Honolulu Heart Program. Stroke 1989; 20: 1460-5.

Yiyohara Y, Ueda K, Hasuo Y *et al.* Haematocrit as a risk factor of cerebral infarction: long-term prospective population survey in a Japanese rural community. Stroke 1986; 17: 687-92.

# CHAPTER 3

## CURRENT SERVICE PROVISION FOR STROKE

*Roger Beech*

**Chapter outline**

## Introduction

Various 'models of good practice' have been proposed for the management and organisation of stroke services (see Chapter 17). The underlying aim of these models is to improve the quality and effectiveness of stroke care. However, when considering such models they need to be set in the context of current service provision. There are several reasons why an understanding of current service provision is desirable:

• It helps expose current service deficiencies and therefore clarifies and quantifies the need for change.

• It gives an indication of the scale of change required.

• By using economic data and data on the effectiveness of proposed innovations in services, it allows an assessment of the likely overall cost and cost-effectiveness of service developments.

This chapter draws on data from the scientific literature, published sources and data being collected as part of a European Union Biomed project on stroke care. These data indicate the current provision of services for stroke care and the way this varies both within England and across the European Union. The likely consequences of current service patterns, in terms of equity, efficiency, effectiveness and cost-effectiveness, are then discussed.

## Current service provision for stroke

It was estimated many years ago that stroke services accounted for at least 4% of the NHS budget but that figure did not take into account social service and carer costs. Services available for stroke management span primary and secondary care settings and long-term care in a variety of public and private sector settings. The routine data available on such a high resource user as stroke are surprisingly scarce. There are no routine data that can be readily accessed for primary prevention. Contacts with general practitioners are documented through spotter practices around the country on a routine basis which provide only a brief insight into the burden of stroke patients in the community. Hospital Episode Statistics (HES) provide some information on stroke admissions to hospital but there are no data on the use of rehabilitation services by stroke patients other than through contract specification information or through audits and research projects. Routine information from social services, nursing homes and other organisations is not available on a regular basis or in a standardised manner. However, in spite of these deficiencies in the data, it is possible to generate a picture of current service provision for stroke and this is given below.

**Primary health care**

Primary preventive services vary considerably around the country and are usually incorporated into the cardiovascular disease preventive programmes developed as part of The Health of the Nation strategy. The provision and uptake of these services is monitored by Family Health Services Authorities and the models of service provision are clearly laid out in The Health of the Nation Handbook on Coronary Heart Disease and Stroke.

Stroke is estimated to account for 7% of emergency calls seen out of hours (Riddell 1980). The morbidity survey in general practice (OPCS 1995) estimates that circulatory diseases account for 9% of consultations, 36% of which are "serious" with the most common reason being for essential hypertension. Overall cerebrovascular disease prevalence was estimated at 5-8 per 1000 individuals. Nearly all patients who consulted for cerebrovascular disease did so for transient cerebral ischaemia or for acute but ill-defined cerebrovascular disease. Comparison of prevalence rates for 1971/2 and 1991/2 shows an overall 64% increase in consultation rates. The number of contacts for follow-up of a stroke would appear from the statistics to be low.

There have been audits of services received by patients discharged from stroke units but these are biased as they do not detail the resources available to, or consumed by, non-admitted patients. Ebrahim *et al.* (1987) audited services six months after discharge from hospital. Eighty four per cent of the survivors were at home. Of those interviewed, just over half had seen their GP, 30% a district nurse, 25% a home help and 21% meals on wheels. Outpatient therapy had been received by 42%, primarily disabled patients. Barer (1991) contacted district nurse services in Nottinghamshire and identified 369 patients in the community receiving help from the district nursing services. He estimated that only 20% of the expected prevalent cases of severely disabled stroke patients were receiving nursing assistance. In Bristol, Legh-Smith *et al.* (1986) assessed 436 patients one year after their stroke and 88% were at home. The GP had been to see 44% recently, the district nurse had visited 19%, 15% were attending a day centre or day hospital, and meals on wheels were delivered to 8%. Services appeared to be reaching all those who required them.

**Secondary health care**

Secondary care services for stroke management span many specialties (care of the elderly, acute medicine, neurology, neurosurgery, rehabilitation) and the patterns of care vary considerably around the country depending on a variety of local influences such as historic patterns of care, priority of purchasers and providers to modify traditional service provision, and local enthusiasm and expertise in the management of stroke patients. The balance of care between the different professional groups involved in the management of the stroke patients varies considerably as does the philosophy of care (therapists, nurses, medical practitioners, psychologists).

Although stroke care usually involves hospitalisation, wide variations have been reported between English districts in the proportion of stroke cases which are admitted to inpatient care: the hospitalisation rate. A study in Oxford estimated a hospitalisation rate of 55% (OCSP 1983) and a study of three health authorities in southern England - West Lambeth; Lewisham and North Southwark (both inner-city); and Tunbridge Wells (rural) - found an overall rate of 71% with no significant difference between districts (Wolfe *et al.* 1993). It is impossible to accurately assess hospitalisation rates without the use of registers such as those established in Oxford and southern England. These were introduced for research purposes and their results may not be typical. In his 'needs assessment for stroke', Wade estimated that between health authorities, hospitalisation rates currently vary from 50 to 90% (Wade 1994). He went on to argue that although it is the less severe stroke cases who tend to remain at home, this is not always the case. The implication appears to be that the variation in hospitalisation rates that exist across the country is to a large extent due to variations in local practice and the availability of resources rather than due to variations in case mix.

Routine HES data can be used to estimate the overall number of admissions for stroke but these data do not distinguish first from recurrent stroke and no data are available on the non-admitted patients. It is also impossible to establish with certainty the reason for admission or the validity of the ICD code assigned to the patient and therefore it is wisest to consider all stroke admissions, with the possible exception of subarachnoid haemorrhage, as one group (Department of Health 1995). HES data for 1993/4 indicate that in England and Wales there were around 5,000 admissions for subarachnoid haemorrhage and around 58,000 for other stroke types. It would therefore appear that a larger proportion of patients with a subarachnoid haemorrhage are admitted relative to the overall incidence of stroke subtypes (see Chapter 1).

It is estimated that in terms of acute stroke services patients consume the following resources: 20% of acute beds, 25% of all long-term beds, including nursing home places (Wade 1994). In The Stroke Association survey 67% of physicians indicated that they routinely cared for patients with acute stroke and around 40% of patients were treated by geriatricians (Lindley *et al.* 1995). Few (5%) had access to an acute stroke unit and a majority (51%) of consultants were uncertain of the benefits of such units. Less than half (44%) had access to a specialized stroke rehabilitation unit, although a majority (68%) were certain of the benefits of stroke rehabilitation units. About one-third of all UK stroke patients were admitted to a hospital without on-site computed tomography (CT) facilities. There are few studies on institutional care and stroke. Barer surveyed nursing homes in Nottingham and estimated that a quarter of beds were occupied by stroke patients and that these patients had a high level of emotional distress and felt lonely (Barer 1991, Gladman *et al.* 1991).

### Between-hospital variations in stroke services

Global statistics provide an incomplete picture of stroke care. Once in hospital, there are variations between hospitals in the types of services that a patient who has suffered a stroke can expect to receive. These variations appear to exist both between hospitals and even within the same hospital. Exposing the scale and nature of these variations in order to assess how they might be leading to differences in outcomes and costs between hospitals has been a theme of ongoing research by colleagues within the Department of Public Health Medicine, UMDS.

Initial research focused on stroke patients' use of rehabilitation services in three health authorities of southern England: West Lambeth; Lewisham and North Southwark; and Tunbridge Wells (Wolfe *et al.* 1993). The study covered all first-time strokes occurring in these authorities during the year commencing August 1989. Significant differences were found between authorities in the percentage of patients receiving inpatient physiotherapy, ranging from 59% in one authority to 91% in another. Overall only 33% of patients received outpatient physiotherapy with no significant differences between districts. There were also differences between authorities in the percentage of patients who received inpatient occupational therapy, ranging from 46% to 62%, and inpatient speech therapy, ranging from 41% to 58%. Although these differences were not significant, the proportion of patients receiving therapy was considered to be low in comparison to the percentage who might have benefited from such therapy. The percentage of patients receiving outpatient occupational and speech therapy was also low, the overall percentages being 12% and 16% respectively.

Patients with paralysis and those with longer stay were more likely to receive inpatient physiotherapy; those with longer lengths of stay and those with paralysis but no incontinence were more likely to receive occupational therapy; and those with a speech impairment were more likely to receive speech therapy. However, concerns were raised both about the proportion of patients who received no therapy and about there being inconsistency within the same hospitals in the ways in which patients were assigned to therapy. These concerns about inconsistency led one of the hospitals included in the study to institute a weekly multidisciplinary meeting to plan stroke care (West Lambeth Health Authority Stroke Steering Group, 1992).

A later study compared the direct cost of stroke care in two of these health authorities, West Lambeth and Tunbridge Wells (Wolfe *et al.* 1995). The cost per inpatient case was estimated as £3555 in West Lambeth and £2466 in Tunbridge Wells. Although some of this difference in cost was due to differences in the sophistication of the cost data available in the two settings, the difference also reflected differences in local policies regarding stroke management and use of services. As later chapters on the effectiveness and cost-effectiveness of stroke care will illustrate, it is difficult at present to assess which of the above costs represents the best value for money.

Within the South Thames Region a stroke group has been set up to foster networks between provider and research units and this has revealed a whole spectrum of models of care which are not similar in any two districts. The results from a European study are now discussed and these illustrate the heterogeneity of models of stroke service in operation.

# A European perspective on resource use for acute stroke care

A current project funded by the European Commission (Wolfe *et al.* 1995) is exploring, both within England and across Europe, variations in services provided for stroke care, the resources and costs of this care, and the subsequent outcomes of care. The results of this research will help indicate which pattern of services appears to be the most effective and hence which represents the best value for money. The study covers 22 hospitals in eight European states and the data being collected in each site include: the baseline characteristics of patients (age, sex etc.); their clinical state at time of maximum impairment (level of consciousness, existence of speech or swallowing problems etc.); their use of inpatient and outpatient services (lengths of stay by bed type, use of major diagnostic and therapeutic interventions, use of rehabilitation services etc.); and their three-month and 12-month outcome from stroke in terms of mortality, handicap, functional ability and clinical state. The study is still to be completed but preliminary results are available which allow a comparison of inpatient service use by stroke patients by hospital.

Tables 1-4 present these results for the five English hospitals covered by the study and for a small sample of similar hospitals from elsewhere in Europe. The non-English hospitals have been included because of their location in regions of Europe that might be considered similar to England in terms of their social and economic make-up: France, Germany and Northern Italy. For the majority of the hospitals the data presented in the tables relate to all stroke admissions during the year commencing September 1993. The data for Hospital 5 and the Rhineland hospital cover a slightly earlier period. In general the data were extracted, during the period of a patient's inpatient stay, from case notes and other hospital records.

Table 1 compares key casemix variables for the sample of patients admitted to each hospital. The hospitals have a similar mix of admissions in terms of their age and diagnosis. They also appear to be similar in terms of the percentage of their admissions who are fully conscious at the time of their maximum impairment. The exceptions are Hospital 8 in Hamburg, which has a very high percentage of fully conscious cases, and Hospitals 3 and 4 in England, where the high percentage of admissions where these data are missing make the results difficult to interpret. In terms of the percentage of patients who were incontinent during the seven days following their stroke, there are large differences between the hospitals. However, the general impression is that variations in casemix are unlikely to fully account for any between-hospital variations in use of services by stroke patients that are revealed by Tables 2-4.

Table 2 indicates for each hospital the type of bed that stroke cases are first admitted to and the mean and median lengths of stay of these admissions inclusive of those who died in hospital. These lengths of stay are also inclusive of any subsequent bed transfers that these admissions may have had during their time in hospital. Admission to an acute medical bed is by far the most common method in all but one of the hospitals. The exception is Hospital 8 in Hamburg which admits just under half of its stroke admissions to neurology beds. Hospital 6 in Dijon is also a frequent user of neurology beds and Hospital 3 admits around a quarter of its cases to rehabilitation beds.

There are large variations between hospitals in the mean and median lengths of stay of stoke admissions. Mean stays range from 14.27 days to 37.30 days and median stays from 12.00 to 22.00 days. Previous research has demonstrated that for elderly acute cases lengths of stay are highly influenced by the presence of facilities which provide lower levels of care, such as nursing homes and convalescent hospitals, in the vicinity of the main acute site (Beech *et al.* 1995). The presence of such facilities increases the number of options available when decisions about patient discharge are being made. The lack of them may mean patients have to stay longer in an acute setting until they are ready to return to their homes. The final row of Table 2 indicates, for those patients who did not die in hospital and for whom a discharge destination was recorded, the number of patients discharged to their home. The residual percentage covers those discharged to non-acute forms of institutional care.

In the hospitals from mainland Europe there does seem to be a possible link between length of stay and the percentage of patients discharged to their home: Hospital 8 has the longest mean stay and the highest percentage of patients going home and Hospital 6 one of the shortest stays and the lowest percentage of patients discharged to their home. In England Hospital 1 does have the longest length of stay and the greatest percentage of patients discharged to their home. In general though the link is rather messy and this demonstrates that variations in local hospital practice styles are also important. For example, Hospital 5 has a low percentage of patients going home and a long length of stay and Hospital 10, Florence, a high percentage of patients going home but the shortest mean stay of all of the hospitals.

In practice, some of the factors which control patient stay are within the direct control of staff within the acute hospital, such as local policies for clinical management. Others, such as the presence of nursing homes, are beyond the staff's direct control and are influenced by factors such as government policy. However, it is important that the factors which are contributing to the current lengths of stay achieved by a hospital are understood and, where possible, factors which are inappropriately prolonging stay are avoided. This is because inpatient hospital care is expensive and, in terms of costs to the health service, inpatient costs account for by far the greatest proportion of spending on the overall care of stroke patients (Wolfe *et al.* 1995). Avoiding some of these costs creates the opportunity to re-invest the funds in other forms of stroke care.

**Table 1: CHARACTERISTICS OF STROKE CASES ADMITTED TO A SAMPLE OF EUROPEAN HOSPITALS**

| PATIENT CHARACTERISTIC | HOSPITAL | | | | | | | | | |
|---|---|---|---|---|---|---|---|---|---|---|
| | Hospital 1 Urban | Hospital 2 Urban | Hospital 3 Urban | Hospital 4 Urban | Hospital 5 Rural | Hospital 6 Dijon France | Hospital 7 Hamburg Germany | Hospital 8 Hamburg Germany | Hospital 9 Rhineland Germany | Hospital 10 Florence Italy |
| Total admissions | 216 | 160 | 220 | 172 | 256 | 213 | 261 | 275 | 96 | 354 |
| Mean age | 71.48 | 75.45 | 75.25 | 76.12 | 75.11 | 74.82 | 78.41 | 70.34 | 73.82 | 74.14 |
| **Stroke diagnosis:** | | | | | | | | | | |
| Subarachnoid n (%) | 5 (2.31) | 1 (0.62) | 0 (0.00) | 0(0.00) | 16(6.25) | 3(1.41) | 0(0.00) | 0(0.00) | 1(1.04) | 4(1.13) |
| Other n (%) | 195(90.28) | 139(86.88) | 182(82.73) | 139(80.81) | 239(93.36) | 205(96.24) | 159(60.92) | 237(86.18) | 94(97.92) | 318(89.83) |
| Missing n (%) | 16(7.41) | 20(12.50) | 38(17.27) | 33(19.19) | 1(0.39) | 5(2.35) | 102(39.08) | 38(13.82) | 1(1.04) | 32(9.04) |
| **Level of consciousness:** | | | | | | | | | | |
| Fully conscious n (%) | 142(65.74) | 95(59.38) | 48(21.82) | 39(22.68) | 138(53.91) | 147(69.01) | 150(57.47) | 237(86.18) | 54(56.25) | 218(61.58) |
| Somnolent/ semi-conscious n (%) | 59 (27.31) | 50(31.25) | 27(12.27) | 10(5.81) | 79(30.86) | 43(20.19) | 90(34.48) | 33(12.00) | 34(35.42) | 99(27.97) |
| In coma (%) | 12 (5.56) | 10(6.25) | 6(2.73) | 14(8.14) | 38(14.84) | 22(10.33) | 16(6.13) | 2(0.73) | 6(6.25) | 37(10.45) |
| Missing n (%) | 3 (1.39) | 5(3.12) | 139(63.18) | 109(63.37) | 1(0.39) | 1(0.47) | 5(1.92) | 3(1.09) | 2(2.08) | 0(0.00) |
| **Incontinence present:** | | | | | | | | | | |
| Yes n(%) | 63 (29.17) | 64(40.00) | 137(62.27) | 88(51.16) | 164(64.06) | 51(23.94) | 119(45.59) | 48(17.45) | 60(62.50) | 154(43.50) |
| No n(%) | 147(68.05) | 89(55.63) | 77(35.00) | 73(42.44) | 87(33.98) | 161(73.59) | 142(54.41) | 227(82.55) | 36(37.50) | 200(56.50) |
| Missing n(%) | 6 (2.78) | 7(4.37) | 6(2.73) | 11(6.40) | 5(1.96) | 1(0.47) | 0(0.00) | 0(0.00) | 0(0.0) | 0(0.00) |

**Table 2:  USE OF SERVICES FOR STROKE CASES ADMITTED TO A SAMPLE OF EUROPEAN HOSPITALS**

HOSPITAL

| SERVICE CATEGORY | Hospital 1 Urban | Hospital 2 Urban | Hospital 3 Urban | Hospital 4 Urban | Hospital 5 Rural | Hospital 6 Dijon France | Hospital 7 Hamburg Germany | Hospital 8 Hamburg Germany | Hospital 9 Rhineland Germany | Hospital 10 Florence Italy |
|---|---|---|---|---|---|---|---|---|---|---|
| Bed type on admission: | | | | | | | | | | |
| Acute medical n (%) | 198(91.67) | 155(96.88) | 154(70.00) | 154(89.54) | 246(96.10) | 151(70.89) | 256(98.09) | 142(51.64) | 93(96.88) | 347(98.02) |
| Neurology  n (%) | 4(1.85) | 1(0.63) | 1(0.45) | 2(1.16) | 0(0.00) | 40(18.78) | 1(0.38) | 125(45.45) | 0(0.00) | 1(0.28) |
| Intensive care n (%) | 5(2.31) | 1(0.63) | 5(2.27) | 1(0.58) | 5(1.95) | 5(2.35) | 0(0.00) | 4(1.46) | 3(3.12) | 2(0.56) |
| Surgery n(%) | 1(0.46) | 1(0.63) | 4(1.82) | 8(4.65) | 0(0.00) | 3(1.41) | 0(0.00) | 1(0.36) | 0(0.00) | 4(1.13) |
| Rehabilitation n(%) | 5(2.31) | 0(0.00) | 56(25.45) | 2(1.16) | 0(0.00) | 0(0.00) | 0(0.00) | 0(0.00) | 0(0.00) | 0(0.00) |
| Private/other n(%) | 2(0.93) | 0(0.00) | 0(0.00) | 0(0.00) | 5(1.95) | 9(4.22) | 0(0.00) | 0(0.00) | 0(0.00) | 0(0.00) |
| Missing n(%) | 1(0.46) | 2(1.23) | 0(0.00) | 5(2.91) | 0(0.00) | 5(2.35) | 4(1.53) | 3(1.09) | 0(0.00) | 0(0.00) |
| Length of stay: | | | | | | | | | | |
| Mean (days) | 37.30 | 31.32 | 30.43 | 27.62 | 36.39 | 16.17 | 23.57 | 25.61 | 21.44 | 13.74 |
| Median (days) | 18.00 | 20.00 | 18.00 | 16.00 | 21.00 | 12.00 | 20.00 | 21.00 | 18.50 | 11.00 |
| Percentage of patients discharged to their home (excludes deaths in hospital) | 87.40 | 36.98 | 67.10 | 72.22 | 49.49 | 56.81 | 66.93 | 86.18 | 60.60 | 74.57 |

The results in Table 3 indicate for each hospital the percentage of patients receiving major diagnostic tests and interventions. Brain imaging, usually in the form of CT scans, is now done on a high percentage of patients, particularly in the mainland Europe hospitals, with four out of five of them have a percentage close to or above 90%. In comparison to the other hospitals, a very low percentage of patients receive brain imaging in Hospital 5. This hospital did have a CT scan machine but stroke patients were not given a high priority. Later chapters of this review will reveal that although there is currently a strong consensus that stroke patients should receive CT scans (Kings Fund Consensus Statement 1988; Royal College of Physicians 1989) the scientific evidence is inconclusive (Sotaniemi *et al.* 1990). Hence the efficacy of the policy adopted by Hospital 5 is also unclear. The results of trials of thrombolysis or anticoagulation may change this.

There were wide variations across the sites in the percentage of patients who underwent secondary preventive investigations such as carotid Doppler tests and echocardiograms. For the use of Doppler, percentages ranged from 0% to 97.09% and for echocardiograms percentages ranged from 0.39% to 74.07%. Across all hospitals there was a low rate of use for the other potential interventions for stroke care listed in Table 3.

**Table 3: USE OF SERVICES FOR STROKE CASES ADMITTED TO A SAMLE OF EUROPEAN HOSPITALS (continued)**

HOSPITAL

| SERVICE CATEGORY | Hospital 1 Urban | Hospital 2 Urban | Hospital 3 Urban | Hospital 4 Urban | Hospital 5 Rural | Hospital 6 Dijon France | Hospital 7 Hamburg Germany | Hospital 8 Hamburg Germany | Hospital 9 Rhineland Germany | Hospital 10 Florence Italy |
|---|---|---|---|---|---|---|---|---|---|---|
| Percentage of patients having inpatient investigations: | | | | | | | | | | |
| Brain imaging | 73.11 | 67.31 | 71.36 | 80.23 | 29.92 | 96.71 | 72.03 | 98.18 | 95.83 | 88.14 |
| Angiography | 4.24 | 3.87 | 0.91 | 0.00 | 1.17 | 17.84 | 0.38 | 8.00 | 0.00 | 3.39 |
| Doppler | 23.70 | 9.03 | 8.22 | 9.38 | 0.00 | 81.69 | 22.22 | 97.09 | 21.88 | 36.16 |
| Echocardiogram | 36.49 | 21.94 | 2.28 | 19.48 | 0.39 | 55.87 | 68.35 | 74.07 | 5.21 | 18.36 |
| Neurosurgery | 0.50 | 0.00 | 0.45 | 0.00 | 0.00 | 0.94 | 0.38 | 1.09 | 0.00 | 1.41 |
| Carotid surgery | 0.00 | 0.00 | 0.00 | 0.00 | 0.00 | 3.76 | 0.00 | 2.91 | 0.00 | 0.56 |
| Other vascular surgery | 0.47 | 0.65 | 0.00 | 0.00 | 0.00 | 2.82 | 0.00 | 0.36 | 0.00 | 0.56 |

Finally, the results in Table 4 compare hospitals in terms of the percentage of patients receiving inpatient rehabilitation services. Wide variations in the percentage of patients who received these services and in the number of sessions they received are revealed. Some of this variation will be due to variations in the characteristics of patients across the hospitals and some to slight variations in the way the data were collected across sites. However, some of the variation is also likely to be due to variations in local policies for clinical management and some due to variations in the availability of resources for rehabilitation.

Patients were also followed up three months after their stroke. For those patients who had been discharged from the acute hospital, the final section of Table 4 indicates the percentage of patients who received further rehabilitation services. Potential settings where this rehabilitation could have occurred include a non-acute institution, during an outpatient appointment, or in the patient's home. In two of the English hospitals very few patients received rehabilitation after discharge. It is also noticeable that in the hospitals of mainland Europe, a consistently higher proportion of patients receive therapy after discharge.

This programme of research into stroke care is on-going. Later analysis will investigate the link between the variations in service use across the hospitals and the subsequent outcomes of stroke care. In this way the results will help to demonstrate which patterns of management are most effective. The cost and resource implications that result from this variation in service use will also be identified. Funding has also been secured for a further Biomed study. This will study in greater detail the variation across Europe in the care provided for stroke patients in the community by health service agencies and by family members and other informal carers.

**Table 4: USE OF SERVICES (continued)**

| SERVICE CATEGORY | HOSPITAL | | | | | | | | | |
|---|---|---|---|---|---|---|---|---|---|---|
| | Hospital 1 Urban | Hospital 2 Urban | Hospital 3 Urban | Hospital 4 Urban | Hospital 5 Rural | Hospital 6 Dijon France | Hospital 7 Hamburg Germany | Hospital 8 Hamburg Germany | Hospital 9 Rhineland Germany | Hospital 10 Florence Italy |
| Percentage of patients having inpatient rehabilitation | | | | | | | | | | |
| Physiotherapy | 78.24 | 33.75 | 82.33 | 52.63 | 60.55 | 69.01 | 97.72 | 86.60 | 55.21 | 39.55 |
| Speech therapy | 30.56 | 11.88 | 42.92 | 27.03 | 22.66 | 34.74 | 90.82 | 62.79 | 2.08 | 0.00 |
| Occupational therapy | 61.57 | 13.13 | 36.07 | 23.68 | 33.59 | 30.52 | 12.12 | 65.67 | 0.00 | 0.00 |
| Mean sessions received for those having therapy: | | | | | | | | | | |
| Physiotherapy | 19.01 | 13.00 | 19.99 | 19.65 | 20.37 | 7.45 | 15.15 | 16.65 | 13.94 | 7.30 |
| Speech therapy | 12.51 | 7.26 | 3.98 | 7.00 | 4.66 | 6.41 | 13.28 | 14.53 | 1.50 | 0.00 |
| Occupational therapy | 10.97 | 3.00 | 8.82 | 5.94 | 14.48 | 5.41 | 18.75 | 14.32 | 0.00 | 0.00 |
| Percentage of patients having rehabilitation after their discharge from the study hospital (excludes those who died in hospital) | 6.87 | 45.95 | 24.32 | 8.82 | 20.29 | 58.76 | 50.54 | 47.53 | 21.69 | 46.67 |

## Executive summary

The previous section has revealed that there are wide variations between and within hospitals in the types of services that stroke patients receive for their care. In 1988 a King's Fund Consensus Statement described stroke services in the United Kingdom as haphazard, fragmented and poorly tailored to the needs of patients (King's Fund Consensus Statement 1988). Five years later The Stroke Association survey of consultant opinion of hospital services for acute stroke in the United Kingdom demonstrated that stroke services were still poorly organised (Lindley *et al.* 1995). For example, access to CT scan was improving but still inefficient. Indeed, in his recent needs assessment Wade (1994) reiterated the point that stroke services have developed in an unplanned manner in the United Kingdom. Perhaps this is inevitable given the shortage of evidence about which pattern of services is the most effective. However, the overall pattern of stroke care that has evolved does have major implications:

• Firstly, even though the efficacy of many of the interventions may be unclear, there is currently geographic inequity in the services that stroke patients receive. The previous section demonstrated that the services that stroke patients can expect to get vary according to their acute hospital of admission. For example, in a sample of English hospitals the earlier results indicated a range from 29.92% to 80.23% in the percentage of admissions who had a CT scan.

• Secondly, the current overall pattern of services cannot be cost-effective. Although the effectiveness of many of the potential interventions for stroke care is still to be clarified, the current variation in service provision implies that in some areas there is over provision of ineffective services and in others under provision of effective services.

• These implications demonstrate the need for developments in stroke care and for continuing research to identify which patterns of care are the most effective and cost-effective. Studies comparing resource use, patterns of care and outcome in contrasting settings can provide guidance for the development of models of care.

Wade (1994) posed a number of issues that health care purchasers and providers should consider. These included questions related to: the proportion of stroke cases who should be cared for at home rather than in hospital; the role of well coordinated specialised units or wards for stroke care as opposed to care in general acute wards; the scope for transferring a greater proportion of care to non-acute inpatient settings through, for example, developments in nursing home care and community rehabilitation services. Later chapters of this review will detail current evidence on the effectiveness and cost-effectiveness of such service developments. Alternative models that have been proposed for the overall provision of care will also be outlined. As will become apparent, although the need for developments and improvements in stroke care is accepted, the precise way forward is only gradually emerging. This chapter has clarified the baseline from which these developments and improvements will be made and hence the cale of change that is required.

# References

Bamford J, Sandercock P, Warlow C, Gray M. Why are patients with acute stroke admitted to hospital? BMJ 1986; 292: 1369-72.

Barer DH. Stroke in Nottingham: the burden of nursing care. Clin Rehab 1991; 5: 103-10.

Beech R, Withey C, Morris R. Understanding variations in lengths of stay between hospitals for fractured neck of femur patients and the potential consequences of reduced stay targets. J Pub Health Med 1995; 17(1): 77-84.

Department of Health. Hospital Episode statistics. Volumes 1 and 2. Financial year 1993-94. Leeds: Department of Health, 1995.

Ebrahim S, Barer D, Nouri F. An audit of follow-up services for stroke patients after discharge from hospital. Int Disability Stud 1987; 9: 103-5.

Gladman J, Albazzaz M, Barer D. A survey of survivors of acute stroke discharged from hospitals to private nursing homes in Nottingham. Health Trends 1991; 23: 158-60.

King's Fund Consensus Statement. The treatment of stroke. BMJ 1988; 297: 126-8.

Legh-Smith J, Wade DT, Langton-Hewer R. Services for stroke patients one year after stroke. J Epidemiol Community Health 1986; 40: 161-5.

Lindley RI, Amayo EO, Marsall J, Sandercock PAG, Dennis M, Warlow CP. Hospital services for patients with acute stroke in the United Kingdom: the Stroke Association survey of consultant opinion. Age Ageing 1995; 24: 525-32.

Office of Population Censuses and Surveys. Morbidity statistics from general practice 1991-1992. London: HMSO, 1995.

Oxfordshire Community Stroke Project. Incidence of stroke in Oxfordshire: first year's experience of a community stroke register. BMJ 1983; 287: 712-7.

Riddell JA. Out-of-hours visits in a group practice. BMJ 1980; 1: 1518-20.

Royal College of Physicians of London. Stroke - towards better management. London: RCP 1989.

Sotaniemi KA, Pyktinen J, Myllya VV. Correlation of clinical and computed tomographic findings in stroke patients. Stroke 1990; 21: 1562-6.

West Lambeth Health Authority Stroke Steering Group. Setting district stroke standards and objectives: a report of the West Lambeth Health Authority Stroke Steering Group. Journal of the Royal College of Physicians of London 1992; 26(2): 172-6.

Wade DT. Stroke (acute cerebrovascular disease). In: Stevens A, Raftery J (eds), Health Care Needs Assessment: The Epidemiology Based Needs Assessment Reviews. Oxford: Radcliffe Medical Press 1994; 1:111-255.

Wolfe CDA, Beech R, Ratcliffe M, Rudd AG. Stroke care in Europe: can we learn lessons from the different ways stroke is managed in different countries? J Roy Soc Health 1995; 115: 143-7.

Wolfe CDA, Taub N, Bryan S, Beech R, Warburton F, Burney PGJ. Variations in the incidence, management and outcome of stroke in residents under the age of 75 in two health districts of southern England. J Pub Health Med 1995; 17 (4): 411-8.

Wolfe CDA, Taub NA, Woodrow J, Richardson E, Warburton FG, Burney PGJ. Patterns of acute stroke care in three districts of southern England. J Epidemiol Community Health 1993; 47: 144-8.

# CHAPTER 4

# THE ACUTE MANAGEMENT OF STROKE

*Tony Rudd*

**Chapter outline**

# Introduction

This chapter discusses the research evidence concerning the management of stroke in the first few days after the acute event. Rehabilitation issues which need to be considered concurrently will be reviewed in later chapters.

At least one million new cases of stroke occur each year in the United States and European Union combined. There is so far little evidence to suggest that any acute intervention will produce significant benefit, except for some small subgroups of patients. The lack of progress in making a significant breakthrough in stroke management is not due to a lack of effort, although it could be argued that the quality of research in many areas has been poor. It is only recently that well organised randomised controlled trials have begun to answer some of the critical questions about the efficacy of treatments that have been tried half-heartedly for years such as anticoagulation, thrombolysis and steroids.

One of the barriers to progress in acute stroke research may have been the failure to organise care in specialised units. Stroke, particularly in the United Kingdom, has been regarded as a disease to be managed by non-specialist clinicians on general medical wards. While stroke rehabilitation is now recognised as being more effectively carried out in stroke units, the same has not been shown to be the case in the early stages of the disease (Langhorne *et al.* 1993). Development of a coherent structure for acute stroke research in the United Kingdom may be the single most important task for funding organisations over the next few years. Bringing together the skills of clinical pharmacologists, neurologists, angiologists and many other clinicians and basic scientists into units running effective clinical services will be essential to develop, test and implement new treatments for a disease that is the third commonest cause of death in the developed world and the commonest cause of long-term disability.

This review summarises the main areas where research is currently being undertaken and highlights the areas where clearly more research is needed. It is not intended to duplicate the thorough analyses already completed in some areas by the Cochrane Database. Where such reviews are available they have been used to inform the discussion.

# Process of care

### Acute stroke units

Stroke units can be established with the intention of performing a variety of roles. Units primarily intended to provide rehabilitation will be discussed in a later chapter. The place of specialist units to provide intensive care for stroke in the acute phase of the illness has received less attention. There have been several non-randomised studies of acute stroke units (Kennedy *et al.* 1970; Drake *et al.* 1973; Pitner and Mance 1973) but none has so far shown that they improve outcome. A trial is needed of such a unit where clear protocols for the management of disorders of swallowing, pressure care, infection and shoulder care are implemented. If and when therapy for acute stroke is discovered, the need for such units may become apparent, particularly if patients need intensive monitoring.

### Hospital or home

Little is known about the criteria for admission to hospital. Different districts have widely differing admission rates. The three major community stroke register studies in the UK have been the Oxford study where 60% (Bamford *et al.* 1990) of incident cases were admitted to hospital, the Southern England study (Wolfe *et al.* 1993) of three districts where in both the rural district and the two urban districts the admission rate was nearer to 80%, and the Frimley study by Weddell and Beresford (1979) where the majority were admitted to hospital. No data are available to indicate that for patients with similar pathology, admission to hospital confers benefit over treatment at home, in the acute phase of the illness. What Wolfe *et al.* did observe was that rehabilitation services to patients managed at home were extremely scanty; whether this was due to lack of availability or lack of need was not established.

Wade *et al.* (1985) performed a randomised controlled trial of a community therapy team available to general practitioners to substitute for hospital admission. No reduction in admission rates was obtained and no differences in outcome between the two groups observed. More research is needed on the issue as to when hospital admission is necessary and the sorts of care that can be effectively developed in a community setting.

# Investigation of stroke

The range of investigations for stroke has increased enormously over the last 20 years, with the development of CT scanning, MRI scanning, PET scanning, magnetic resonance angiography, Doppler ultrasound scanning of carotids and transcranial Dopplers. Clinical diagnosis on history and examination alone is not adequate to differentiate between different pathologies (Weir *et al.* 1994). The benefits of investigations as research tools is beyond dispute but there remains controversy as to their role in routine medical practice (Sandercock *et al.* 1985; Sotaniemi *et al.* 1990). Theoretical arguments as to the importance of accurately differentiating between haemorrhage and infarction, large infarcts and lacunar infarcts, single isolated lesions and diffuse cerebrovascular disease are used to justify routine CT scanning and yet unfortunately it still has to be proven with a randomised trial that such a policy is effective at influencing outcome (Wardlaw 1994; Allison 1994). Whether, at a cost of only £120 per scan compared to £300-400 per day for a hospital bed (local prices), it is the most important question to answer is debatable. Certainly the question produces considerable emotion and is responsible for dominating the discussion at many meetings on stroke. The question will need to be reviewed in the light of trials of thrombolysis and heparin.

Dunbain and Sandercock (1991) list the general aims of investigation as confirming the diagnosis, clarifying pathology, discovering the cause, guiding prognosis and treatment and to make or save money. Included in this list should be the education of physicians, therapists, nurses, patients and carers. Many of the tests patients have almost routinely on admission to hospital such as haematology and biochemistry are cheap and relatively non-invasive. It is likely that they will be performed anyway for reasons unrelated to the stroke at some stage during the admission and although overall expenditure on such 'simple' investigations may be high there is probably not much scope for cost reduction. It seems unlikely that formal research to investigate their value is justified. The more costly and invasive investigations do need evaluation and this particularly applies to new technology. Care in the development of protocols for such studies should be taken to ensure that 'change in clinical practice' includes attitudes of patients and carers and that 'cost-effectiveness' is not interpreted in too narrow a way.

**Treatment of cerebral infarction**

Regarding cerebral infarction as a single disease which can be managed in a generic way regardless of aetiology, size and site of lesion may explain why so many of the research studies into stroke have yielded disappointing results. Classification of stroke clinically is notoriously difficult even when very crude methods such as the PACI, TACI, POCI, LACI (partial anterior cerebral infarct, total anterior cerebral infarct, posterior cerebral infarct, lacunar infarct) system are used. The significance of silent infarction detected only on radiological investigation needs clarification. The extent of small vessel disease or other co-existing cerebral pathology such as Alzheimer's disease underlying the acute infarction is inevitably going to influence outcome. These changes therefore need recording and consideration in the evaluation of patients before and after treatment. Too many studies exclude patients with recurrent stroke who make up a significant proportion of stroke cases. For example, cerebral infarction resulting from hypertension may be a different entity with a different natural history to cerebral infarction caused by cardioembolic disease. Classification, and studies of the natural history of stroke subtypes should be an urgent priority for stroke research.

*(a) Thrombolysis*

Meyer *et al.* in 1963 undertook a randomised controlled trial of streptokinase in 73 patients with stroke. Treatment was given intravenously with and without anticoagulation within three days of the onset of the illness. The trial was abandoned early because 10 patients died and some others sustained intracerebral bleeding. It took until the 1990s and the success of thrombolysis in myocardial infarction before treatment was again seriously reconsidered in stroke. The Cochrane Database (1995, Issue 1) reviews eight trials with a total of 899 patients (Abe *et al.* 1981; Atarashi *et al.* 1985; Haley *et al.* 1993; Yamaguchi *et al.* 1993; Meyer et el. 1963; Mori *et al.* 1992; Ohtomo *et al.* 1985). There was a non-significant reduction of 37% in the odds of death (95% confidence interval 68% reduction to 24% excess) and a significant reduction of 40% in the odds of death or deterioration (95% CI 62% to 5% reduction) following thrombolysis. There was a low incidence of haemorrhagic change in the treated groups, but the overall number of these events was very small. The eight trials reviewed varied considerably in methodology, reducing the value of the meta-analysis.

The third edition of the Cochrane database due to be published in spring 1996 should include an updated analysis of thrombolysis trials to include the results of MAST-I, MAST-E, ASK and ECASS (Sandercock 1995). Sandercock cites a personal communication with Wardlaw J *et al.*, based on 11 trials reporting mortality data, that patients treated with thrombolytics showed a significant excess of deaths (23.1% versus 18.8%).

It is disappointing that three of the large trials, MAST-E and ASK and MAST-I have been stopped early because of significantly adverse outcomes in the treatment groups (Hommel *et al.* 1995; Donnan *et al.* 1995; MAST-I 1995). These results do not necessarily mean that thrombolysis is not an effective treatment in any form. Donnan *et al.* (1995) on behalf of the steering committees of ASK and MAST-E comment that time windows, drug doses and stroke populations in different protocols may lead to different outcomes.

Dispute within the steering committee of MAST-I has led to two different interpretations of the data. Early mortality was higher in the groups treated with streptokinase either with or without aspirin. A non-significant reduction in six-month case fatality and severe disability with streptokinase plus or minus aspirin or with aspirin alone is interpreted by part of the MAST-I group as an important finding. Concern about over-interpretation of subgroup analysis is the reason for the 'alternative' report (Tognoni and Roncaglioni 1995). The National Institute of Neurological Disorders and Stroke rt-PA Stroke Study Group (1995) found no increase in early mortality although there was a significant increase in early symptomatic cerebral haemorrhage. At three months, however, patients treated with rt-PA were 30% more likely to have minimal or no disability than untreated patients. The results from the remaining trials (Boehringer, JTSII, PROACT) and the subsequent meta-analysis are awaited with considerable interest.

Apart from the trials included in the meta-analysis, there have been many other smaller, often uncontrolled studies, both in animals and man (Hedershee *et al.* 1990; Zivin *et al.* 1992; Brott *et al.* 1992; Castro 1992; von Kummer 1992; Haley *et al.* 1992; Zeumer *et al.* 1993; Fitt *et al.* 1993; Baird *et al.* 1994; Overgaard 1993; Barr *et al.* 1994; Bollaert *et al.* 1995). Results from these trials are not encouraging. Dramatic improvements in results are not seen and in many of the studies very large numbers of patients were excluded from the trials, often because of delay in presentation. If only small percentages of patients are suitable from centres participating in thrombolysis research then even fewer will be treated in district general hospitals. Uncontrolled studies where outcomes are often radiographic clearance of thrombus are of very little value. Without intervention the evidence is that emboli clear spontaneously in the majority of cases by 48 hours (Fieschi *et al.* 1989; Dalal *et al.* 1965; Lhermitte *et al.* 1968) with 76% clearing by one week and 89% by 2-3 weeks (Ringelstein *et al.* 1992).

No randomised study has yet been performed on local thrombolysis after stroke. There have been some small-scale studies reporting some encouraging results (Zeumer *et al.* 1993; Higashida *et al.* 1989) and it may be that if evidence grows that conventional thrombolysis is ineffective then local intra-arterial therapy should be evaluated.

The major problems with research in this area are therefore the scarcity of results so far from randomised controlled trials, very low recruitment rates, the likelihood that intervention, if it is successful, will need to be given very early in the course of the ischaemia and only after CT scanning, and the high haemorrhagic transformation rate in some studies. Before further research is commissioned the results from current studies should be awaited. There is however perhaps value in a trial of thrombolysis in patients with stroke in evolution. This is a group for whom prognosis is currently poor and thrombolysis theoretically should offer considerable benefits.

### (b) Anticoagulation

Anticoagulants have been shown to have considerable value in the management of unstable angina pectoris and myocardial infarction and it is therefore reasonable to suppose that there may be similar benefits for acute brain ischaemia. The incidence of deep venous thrombosis (DVT) is also very high in stroke, with some studies reporting up to 75% of hemiparetic limbs developing clot. The incidence of pulmonary embolism has not been studied prospectively. Anticoagulation may therefore not only reduce death by limiting cerebral infarct size but also by preventing pulmonary embolism. The Cochrane Database (1995 Issue 1) found 12 trials to subject to meta-analysis. No significant effect on the odds of death during the period of treatment was shown, although the numbers in treated and untreated groups were small (44/100 anticoagulated and 31/364 not anticoagulated). Similarly there was no difference in death rate during the follow-up period. There was no difference between the groups in vascular deaths, although there were very wide confidence intervals. There was a highly significant reduction in the rates of DVT but the data for pulmonary embolism were inadequate. Not enough data were found to assess the effect of anticoagulation on stroke recurrence, myocardial infarction or functional outcome.

There is therefore an urgent need for trials to determine the role of anticoagulation in stroke. The largest single trial in progress at the moment, The International Stroke Trial (IST), compared medium-dose unfractionated heparin (UFH) (12500 IU given subcutaneously 12 hourly), low dose UFH (5000 IU subcutaneously 12 hourly and no treatment) with or without aspirin. Preliminary results of IST have shown a significant increase in mortality in patients treated with low-dose heparin. The results suggested that immediatetreatment with aspirin may produce a small benefit on 14-day outcome although definite conclusions cannot be drawn until the longer-term outcome outcome data become available in 1997. Kay *et al.* (1995) report a trial of either high or low-dose low molecular weight heparin versus placebo given within 48 hours of stroke to 312 patients. A significant reduction in death and dependency was obtained in the treated groups (45% vs. 52% vs. 65% dead or dependent in high-dose, low-dose and placebo respectively) at six months. This trial excluded elderly patients (over 80 years), hypertensives, and previous stroke victims. Larger-scale trials to confirm these results and to determine optimal dosage and duration of treatment are needed. There is also a need to determine the effect of anticoagulation on the frequency of pulmonary embolism, both fatal and those of less severity but possibly sufficient to limit rehabilitation by reducing cardio-respiratory reserve and exercise tolerance.

### (c) Ancrod
Reduction of blood viscosity and also, potentially, alteration of blood coagulability may be achieved by the use of substances that reduce fibrinogen levels. Fibrinogen is an important contributor to blood viscosity and high fibrinogen levels have been noted to predict stroke recurrence in high-risk patients (Grotta *et al.* 1982). Ancrod is a substance extracted from the venom of the Malayan pit viper and has a potent thrombin-like enzymatic effect. The Ancrod Stroke Study Investigators (1994) conducted a double blind randomised controlled trial in 64 patients and 68 controls but failed to demonstrate any difference between the groups. Unfortunately the dose of ancrod used proved ineffective at reducing fibrinogen levels significantly, rendering the trial

inconclusive. Previous studies have shown that it is feasible to lower fibrinogen levels in acute brain ischaemia using ancrod (Olinger *et al.* 1988). A further large multicentre trial is just beginning and there seems little value in pursuing further studies in this field until the results of this trial are available.

**Improving the survival of ischaemic brain**

Improving the survival of neurones in the ischaemic penumbra is the alternative strategy to improving cerebral perfusion. Increasing understanding of the cellular processes that occur in the brain after an acute ischaemic insult has led to many new exciting areas where pharmacological intervention may produce benefit. One of the areas receiving most attention is the observation that some neurotransmitters, in particular glutamate, released at sites of ischaemia might overexcite neurones and cause toxic damage, thereby increasing the effects of the ischaemia. Attention has also been paid to calcium flux after stroke. Preventing the massive influx of calcium into ischaemic cells and normalising the extracellular-to-intracellular calcium gradient has been suggested as a potentially useful strategy for limiting ischaemic damage.

*(a) Calcium antagonists*

As a result of membrane depolarisation and release of excitatory neurotransmitters calcium enters neurones through both voltage-operated and receptor-operated channels. This leads indirectly to the production of nitric oxide and the generation of free radicals. It is therefore suggested that inhibiting the influx of calcium may prevent subsequent cytotoxic reactions. Calcium antagonists have been found to be effective in cerebrovascular conditions where vasospasm is a prominent feature such as subarachnoid haemorrhage. Trials of nimodipine in acute cerebral infarction have given conflicting results but overall the impression is not one to suggest overwhelming benefit. Gelmers *et al.* (1988), in a randomised trial of 186 patients, demonstrated a significant reduction in mortality (9 vs. 20%) in the nimodipine group although this was mainly due to a reduction in cardiac endpoints. A large European study (Trust Study Group 1990) of 1215 patients failed to demonstrate any benefit for nimodipine. Kaste *et al.* (1994) randomised 350 patients and actually demonstrated a higher case fatality rate in the treated group. Giving the drug intravenously (Wahlgren *et al.* 1994) also produced no benefit and caused hypertension. Post hoc analysis of a large United States study (American Nimodipine Study Group 1992) of three doses of nimodipine did however show that patients treated within 12 hours with 60 or 120 mg of nimodipine daily had statistically significant better outcome than the placebo group. A meta-analysis of all patients recruited early into nimodipine trials for cerebral infarction arrived at the same conclusion (International Nimodipine Study Group 1992).

It is difficult at present to draw clear conclusions from these results. Nimodipine should not be dismissed altogether. There may well be important differences in response according to the timing of the intervention and the dose used. More studies to establish the precise role of nimodipine should be performed.

### (b) Gangliosides

The principle of treatment with gangliosides is that gangliosides are normal components of neural membranes. Giving exogenous ganglioside such as monosialoganglioside GM1, which enters neural plasma membranes, might result in increased intracellular levels and be cytoprotective. An early trial (Argentino *et al.* 1989) gave inconclusive results. The SASS Trial (1994) was a randomised controlled trial limited by the poor recruitment rate. Of 5000 patients screened only 287 were entered into the trial and 217 completed the course. No differences between the groups were found except on post hoc analysis where a slight improvement in some of the motor components of some of the disability scales were found. Lenzi *et al.* (1994) in the Early Stroke Trial (EST) treated 805 patients. Survival was similar in both arms of the trial. Marginal improvements in the Canadian neurological score were found. The evidence for the effectiveness of ganglioside therapy is flimsy (Svennerholm 1994) and at present there seems little to commend more drug trials.

### (c) NMDA receptor antagonists

The excitotoxin hypothesis suggests that following an infarction, hypoxia in the ischaemic penumbra causes the release of large amounts of glutamate into the tissues (Rothman and Olney 1986; Choi *et al.* 1987). Glutamate is then taken up by receptors, exciting the cells with huge waves of depolarisation. The cells already depleted of blood are unable to cope with the massive increase in metabolic activity and are irreversibly damaged.

A number of experimental studies on animals of NMDA receptor antagonists have shown encouraging results in reducing the size of infarcts produced by occlusion of major cerebral arteries (Buchan *et al.* 1992; Cohen *et al.* 1994; Park *et al.* 1994; Wahlestadt *et al.* 1993). AMPA receptor antagonist may also prove valuable (Buchan *et al.* 1993). Development of drugs suitable for use in man is being undertaken by many drug companies (Table 1) who see enormous financial possibilities for such treatments.

Trials in man are awaited but experience suggests that animal work is often an unreliable guide to human stroke (De Zoppo 1995). Animal experiments are always very carefully controlled for environmental factors and size of infarct. Outcome endpoints are usually infarct size rather than disability or other functional measures. Drug treatment is given at well controlled times after the ischaemic event and in some studies is actually given before the ischaemia which rather lessens the relevance to real life (Grotta 1995). Animal studies may also be particularly prone to publishing bias.

**Table 1 (from Financial Times July 29 1994)**

| Company | Drug | Launch date |
|---|---|---|
| Upjohn | Freedox | 1994 |
| Ciba | Selfotel | 1997 |
| Alkermes | Calpain inhibitor | ? |
| Cambridge Neuroscience | Cerestat | 2000? |
| Cephalon | Calpain inhibitor | ? |
| Cocensys | Acea 1021 | ? |
| Fisons | Remacemide | ? |
| Gensia | Adenosine inhibitor | ? |
| Guilford | PARS inhibitor | ? |
| Wellcome | 619C89 | 2000? |
| Sandoz | SDZ EEA 494 | ? |
| Synthelabo | Eliprodil | 2000? |

It may well be that one of the drugs listed will prove to be a major advance in stroke management. Development of a drug that can be given safely by the first doctor or paramedic to come into contact with the patient without having to first get a brain scan would, even if its benefit was small, have a greater impact on the whole stroke population than risky but possibly highly effective treatments only accessible to a few. It seems likely that the drugs companies will finance future research in this field and that The Stroke Association will be able to direct its funds elsewhere.

### (d) Reducing oedema

Both cerebral haemorrhage and cerebral infarcts are associated with considerable oedema. There are two types of oedema known, vasogenic and cytotoxic. Oedema associated with tumours is usually vasogenic and is known to be highly sensitive to steroid treatment. Oedema associated with vascular disease is predominantly cytotoxic, caused by swelling of cells themselves. Reduction of oedema after stroke could very significantly reduce mortality and morbidity and several techniques have been employed in an attempt to achieve this.

### (e) Steroids

The use of steroids in stroke will be the subject of a meta-analysis by the Cochrane Database of Systematic Reviews (1995, Issue 1). Mulley *et al.* (1978) in a trial of dexamethasone in acute stroke failed to demonstrate any significant benefit for steroids and there has been no convincing evidence since then to support their use. Despite this they remain one of the most widely used pharmacological interventions in acute stroke. A recent study in cats (de Courten-Meyers 1994) has shown a six-fold reduction in infarct size following middle cerebral artery occlusion when the animals were given high dose methylprednisolone. Norris and Hachinski (1986), giving high-dose dexamethasone in a double blind randomised controlled trial to 113 patients with acute cerebral infarction within 48 hours, failed to demonstrate a significant benefit in mortality or disability in the treated group. It seems unlikely therefore that steriods have any role in acute stroke management.

### (f) Hyperosmolar agents

Both mannitol and glycerol have been used in haemorrhagic and ischaemic stroke (O'Brien 1979). Trials of intravenous glycerol have been reviewed by the Cochrane Database. Eight trials met their entry criteria (Bayer *et al.* 1987; Fawer *et al.* 1978; Frei *et al.* 1987; Friedli 1979; Frithz and Werner 1975; Larsson *et al.* 1976; Mathew *et al.* 1972; Yu *et al.* 1993). The pooled data revealed that treatment reduces the odds of death in the first two weeks by 42% (95% CI 9-64%). No significant reduction in long-term case fatality was found however. Meta analysis of functional outcome proved impossible because of widely differing outcome measures. Half of the trials showed no difference between functional outcome in the glycerol-treated and the control groups, but some of the trials did report improvement, particularly in the group of patients with moderate deficits. Several of the trials had serious flaws and the issue as to whether glycerol should be used routinely in ischaemic stroke remains unclear. A well conducted, large randomised trial is justified.

## (g) Prostacyclin

Prostacyclin has vasodilating, antiplatelet, antileucocyte, fibrinolytic and cytoprotective effects. These actions, taken together with the observation that prostacyclin synthesis is reduced in acute stroke, make the substance a candidate for use therapeutically. Four trials (Hsu *et al.* 1986; Huczynski *et al.* 1985, 1988; Hamdy *et al.* 1984) have been included in the meta-analysis performed by the Cochrane Database (1995 Issue 1). The total number of patients in the four trials was only 168 and no significant effect of treatment was found. Confidence intervals were wide reflecting the small numbers of patients studied and again major methodological flaws in diagnosis and randomisation were evident. The place of prostacyclin in acute ischaemic stroke remains unclear and needs further research, although it seems unlikely to have a major role in the future.

## (h) Haemodilution

An inverse relationship between haematocrit and cerebral infarction volume (Harrison *et al.* 1981) and an inverse correlation between blood flow and haematocrit (Wood *et al*, 1984) suggest the possibility that reducing the haematocrit may produce beneficial effects in patients with ischaemic stroke. Dextran has been the most widely used agent. Results have been disappointing. The Scandinavian Stroke Study Group (1987), in a trial of 183 patients receiving isovolumic haemodilution relative to 180 control patients, failed to demonstrate any benefit. Similarly, the Italian Acute Stroke Study Group (1988) failed to demonstrate improvement in six-month mortality or any improvement in disability. Alternative methods of haemodilution may be worth studying but the prospect of a major impact on outcome seems unlikely. Specific studies on patients with polycythaemia are needed to give clear direction as to the role of venesection in acute stroke and the same applies to the management of patients with hyperviscosity syndromes such as myeloma and Waldenstrom's macroglobulinaemia.

## Interventional radiology

### Balloon angioplasty

Interventional radiology is beginning to transform the management of cardiovascular and peripheral vascular disease. The potential for its use in cerebrovascular disease remains relatively unexplored because of concerns about the risks of distal embolisation. Balloon angioplasty was first reported in the early 1980s (Sundt *et al.* 1980; Bockenheimer and Mathias 1983). Further reports (Higashida 1993), although still preliminary, have demonstrated safety and given some indication that the technique may have long-term efficacy. There is a randomised trial currently underway in the United States and one recently funded by The Stroke Association in the UK but no data has yet been presented.

## Surgery

There is no evidence to indicate any role for surgical intervention after acute cerebral infarction. Occasionally, surgical decompression after cerebellar infarction has been performed where there is risk of herniation due to raised intracranial pressure (Feely 1979; Shenkin 1982) but the need for this is relatively rare. The EC-IC Bypass study group (1985) failed to demonstrate any benefit for intracranial extracranial anastamosis which at the time was a very popular operation for stroke prevention in North America. This trial evaluated the surgery at a mean of six weeks after stroke and it may be that the operation performed earlier in the illness would be beneficial, as a way of limiting ischaemia. This needs evaluation.

# Treatment of cerebral haemorrhage

Approximately 10 to 15% of stroke is due to cerebral haemorrhage with the higher incidences seen in areas with large populations of subjects with a high incidence of hypertension, such as Afro-Caribbeans. Early mortality is high but if patients survive the initial acute phase of the illness recovery may be more satisfactory than for a cerebral infarction of equivalent size.

## Medical care

The principle concern in the acute stage of an intracerebral bleed is the rise in intracranial pressure. 'Medical decompression' with corticosteroids, mannitol or glycerol is widely used in these patients but there is precious little evidence in the research literature to support their use. Langfitt (1977) reported benefits with mannitol and forced hyperventilation to reduce intracranial pressure but this was not validated with a formal randomised trial.

The management of hypertension in the acute phase of an intracerebral bleed also remains unclear, as it does in cerebral infarction. Undoubtedly more damage has been done in the past by overenthusiastic treatment of hypertension than by undertreatment but clear guidance is needed to define the precise level at which hypertension becomes dangerous rather than helpful at maintaining cerebral perfusion.

Studies to define the optimal control of hypertension will require the use of dynamic scanning using either SPECT or PET to determine changes in cerebral perfusion and metabolism in association with changes in the level of systolic and diastolic pressure. Such studies need to be performed both in patients with cerebral haemorrhage and cerebral infarction. Continuous monitoring of blood pressure during the acute phase of stroke has been performed (Sander *et al.* 1994; Harper *et al.* 1994) and shows significant variations in blood pressure in both the first few hours after stroke and over the subsequent six weeks. It may well be that the peak and trough pressure is of more relevance to outcome than the mean pressure and this needs evaluation.

## Surgery

Attitudes towards surgical evacuation of cerebral haematomas in the United Kingdom are generally conservative compared to some other parts of Europe and the United

States (Heiskanen 1993). Most, although not all, (Kaufman 1993) accept that evacuation of basal ganglia and pontine haematomas offers little benefit. The discussion centres around the cortical and shallow subcortical haematomas. Caplan (1993) suggests surgery wherever there is evidence of significantly raised intracranial pressure or compression of the ventricular system. Where the aetiology is congophilic angiopathy or associated with abnormal clotting, Caplan thinks surgery should be avoided. Surgery is more easily performed within the first 36 hours, while haematomas are still liquid. There is clearly a need for further research to establish whether surgery is appropriate, and for which groups; large or small haematomas, deep or superficial, early or late and by aetiological group e.g. hypertensive vascular disease, congophilic angiopathy, arteriovenous malformation.

**Cerebellar haemorrhage**

Mathews and Teasdale (1994) have reviewed the literature on the role of neurosurgery in the management of posterior fossa stroke. There is much stronger evidence to support neurosurgical intervention in cerebellar haemorrhage than cortical haemorrhage, particularly if there is evidence of hydrocephalus or deteriorating consciousness level (Auer *et al.* 1986). The majority of patients do not fall into these groups and are, on the evidence available at present, better managed conservatively.

**Subarachnoid haemorrhage**

Approximately 6% of the population have intracerebral aneurysms (McCormick 1978). The annual incidence of rupture of saccular aneurysms is however low at 10-12/100,000. Subarachnoid haemorrhage accounts for 5-10% of all strokes with a higher incidence in the younger stroke population. Mortality is high with a third dying before reaching medical attention and a further 20% dying in hospital, often from rebleeding. Management is directed at :

1. Reducing the impact of the initial haemorrhage

2. Preventing recurrence

3. Rehabilitation of neurological deficits.

## Initial treatment

a) The management of hypertension is as problematic as with the other causes of stroke. There is little guidance in the literature and management at present is therefore guided by clinical intuition alone. Guidelines for management need to be developed.

b) Prevention of vasospasm. It is suggested that subarachnoid haemorrhage results in the release into the CSF of substances, possibly oxyhaemaglobin, which result in widespread vasospasm within the brain. This occurs within 3-5 days of the initial haemorrhage and lasts for up to six weeks. Calcium channel blockers have now been accepted as being useful, perhaps working by preventing vasospasm, although the precise mechanism is unclear. Nimodipine (Pickard *et al.* 1981), in a randomised controlled trial, reduced delayed ischaemia and infarction. There has been some doubt as to whether nimodipine actually improves outcome and this needs further study, particularly comparing it with the alternative strategy suggested of liberal volume expansion to prevent hypovolaemia.

## Prevention of re-bleeding

Conventional management uses bedrest, pain control, prevention of straining by the use of laxatives, and adequate blood pressure control in an attempt to prevent re-bleeding. Whether it is justified to put these practices to the test in a research study is doubtful.

Antifibrinolytic drugs such as epsilon aminocaproic acid (amica) have been used to try to prevent rebleeding. It is said to work by inhibiting plasmin by blocking the conversion of plasminogen to plasmin and by binding with the receptor protein on the portion of the plasmin that binds fibrin. Kassell *et al.* (1984) reviewed the evidence for their use and concluded that any benefit in preventing re-bleeding was offset by an increase in thrombophlebitis, pulmonary embolism and ischaemic deficit.

Surgical clipping of the aneurysm is the 'definitive' treatment. There is little doubt that patients who survive the surgical procedure do better in the long-term than those treated medically. The unanswered questions remain the best timing for surgery and the most appropriate selection criteria for surgery. Many hospitals in the United Kingdom select in part by age, excluding patients over 60 or 65 years. There is no clear evidence to support this policy in the literature and it needs confirmation.

# Complications in the acute phase of stroke

## *Deep venous thrombosis (DVT) and pulmonary embolism (PE)*

Deep venous thrombosis occurs in 25-75% of patients with stroke (McCarthy *et al.* 1977; Warlow *et al.* 1972; Oczkowski *et al.* 1992) and pulmonary embolism in 5-50% (Noel *et al.* 1991). There is good evidence, although mainly from non-stroke patients, that low-dose heparin is effective at preventing DVT and PE (Sandercock *et al.* 1993). The safety of giving low-dose heparin to patients with stroke who have not had CT scan to exclude cerebral haemorrhage may be answered when data from the IST trial becomes available. The use of compression stockings has again been shown to be effective for non-stroke patients but needs evaluating specifically in stroke. Management of established DVT and PE with warfarin needs further study; the ideal level of anticoagulation that minimises the risk of further thromboembolism and haemorrhagic transformation of infarction has not been defined.

The consequences of 'silent' DVT and PE have not been established. It may be that many patients are having undiagnosed thromboembolism. These could result in slower rehabilitation due to pain or increased spasticity in the affected limb and reduced exercise tolerance due to anoxia when the patient is exercised in the gymnasium. A prospective study of the frequency of PE would be justified using ventilation perfusion scanning and the consequences on respiratory physiology and rehabilitation outcomes.

## *Pressure sores*

This subject is discussed in the section on nursing and stroke.

## *Epilepsy*

Between 7 and 20% of patients will develop epilepsy in the first six months after stroke. Over half of these will present in the first month with a significant proportion in the first 24 hours. They are particularly likely to occur after large cortical infarcts. Management is not usually a problem as single anticonvulsant treatment is usually effective. There are sometimes problems in the differential diagnosis between a further cerebral ischaemic event and an epileptic fit which is not always resolved using EEG. The consequences of repeated post stroke fits are worthy of study. One study (Bogousslavsky *et al.* 1992) suggests that there can be permanent worsening of neurological signs following seizures and early seizures can indicate a significant risk of seizure recurrence (Kilpatrick *et al.* 1992)

## Cardiac abnormalities

In stroke survivors, myocardial infarction is the commonest cause of death. Electrocardiographic changes are a frequent accompaniment of stroke with both dysrhythmias and ischaemic changes. Levels of catecholamines in stroke have been shown to be high and may be the cause of myocardial damage (Meyers *et al.* 1981). Barer *et al.* (1988) reported a trial of atenolol, propranolol or placebo for three weeks following hemispheric stroke. More deaths occurred among the patients allocated to receive beta-blockers but this was explained by differences in case mix between the groups. A further group of 60 patients, already on beta-blockers at the time of their stroke, had better outcomes, raising the possibility that prior treatment might be protective. More work is needed in this field.

## Respiratory dysfunction

Abnormal respiratory patterns do not appear uncommon after stroke. Some work has been reported on respiratory function (Lane *et al.* 1971; Rout *et al.* 1971; Lee *et al.* 1974; Korczyn *et al.* 1969) but the frequency, mechanisms and consequences of abnormal breathing patterns still need much closer attention. New technology, including pulse oximeters and devices for continuous non-invasive monitoring of chest wall and diaphragmatic movements, EEG and eye movements, make closer more detailed assessment of sick patients after stroke feasible. Maintenance of adequate oxygenation after stroke is critical and we still do not know the best way to achieve this.

## Arousal and sleep disturbance

Sleep dysfunction with a reduction in rapid eye movement phases has been demonstrated as being a common association with middle cerebral artery lesions (Giubilei *et al.* 1992). The severity of the sleep abnormality on day two correlated with clinical outcome and it may be that polysonography could be a useful prognostic tool. Although some research on sleep dysfunction has been performed in brainstem stroke, very little information is available for supratentorial ischaemia. Given that many patients spend the early days after stroke in a very drowsy state, unreceptive to any attempt at active rehabilitation, a better understanding of the underlying mechanisms and possible therapeutic strategies is needed. The incidence of sleep disturbances among stroke patients has been shown to be high, not just in brainstem lesions but also in those with hemispheric strokes (Markand and Dyken 1976; Hachinski *et al.* 1977; Kapen *et al.* 1991). Cerebral oedema is nearly always blamed. This may not be justified.

*Metabolic and nutritional disturbances*

Fluid, electrolyte and nutritional abnormalities may occur during the acute phase of stroke. Inappropriate ADH secretion has been frequently reported and may result in hyponatraemia, which could cause deterioration of neurological function. The role of fluid restriction or drug treatment in these cases needs evaluation. The role of atrial natriuretic factor in producing hyponatraemia has also been questioned and needs assessment.

Undernutrition in the early stage of stroke has not been examined. Studies have been initiated to examine the benefits of gastrostomy feeding earlier than conventionally used, but even these will not intervene with supplementary feeding before the end of the first week. Study is needed to look at the consequences of early starvation. Allison *et al.* (1992) have demonstrated that percutaneous gastrostomy feeding improves late rehabilitation outcome and a recently reported randomised controlled trial (Norton *et al.* 1996) of percutaneous endoscopic gastrostomy feeding showed significantly better outcomes in mortality and discharge rate when compared to a group treated with nasogastric feeding.

*Infections*

Dysphagia and aspiration leading to pneumonia are very common after stroke. Management of swallowing disorders is discussed in the section on speech therapy. Pneumonia after stroke is of course not only due to aspiration; problems of stasis, poor respiratory and diaphragmatic function and impaired immune function all contribute. The role of physiotherapy or nursing techniques in preventing and treating pneumonia should be researched.

Urinary tract infections are common and may in part be due to a high rate of use of urinary catheters and abnormalities in bladder and sphincter dysfunction. Management of incontinence is discussed in the nursing section. The role of cystometry, the mechanism of bladder dysfunction and the use of drugs in modifying urinary function after stroke all need further research.

## Stroke in children and young adults

The aetiology of stroke in the young is often different to the older population with a higher frequency of haemorrhage from aneurysms and arteriovenous malformations. Nencini *et al.* (1988), in an incidence study in Florence, found 60% of stroke in the young was due to haemorrhage. Geographical, socio-economic and environmental factors play a more significant role in stroke aetiology in the young compared to the old (Chopra and Prabhakar 1979). Illicit use of drugs such as cocaine may contribute to some cases while prescribed drugs such as oral contraceptives or anticoagulants explain others. Trauma not infrequently contributes to ischaemia with Hilton-Jones and Warlow (1985) finding evidence of some head and neck trauma prior to the stroke in 13 out of 75 cases. Cardial dissection was one of the consequences of trauma. There is also a higher incidence of congenital cardiovascular abnormalities, with Lechat *et al.* (1988) demonstrating that 40% of young stroke victims had a patent foramen ovale compared to 10% of age-matched controls. Because of the differences in causation, investigation of stroke in the young also needs to be different. Little specific research on the management of stroke in the young has been reported. There may be no important differences but the question needs to be asked.

## Executive summary and priorities for research

There is little evidence that any form of acute intervention after stroke produces significant benefit except for small subgroups of patients. This reflects both the lack of a major pharmacological breakthrough and the generally poor quality of stroke research in this area. Improvement in the systems for stroke classification and a better understanding of the natural history of stroke subtypes are needed if coherent trials of treatment are to be conducted. Silent infarcts, multiple infarcts, diffuse small vessel disease and patients with multiple pathology should no longer be excluded from study.

The value of acute stroke units for the intensive care of patients in the immediate aftermath of stroke has not been demonstrated and needs further evaluation.

Provision of care at home as an alternative to admission to hospital is already provided for a significant proportion of patients. Evidence is needed to determine what role domiciliary care has in the management of stroke.

Investigation of stroke in routine clinical practice, particularly the role of neuroimaging, remains controversial. It is likely that purchasers of health care will demand evidence of cost-effectiveness for such investigations, which at present is not available.

Thrombolysis trials that have reported so far have not indicated a role in stroke care. More results are awaited and there would be a considerable interest in a trial of thromboylsis for patients with evolving stroke.

The role for calcium antagonists looks unpromising but may be worthy of further study. Pharmaceutical companies are investigating drugs to reduce the ischaemia in the stroke penumbra and this is an area where a major development may occur.

Reduction of cerebral oedema should improve outcome after infarction. Further trials of high-dose steroids and glycerol and other hyperosmolar agents could be performed. Trials of prostacyclin and haemodilution although inadequate do not give much cause for optimism and further studies should not be a high priority.

Results are awaited from a trial of balloon angioplasty compared to carotid endarterectomy. The use of angioplasty acutely after stroke also needs assessment. EC-IC bypass in the acute phase of stroke could also be evaluated.

The management of cerebral haemorrhage has received even less attention than cerebral infarction. The medical management of hypertension and cerebral oedema is unclear. A trial of surgical evacuation of intracerebral haematomas is justified.

Research into the prevention and treatment of the complications of stroke could well yield greater benefits than attempts to reduce cerebral damage. Deep venous thrombosis, pulmonary embolism, epilepsy, respiratory dysfunction and pneumonia, and problems with reduced arousal in the immediate aftermath of stroke are all topics where major questions remain unanswered.

The particular problems of the acute and longer-term management of stroke in children and young adults, although small in number, should not be neglected.

**The priorities for research are therefore:**

1. A trial of thrombolysis for stroke in evolution.

2. Assessment of the extent and consequences of respiratory dysfunction after stroke and the effect of respiratory support when required to reduce potential hypoxic damage and chest infection.

3. Development of guidelines for the management of hypertension following both infarction and haemorrhage, based on studies of cerebral perfusion and clinical outcome of treatment.

4. A trial of domiciliary therapy compared to hospital treatment in subtypes of stroke.

5. A trial of surgical evacuation of intracerebral haematomas.

6. Evaluation of the clinical effects of introducing protocols for care and critical care pathways and evaluation of the consequences of introducing acute stroke units.

# References

Abe T, Kazama M, Naito *et al*. Clinical evaluation for efficiency of tissue cultured urokinase (TCUK) on cerebral thrombosis by means of a multi-centre double blind study. Blood Vessel 1981; 12: 321-41.

Allison MC, Morris AJ, Park RH, Mills PR. Percutaneous endoscopic gastrostomy feeding may improve outcome of late rehabilitation following stroke. J Roy Soc Med 1992; 85: 147-9.

Allison SP. Costs outweigh benefits. Br Med J 1994; 309: 1499-500.

American Nimodipine Study Group. Clinical trial of nimodipine in acute ischemic stroke. Stroke 1992; 23: 3-8.

Ancrod Stroke Study Investigators. Ancrod for the treatment of acute ischemic brain infarction. Stroke 1994; 25: 1755-9.

Argentino C, Sacchetti ML, Toni D *et al*. GM ganglioside therapy in acute iscahemic stroke Stroke 1989; 20: 1143-9.

Atarashi J, Ohtomo E, Araki G, Itoh E, Togi H, Matsuda T. Clinical utility of urokinase in the treatment of acute stage cerebral thrombosis: Multi-centre double blind study in comparison with placebo. Clin Eval 1985; 13: 659-709.

Auer LM, Auer TH, Sayoma I. Indication for surgical treatment of cerebellar haemorrhage and infarction. Acta Neurochirurg 1986; 79: 74-9

Baird AE, Donnan GA, Austin MC, Fitt GJ, Davis SM, McKay WJ. Reperfusion after thrombolytic therapy in ischaemic stroke measured by single-photon emission computed tomography. Stroke 1994; 25: 79-85.

Bamford J, Sandercock P, Dennis M, Burn J, Warlow C. A prospective study of acute cerebrovascular disease in the community: The Oxfordshire Community Stroke Project 1981-1986. 2. Incidence, case fatality rates and overall outcome at one year of cerebral infarction, primary intracerebral and subarachnoid haemorrhage. J Neurol Neurosurg Psychiat. 1990; 53: 16-22.

Barer DH, Cruikshank JM, Ebrahim SB, Mitchell JR. Low dose beta blockade in acute stroke (ÒBESTÓ trial): an evaluation. Br Med J 1988; 296: 737-41.

Barr JD, Mathis JM, Wildenhain SL, Wechsler l, Jungreis CA, Horton JA. Acute stroke intervention with intraarterial urokinase infusion. J Vascul Intervent Radiology 1994; 5: 705-13.

Bayer AJ, Pathy MS, Newcombe R. Double-blind randomised trial of intravenous glycerol in acute stroke (plus letters). Lancet 1987; 1: 405-8.

Bockenhemier SA, Mathias K. Percutaneous transluminal angioplasty in arteriosclerotic internal carotid artery stenosis. AJNR 1983; 4: 791-2.

Bogousslavsky J, Martin R, Regli F, Despland P-A, Bolyn S. Persistent worsening of stroke sequelae after delayed seizures. Arch Neurol 1992; 49: 385-8.

Bollaert P-E, Bracard S, Boulanger T, Picard L, Larcan A. Early local intra-arterial thrombolysis for severe middle cerebral artery stroke. Cerebrovascular Disease 1995; 5: 292-6.

Brott TG, Haley EC, Levy DE, Barsan W, Broderick J, Sheppard GL, Spilker J, Kongable GL, Massey S, Reed R, Marler JR. Urgent therapy for stroke. Part I. Pilot study of tissue plasminogen activator adminstered within 90 minutes. Stroke 1992; 23: 632-40.

Buchan AM, Lesiuk H, Barnes KA, Li H, Huang ZG, Smith KE, Xue D. AMPA antagonists: do they hold more promise for clinical stroke trials than NMDA antagonists? Stroke 1993; 24; 1148-52.

Buchan AM, Slivka A, Xue D. The effect of the NMDA receptor antagonist MK-801 on cerebral blood flow and infarct volume in experimental focal stroke. Brain Research 1992; 574: 171-7.

Caplan LR. Stroke. A clinical approach. 2nd Edition. Butterworth Heinemann. Stonehaem MA USA. 1993.

Castro L, Moschini L, Camerlingo M, Gazzaniga G, Partziguain T, Belloni G, Mamoli A. Local intraarterial thrombolysis for acute stroke in the carotid artery territories. Acta Neurologica Scandinavica 1992; 86: 308-11.

Choi DW, Malulucci Gedde M, Kriegstein MR. Glutamate neurotoxicity in cortical cell culture. J Neurosci 1987; 7: 357-68.

Chopra JS, Prabhakar S. Clinical features and risk factors in stroke in young. Acta Neurol Scand 1979; 60: 289-300.

Cohen RA, Hasegawa Y, Fisher M. Effects of a novel NMDA receptor antagonist on experimental stroke quantitatively assessed by spectral EEG and infarct volume. Neurological Research 1994; 16: 443-8.

Dalal PM, Shah P, Sheth Sl, Deshpande CK. Cerebral embolism: angiographic observations on spontaneous clot lysis. Lancet 1965; 1: 61-4.

de Courten-Meyers GM, Kleinholz M, Wagner KR, Xi G, Myers RE. Efficacious experimental stroke treatment with high-dose methylprednisolone. Stroke 1994; 25: 487-92.

De Zoppo GJ. Why do all drugs work in animals but none in stroke patients? 1. Drugs promoting cerebral blood flow. J Internal Med 1995; 237: 79-88.

Donnan GA, Davis SM, Chambers BR, Gates PC, Hankey GJ, McNeil JJ, Rosen D, Stewart-Wynnes, Tuck RR. Trials of streptokinase in severe acute ischaemic stroke (Letter). Lancet 1995; 345: 578-9.

Drake WE, Hamilton MJ, Carlson M, Kand F, Blumenkrantz J. Acute stroke management and patient outcome: the value of neurovascular care units (NCU). Stroke 1973; 4: 933-45.

Dunbain DW, Sandercock PAG. Investigation of acute stroke: what is the most effective strategy? Postgrad Med J 1991; 67: 259-70.

EC-IC Bypass Study Group. Failure of the extracranial-intracranial arterial bypass to reduce the risk of ischemic stroke. N Engl J Med 1985; 313: 1191-1200.

Fawer R, Justafre JC, Berger JP, Schelling JI. Intravenous glycerol in cerebral infarction: a controlled 4-month trial. Stroke 1978; 9; 484-6.

Feely MP. Cerebellar infaction. Neurosurgery. 1979; 4: 4-11.

Fieschi M, Argentino C, Lenzi G, Sacchetti ML, Toni D, Bozzao L. Clinical and instrumental evaluation of patients with ischemic stroke within the first six hours. Journal of Neurological Sciences. 1989; 91: 311-22.

Fitt GJ, Farrar J, Baird AE, Brooks M, Gilligan A, Donnan GA, Hennessy O. Intra-arterial streptokinase in acute ischaemic stroke. A pilot study. Med J Australia 1993; 159: 331-4.

Frei A, Cottier C, Wunderlich P, Ludin E, Glycerol and dextran combined in the therapy of active stroke. A placebo-controlled, double-blind trial with a planned interim analysis. Stroke 1987; 18: 373-9.

Friedli W, Imbach P, Ghisleni-Steinegger S, Schwarz C, Marie P. Treatment with 10% glycerin in acute ischaemic cerebral infarct. Double blind study. Schweiz Med Wochenschr 1979; 109: 737-42.

Frithz G, Werner I. The effect of glycerol infusion in acute cerebral infarction. Acta Med Scand 1975; 198: 287-9.

Gelmers HJ, Gorter K, deWeerdt C et al. A controlled trial of nimodipine in acute ischemic stroke. N Engl J Med 1988; 318: 203-7.

Giubilei F, Iannilli M, Vitale A, Pierallini A, Sacchetti L, Antonini G, Fieschi C. Sleep patterns in acute ischaemic stroke. Acta Neurol Scand 1992; 86: 567-71.

Grotta J, Ackerman R, Correira J et al. Whole-blood viscosity parameters and cerebral blood flow. Stroke 1982; 13: 296-8.

Grotta J. Why do all drugs work in animals but none in stroke patients? 2. Neuroprotective therapy. J Internal Med 1995; 237: 89-94.

Hachinski V, Manelak M, Norris JW. Sleep morphology and prognosis in acute cerebrovascular lesions. In: Sleep morphology and prognosis in acute cerebrovascular lesions 1977. Hachinski V, Mamelak M, Norris JW (eds) pp 287-91. Amsterdam: Excerpta Medica.

Haley EC, Brott TG, Sheppard GL et al. Pilot randomised trial of tissue plasminogen activator in acute ischaemic stroke. Stroke 1993; 24: 1000-4.

Haley EC, Levy DE, Brott TC, Sheppard GL,Wong MCW, Kongable GL, Torner JC, Marler JR. Urgent therapy for stroke. Part II. Pilot study of tissue plasminogen activator administered 91-180 minutes from onset. Stroke 1992; 23: 641-5.

Hamdy NAT, Martin JF, Nicholl J, Owen P, Bergvall UB, Whittington D, Holroyd AM. Controlled trial of prostacyclin in acute cerebral infarction. Clin Sci 1984; 66: (2),48P.

Harper G, Castleden CM, Potter JF. Facors affecting changes in blood pressure after acute stroke. Stroke 1994; 25: 1726-9.

Harrison MJG, Pollock S, Dentell BE, Marshall J. Effect of haemoatrit on carotid stenosis and cerebral infarction . Lancet 1981; 2: 114-5.

Heiskanen O. Treatment of spontaneous intracerebral and intracerebellar haemorrhages. Stroke 1993; 24 [suppII]: I-94-I-95.

Herderschee D, Limburg M, van Royen EA, Hijdra A, Buller HR, Koster PA. Thrombolysis with recombitant tissue plasminogen activator in acute ischemic stroke: evaluation with rCBF-SPECT Acta Neurol Scand 1991; 83: 317-22.

Higashida RT, Hieshima GB, Halbach VV. Intravascular techniques for angioplasty and thrombolysis. In: Weinstein PR, Fadden AL (eds) Current Neurosurgical Practice, Protection of the Brain from Ischemia. Baltimore, MA: Williams and Wilkins. 1989: 279-84.

Higashida RT, Tsal FY, Halbach VV, Dowd CF, Smith T, Fraser K et al. Transluminal angioplasty for atherosclerotic disease of the vertebral and basilar arteries. J Neurosurg. 1993: 78: 192-8.

Hilton-Jones D, Warlow CP. The causes of stroke in the young. J Neurol 1985; 232: 137-43.

Hommel, M, Boissel JP, Cornu C, Boutitie F, Lees KR, Besson G, Leys D, Amerenco P, Bogaert M. MAST Study Group. Lancet 1995; 345: 57.

Hsu CY, Faught Jn RE, Furlan AJ, Coull BM, Huang EL, Linet OI, Yatsu FM. Intravenous prostacyclin in acute nonhaemorrhagic stroke: A placebo-controlled double-blind trial. Stroke 1986; 18: 352-8.

Huczynski J, Gryglewski RJ, Kosta-Trabka E *et al.* Use of prostacyclin in patients with ischemic stroke. A double-blind method II. Neurol Neurochir Pol 1988; 22: 299-304.

Huczynski J, Kostka-Trabka E, Sotowska W, Bieron K, Grodzinska L, Dembinska-Kiec A, *et al.* Double-blind controlled trial of the therapeutic effects of prostacyclin in patients with completed ischemic stroke. Stroke 1985; 16: 810-4.

International Nimodipine Study Group. Meta-analysis of nimodipine trials in acute ischaemic stroke. Stroke 1992; 3: 148.

Italian Acute Stroke Study Grup. Hemodilution in acute stroke: results of the Italian hemodilution trial. Lancet 1988; 1: 318-21.

Kapen S, Park A, Goldberg J, Wynter J, Park A. The incidence and severity of obstructive sleep apnea in iscaemic cerebrovascular disease. Neurology 1991; 41: 125.

Kassell N, Torner D, Adams H. Antifibrinolytic therapy in the acute period following aneurysmal subarachnoid haemorrhage. J Neurosurg 1984; 61: 225-30.

Kaste M, Fogelholm R, Erila T, Palomaki H, Murros K, Rissanen A, Sarna S. A randomised double-blind, placebo-controlled trial of nimodipine in acute ischemic hemispheric stroke. Stroke 1994; 25: 1348-53.

Kaufman HH. Treatment of deep intracerebral haematomas. A review. Stroke 1993; 24(supp 1) I 101.

Kay R, Wong KS, Yu YL, Chan YW, Tsoi TH, Ahuja AT, Chan FL, Fong KY, Law CB, Wong A, Woo J. Low-molecular-weight heparin for the treatment of acute ischaemic stroke. N Engl J Med 1995; 333: 1588-93.

Kennedy FB, Pozen TJ, Gableman EH, Tuthill JE, Zaentz SD. Stroke intensive care - an appraisal. Am. Heart J 1970; 80: 188-96.

Kilpatrick CJ, Davis SM, Hopper JL, Rossiter SC. Early seizures after stroke: risk of late siezures. Arch Neurol 1992; 49: 509-11.

Korczyn AD, Hermann G, Don R. Diaphragmatic involvement in hemiplegia and hemiparesis. J Neurol Neurosurg Psychiat. 1969; 32: 588-90.

Lane DJ, Rout MW, Williamson DH. Mechanism of hyperventilation in acute cerebrovascular accidents. Br Med J 1971; 3: 9-12.

Langfitt T. Conservative care of intracranial haemorrahge. In: Thompson R, Green J, (eds). Advances in Neurology: Vol 11. Stroke. New York: Raven Press 1977: 169-80.

Langhorne P, Williams BO, Gilchrist W, Howie K. Do stroke units save lives? Lancet 1993; 342: 395-7.

Larsson O, Marinovich N, Barber K. Double-blind trial of glycerol therapy in early stroke. Lancet 1976; 1: 832-4.

Lechat P, Mas JL, Lascault G *et al.* Prevalence of patent foramen ovale in patients with strokes. N Engl J Med 1988; 318: 1148-52.

Lee MC, Klassen AC, Resch JA. Respiratory pattern disturbance in ischemic cerebral vascular disease. Stroke 1974; 5: 612-6.

Lenzi GL, Grigoletto F, Gent M, Roberts RS, Walker MD, Easton JD, Carolei A, Dorsey FC, Rocca WA, Bruno R *et al.* Early treatment of stroke with monosialoganglioside GM-I. Efficacy and safety results of the Early Stroke Trial. Stroke 1994; 25: 1552-8.

Lhermitte F, Gautier JC, Derouesne G, Guiraud B. Ischemic accidents in the middle cerebral artery territory. Arch Neurol 1968; 19: 248-56.

Markand ON, Dyken ML. Sleep abnormalities in patients with brainstem lesions. Neurology 1976; 26: 769-76.

Mathew NT, Rivera VM, Meyer JS, Charney JZ, Hartmann A. Double-blind evaluation of glycerol therapy in acute cerebral infarction. Lancet 1972; 2: 1327-9.

Mathews P, Teasdale GM Role of neurosurgery in the management of posterior fossa stroke. Br J Hosp Med 1994; 52: 588-93

McCarthy ST, Turner JJ, Robertson D, Hawkey CJ. Low dose heparin as a prophylaxis against deep vein thrombosis after stroke. Lancet 1977; 1: 800-1.

McCormick WF. The natural history of intracranial saccular aneurysms. Neurol Neurosurg (Weekly Update) 1978; 1(3): 2.

Meyer JS, Gilroy J Bqarnhart MI *et al.* Anticoagulants plus streptokinase therapy in progressing stroke. J Am Med Assoc 1963; 189: 373.

Meyer JS, Gilroy J, Barnhart MI, Johnson JF. Therapeutic thrombolysis in cerebral thromboembolism. Neurology 1963; 189: 373.

Meyers MS, Norris JW, Hachinski VC *et al.* Plasma norepinephrine in stroke. Stroke 1981; 12: 200-4.

Mori E, Yoneda Y, Tabuchi M, *et al.* Intravenous recombitant tissue plasminogen activator in acute carotid artery territory stroke. Neurology 1992; 42: 976-82.

Mulley G, Wilcox R, Mitcell J. Dexamethasone in acute stroke. Br Med J 1978; 2: 994-6.

Multicentre Acute Stroke Trial - Italy (MAST-I) Group. Randomised controlled trial of streptokinase, aspirin, and combination of both in treatment of acute ischaemic stroke. Lancet 1995; 346: 1509-14.

National Institute of Neurological Disorders and Stroke rt-PA Stroke Study Group. Tissue plasminogen activator for acute ischaemic stroke. N Engl J Med 1995; 33: 1581-7.

Noel P, Gregoire F, Capon A, Lehert P. Atrial fibrillation as a risk facor for deep venous thrombosis and pulmonary emboli in stroke patients. Stroke 1991; 22: 760-2.

Nencini P, Inzitari D, Baruffi MC *et al.* Incidence of stroke in young adults in Florence Italy. Stroke 1988; 19: 977-81.

Norris JW, Hachinski VC. High dose steriod treatment in cerebral infarction. Br Med J 1986; 292: 21-3.

Norton B, Homer-Ward M, Donnelly MT, Long RG, Hommes GKT. A randomised prospective comparison of percutaneous endoscopic gastrostomy and nasogastic tube feeding after acute dysphasic stroke. BMJ 1996; 312: 13-6.

O'Brien M. Ischemic cerebral oedema: a review. Stroke 1979; 10: 623-8

Oczkowski WJ, Ginsberg JS, Shin A, Panju A. Venous thrombosis in patients undergoing rehabilitation for stroke. Arch Phys Med Rehab 1992; 73: 712-6.

Ohtomo E, Araki G, Itoh E, Toghi H, Matsuda T, Atarashi J. Clinical efficiency of urokinase in the treatment of cerebral thrombosis. Multi-centre double-blind study in comparison with placebo. Clin-Eval 1985; 15: 711-31.

Olinger CP, Brott TG, Barsan TG *et al.* Use of Ancrod in acute or progessing ischemic cerebral infarction. Annal Emergency Med. 1988; 17: 1208-9.

Overgaard K, Sperling B, Boysen G, Pederson H, Gam J, Ellemann K, Karle A, Arlien-Soborg P, Olsen TS, Videbaek C, Knudsen JB. Thrombolytic therapy in acute ischemic stroke. A Danish pilot study. Stroke 1993; 24: 1439-46.

Park CK, McCulloch J, Kang JK, Choi CR. Pretreatment with a competitive NMDA antagonist D-CPPene attenuates focal cerebral infarction and brain swelling in awake rats. Acta Neurochirurgica 1994; 127: 220-6.

Pickard JD, Murray GD, Illingworth R *et al.* Effect of oral nimodipine in cerebral infarction and outcome after subarachnoid haemorrhage: British aneurysm nimodipine trial. Br Med J 1981; 298: 636-42.

Pitner SE, Mance CJ. An evaluation of stroke intensive care: results in a municipal hospital. Stroke 1973; 4: 737-41.

Ringlestein MD, Biniek R, Weiller C, Ammeling B, Nolte PN, Thron MD. Type and extent of hemispheric brain infarctions and clinical outcome in early and delayed middle cerebral artery recanalization. Neurology 1992; 42: 289-98.

Rothman S, Olney J, Glutamate and the pathophysiology of hypoxic-ischaemic brain damage. Annal Neurology 1986; 19: 105-11.

Rout MW, Lane DJ, Wollner L. Prognosis in acute cerebrovascular accidents in relation to respiratory pattern and blood gas tensions. Br Med J 1971; 3: 7-9.

Sander D, Klingelhofer J. Changes of circadian blood pressure patterns after hemodynamic and thromboembolic brain infarction. Stroke 1994; 25: 1730-7

Sandercock P. Thrombolytic therapy for acute ischaemic stroke: promising, perilous or unproven (Letter). Lancet 1995; 346: 1504-5.

Sandercock P, Molyneux A, Warlow C. Value of computed tomography in patients with stroke. Oxfordshire Community Stroke Project. Br Med J 1985; 290: 193-7.

Sandercock PA, van den Belt AG, Lindley RI, Slattery J. Antithrombotic therapy in acute ischaemic stroke: an overview of the completed randomised trials. J Neurol Neurosurg Psychiat 1993; 56: 17-25IS

SASS Trial. Ganglioside GM1 in acute ischemic stroke. Stroke 1994; 25: 1141-8.

Scandinavian Stroke Study Group. Multicenter trial of hemodilution in acute ischaemic stroke. Results in the total patient population. Stroke 1987; 18: 691-9.

Shenkin HA, Zavala M, Cerebellar strokes: mortality, surgical indications and results of ventricular drainage. Lancet 1982; 2: 429-31

Sotaniemi KA Pyktinen J, Myllyla VV. Correlation of clinical and computed tomographic findings in stroke patients. Stroke 1990; 21: 1562-6.

Sundt TM, Smith HC, Campbell JK, Vliestra RE, Cucchiara RF, Stanson AW. Transluminal angioplasty for basilar artery stenosis. Mayo Clinic Proc 1980: 55: 673-80.

Svennerholm 1. Gangliosides-a new therapeutic agent against stroke and Alzheimers disease. Life Sciences 1994; 55; 2125-34.

Tognoni G, Roncaglioni MC. Dissent: an alternative interpretation of MAST-I. Lancet 1995; 346: 1515.

Trust Study Group. Randomised, double-blind, placebo-controlled trial of nimodipine in acute stroke. Lancet 1990; 336: 1205-9.

von Kummer R, Hacke W. Safety and efficacy of intravenous tissue plasminogen activator and heparin in acute middle cerebral artery stroke. Stroke 1992; 23: 646-52.

Wade DT, Langton Hewer R, Skilbeck CE, Bainton D, Burns-Cox C. Controlled trial of a home care service for acute stroke patients. Lancet 1985; I: 323-6.

Wahlestedt C, Golanov E, Yamamoto S, Yee F, Ericson H, Yoo H, Inturrisi CE, Reis DJ. Antisense oligodeoxynucleotides to NMDA-R1 receptor channel protect cortical neurons from excitotoxicity and reduce focal ischaemic infarctions. Nature 1993; 363: 260-3.

Wahlgren NG, MacMahon DG, De Keyser J, Indredavik B, Ryman T. Intravenous West European Stroke Trial (INWEST) of nimodipine in the treatment of acute ischaemic stroke. Cerebrovascular Disease 1994; 4: 260(A)

Wardlaw JM. Is routine computed tomography in stroke unnecessary? Br Med J 1994; 309: 1498-9.

Warlow C, Ogston D, Douglas AS. Venous thrombosis following strokes. Lancet 1972; 1: 1305-6.

Weddell JM, Beresford SAA. Planning for stroke patients. A four year descriptive study of home and hospital care. Department of Health and Social Security 1979.

Weir CJ, Murray GD, Adams FG, Muir KW, Grosset DG, Lees KR. Poor accuracy of stroke scoring systems for differential clinical diagnosis of intracranial haemorrhage and infarction Lancet 1994; 344: 999-1002.

Wolfe CDA, Taub NA, Woodrow J, Richardson E, Warburton FG, Burney PGJ. Patterns of acute stroke care in three districts in southern England. J Epidemiol Community Health 1993; 47: 139-43.

Wood JH, Polyzoidis KS, Epstein CM, Giddy GL, Tindall GT. Quantam EDEG alterations after isovolemic haemo-dilutional augmentation of cerebral perfusion in stroke patients neurology. 1984; 43: 764-8.

Yamaguchi T, Japanese Thrombolysis Study Group. Intravenous tissue plasminogen activator in acute thromboembolic stroke: A placebo controlled double blind trial. In: del Zoppo GJ, Mori E, Hacke W, eds. Thrombolytic Therapy in Acute Stroke II New York: Springer Verlag, 1993: 59-65.

Yu YL, Kumana CR, Lauder IJ, Cheung YK, Chan FL, Kou M, Fong KY, Cheung RTF, Chang CM. Treatment of acute cortical infarct with intravenous glycerol. A double blind, placebo-controlled randomised trial. Stroke 1993; 24: 1119-24.

Zeumer H, Freitag HJ, Zanella F, Thie A, Arning C. Local intra-arterial fibrinolytic therapy in patients with stroke: urokinase versus recombitant tissue plasminogen activator (r-TPA). Neuroradiology 1993; 35: 159-62.

Zeumer H. Local thrombolysis in the management of acute cerebral ischemia. Arzneim.-Forsch 1991; 41: 352-4.

Zivin JA, Mazzarella V. Tissue plasminogen activator plus glutamate antagonist improves outcome after embolic stroke. Arch Neurol 1992; 48: 1235-8.

# CHAPTER 5

# STROKE REHABILITATION

*Tony Rudd*

**Chapter outline**

# Introduction

Around 20% of stroke patients die within the first four weeks. Of the survivors, about 50% have significant disability ranging from motor or sensory dysfunction, speech disturbance, perceptual problems or more global cognitive loss. Surveys of patients' views (Stroke Association 1994) show considerable faith in the power of rehabilitation, particularly physiotherapy. This faith is however not strongly supported by scientific evidence of efficacy. At a time when evidence-based medicine is being encouraged from most quarters, this paucity of evidence for rehabilitation is weakening the case for further development of services for stroke patients. Obtaining the evidence will be one of the major challenges for stroke research over the next few years.

*The aims of rehabilitation have been defined by the WHO as:*
1. To aid physical recovery from stroke.

2. To promote physical, psychological and social adaptation to stroke-related disability and handicap.

3. To encourage a return to independence and activities of daily living.

4. To prevent secondary complications of stroke and related conditions, such as pneumonia and depressive illness.

The understanding of the ICD classification of disease into pathology, impairment, disability and handicap, in the process of rehabilitation is crucial in clarifying what benefits might be achieved with particular treatments and how these effects can be measured.

This chapter reviews the evidence for the role of rehabilitation services after stroke and how such services should be organised. It will discuss the problems of undertaking research in rehabilitation and summarise the evidence available from the literature on the role of the four major rehabilitation disciplines: physiotherapy, occupational therapy, speech and language therapy, and nursing. The Effectiveness Bulletin provides a very good summary of the research up until 1992 and this chapter draws heavily upon it and updates it. Detailed reviews of the evidence for the individual therapy specialities are provided in the subsequent chapters.

## Methodological problems in stroke rehabilitation research

Few well conducted randomised controlled trials of stroke rehabilitation have been performed although this is beginning to change. The reasons for this relate in part to the difficulties of conducting research on a group of patients with such variable pathology and impairments and where in many cases the natural history of recovery is poorly defined. Research, and the development of academic skills rather than practical ones, have until recently not been priorities in the schools of physiotherapy and occupational therapy and there is no career structure within these disciplines which allows for such developments.

Funding for research into areas of what is now regarded as routine clinical practice is difficult to obtain, particularly where new clinical services are having to be developed alongside existing services to enable comparisons to be made. The research worker may be funded but the therapists providing the care are much more difficult to obtain.

Some aspects of rehabilitation are now so well established that many people argue that it is unethical to perform randomised controlled trials of therapy versus no therapy. One way to perform such evaluations may now be to use the natural experiments that have developed with the very different styles of care for stroke that exist around the world. Italy and Hungary for example have very few speech therapists and occupational therapists working with stroke patients and although it would be difficult to control for the other variables it might be possible to identify differences in outcome across the European Union. The initial results from the EC-funded BIOMED study expected within the next year (Wolfe, personal communication) may identify whether such studies would be feasible. Trials comparing different types and styles of therapy are of course ethical and should be performed.

Meta-analysis is increasingly being used and sometimes abused as a substitute for large scale clinical trials and stroke rehabilitation research is no exception to this. It is a valid technique but its power is much reduced if it is analysing studies with very variable design and different outcome measures. Attempts have been made to standardise outcome measures, for example by the British Stroke Research Group, with little success. Each study still chooses its own selection of measures, apparently with little regard to similar studies. This is particularly true for studies performed outside the

United Kingdom and one of the roles the WHO could usefully perform would be to get agreement on such outcome measures for the purpose of stroke research. The major development in this field over the last ten years has been the widespread acceptance of the Barthel score. Whatever the flaws in this scale, at least scientists around the world are using one common outcome measure.

## Process of rehabilitation

### Stroke units

The meta-analysis of 10 trials of stroke units (Langhorne *et al.* 1993) clearly showed that organised care for stroke is better than disorganised care. A reduction of 28% was demonstrated in in-patient mortality in the groups managed on a stroke unit and this difference was still present when the one-year mortality statistics were analysed. Further trials have now been added to the meta-analysis under the auspices of the Cochrane Collaboration, confirming the original findings and also showing improvements in length of stay and disability outcomes. A recent very large study from Denmark (Jorgensen *et al.* 1995) showed very significant benefits for a stroke unit at reducing mortality, length of hospital stay, frequency of discharge to nursing homes and cost. Most of the trials analysed did not describe the units in detail but the key feature they had in common was some form of co-ordinated care by staff with an interest in stroke. Dennis and Langhorne (1994) examine the issues that arise out of the meta-analysis. How do stroke units compare with generic rehabilitation units and do the units have to be geographically defined within a hospital? How should people be selected for stroke unit care? Many units have adopted a policy of accepting patients with stroke of intermediate severity, arguing that the mildly impaired patients will get better whatever the care and the severely affected will not improve. A study from the Orpington Unit (Kalra *et al.* 1993) does however show that even the most severely affected patients have a lower mortality and shorter length of stay on a stroke unit. The unit at St Thomas' Hospital operates a policy that accepts all patients except for those expected to die or walk out of hospital within a few days. Even though outcome, as measured by length of stay or discharge destination in the profoundly impaired, may not be affected, there is still potential to reduce handicap by properly co-ordinated care. This observation does however need confirmation.

The other question Dennis and Langhorne pose in their article is what happens in a stroke unit? The evidence is not yet available but there is some evidence that the introduction of protocols for the detection and management of swallowing problems, for example, leads to a lower incidence of chest infections (Depippo *et al.* 1992; Depippo 1994). Pressure sores develop in up to 5% of patients during the weeks following stroke (Brown and Glassenberg 1973) and the effect of stroke unit care on pressure sore rates needs to be assessed. Other adverse outcomes which might also be expected to be less common in patients nursed on stroke units include painful subluxed shoulders, urinary tract infection arising from urinary catheterisation and fixed flexion contractures. Again this has yet to be demonstrated.

More information is required on what actually takes place on a stroke unit that is different from a general ward (Keith and Cowell 1987; Tinson 1989; Pound, personal communication). The Stroke Association is funding a study by Pound which is looking in more detail at exactly what happens on a stroke unit compared to general wards in terms of interactions between staff and patients, and amongst the staff. This may provide useful data to begin to explain the differences in outcome.

**Hospital or home**

Admission rates for patients with stroke vary from around 60% in the Oxford Community Stroke Study to nearly 80% in the SE Thames Community Stroke Study (Wolfe *et al.* 1993). The reasons for admission or non-admission were not reported in these studies. In the Netherlands (Schuling *et al.* 1993), approximately one-third of stroke patients are managed at home. These patients tend to be older, with co-morbidities such as Alzheimer's Disease and with less severe strokes. They were already more likely to be in institutional care. Recovery showed much the same pattern in the hospitalised and non-hospitalised patients.

Wade *et al.* (1985) looked at the provision of a stroke rehabilitation team in the community to assess whether it had an impact on rates of hospital admission and outcome and found little benefit. General practitioners taking part in this study had the choice as to whether to use the rehabilitation team or whether to admit their patients to hospital. The lack of benefit as measured by use of hospital beds or disability may therefore reflect the desires of the patients to be in hospital rather than any intrinsic failures of the team itself. Pound *et al.* (1995), interviewing 40 patients in depth, found important psychological needs during the acute stage of stroke were often met by admission to hospital, with patients gaining benefits from their admission over and above those measured in terms of morbidity or function.

For the majority of patients, remaining at home is not an option. Elderly patients who have a significant stroke while living alone or with frail relatives in poor-quality accommodation have to be admitted to hospital. What may be feasible is a brief admission for initial assessment and treatment and then early discharge with a co-ordinated package of social care and stroke rehabilitation. This model is currently being evaluated in a randomised controlled trial, partly funded by The Stroke Association, at St Thomas' Hospital and results should be available by the end of 1996. A similar study is just beginning in Orpington.

## Rehabilitation after discharge

A trial of day hospital care compared with domiciliary physiotherapy (Young and Forster 1991, 1992) demonstrated a small but significant benefit for home-based care. A similar comparison between hospital outpatient rehabilitation and domiciliary care (Gladman *et al.* 1993) showed little difference in outcomes between the two groups except for some benefit for the elderly in attending a day hospital, even when data were re-analysed at a year (Gladman *et al.* 1994).

A separate issue to the site of rehabilitation is the question as to whether stroke rehabilitation in the community is the role of primary health care services or of secondary outreach services. No study has compared general practitioner and generic therapist input with a consultant and specialist stroke rehabilitation team. The average general practitioner will see approximately four new cases of stroke a year and would therefore find it difficult to maintain expertise. The question is probably comparable to the hospital-based question of care on general wards versus stroke unit. The issue may nevertheless be worthy of a cost-benefit analysis.

## How long should stroke rehabilitation continue?

Stroke rehabilitation should start immediately the stroke is diagnosed. Enormous damage can be done by inappropriate care within the first few hours and days of a stroke. Placing a patient in an unsympathetic environment, in a bed with cot sides, with a catheter, drip and nasogastric tube inserted, in a bare backed night-dress and being handled and positioned badly can lead to a depressed, demoralised, pushing, contracted patient with pressure sores. The concept that acute care can be separated from rehabilitation therefore does not seem to make much sense. Rehabilitation is not what happens to a patient when the admitting physician gets bored.

More difficult is the question as to when to stop rehabilitation (Brocklehurst *et al.* 1978). Many patients think they stop physiotherapy too early and have a belief that the longer they continue, the better they will get (Lewinter and Mikkelsen 1995). Langton-Hewer (1990) considers that progress which continues beyond the first year is highly exceptional and would therefore presumably argue that continued therapy beyond that time was pointless. There have been few studies of long-term rehabilitation but, of note, Dam *et al.* (1993) did show that continuing rehabilitation for up to two years produced benefit in a group of 51 hemiplegic patients who were unable to walk at three months. At the end of the study 74% of the patients had regained the capacity to walk without assistance with an increase in the Barthel score (out of 100) from a mean of 47 to 70. Although this improvement mainly occurred in the first year, a significant change was observed in the second year of treatment. The benefits of continued therapy were also observed by Wade *et al.* (1992), who conducted a trial of physiotherapy between one and two years after stroke and demonstrated that improvements were obtained while therapy continued but that the patients relapsed after therapy was withdrawn. Long-term follow-up studies certainly show a significant proportion of patients are left with disability (Lindmark and Hamrin 1995).

A trial is needed to examine the benefits of continued multidisciplinary involvement in the care of stroke patients. The very long-term outcome of stroke is discussed in a separate chapter. Significant disability remains and there is some evidence that function actually steadily declines even without further discrete neurological events (Wade *et al.* 1992; Nydevik and Hulter-Asberg 1992). Would continued rehabilitation arrest the decline or even result in maintained improvements?

# Current controversies in rehabilitation research

1. What is it about the 'black box' of focused stroke rehabilitation that works? There is now increasing evidence that rehabilitation stroke units are effective at reducing mortality, disability and hospital length of stay. Having identified the effective components, will providing more of them produce further benefits? In other words is there a dose response curve for rehabilitation?

2. What is the best structure for a stroke team and what is the most effective way of running it? The meta-analysis of stroke units includes units that vary considerably in their *modus operandi.*

3. Where is rehabilitation best provided? Is admission to hospital always appropriate and what is the optimal time for discharge? Is the Government policy of encouraging the development of 'intermediate care centres' run by primary health services a model that is appropriate for stroke care? Is community rehabilitation best provided at home, in outpatient departments or in dedicated rehabilitation centres?

4. How long should rehabilitation continue and is there any benefit to be gained from courses of rehabilitation repeated indefinitely?

5. What is the natural history of stroke subtypes such as lacunar infarction, small vessel disease, and deep intracerebral haemorrhage and does the rehabilitation of strokes of different pathologies need to be different?

6. Does the quality of rehabilitation affect the long-term outcome? Could the frequency of falls and subsequent hip fractures, for example, be reduced by continuing with rehabilitation longer to achieve more than just basic mobility with a zimmer frame?

7. What is the potential for improved pharmacological agents to treat spasticity?

8. Can we provide better treatment for post-stroke pain both due to local neuromuscular and skeletal problems and central pain syndromes?

9. For each of the individual therapies, what are the best techniques to employ and how can progress best be measured?

10. To what extent can rehabilitation be provided by unqualified staff or carers? Is there a role for a generic therapist crossing the boundaries of the individual professions?

11. How do patient personality and beliefs affect the rehabilitation process? Are there differences between cultures in the approach to chronic diseases such as stroke and, if so, are there alternative approaches to care that should be adopted depending on the premorbid character of the patient?

12. Is there any justification for adopting a different approach to care depending upon the age of the patient?

13. What is the best treatment for patients with major cognitive impairment or perceptual problems?

14. How does mood disturbance affect rehabilitation outcome and do antidepressants help?

## Executive summary and priorities for research

Physiotherapy, occupational therapy and speech therapy are highly valued by patients but the evidence to prove their scientific worth is scanty.

Rehabilitation research poses major but not insuperable methodological and ethical problems. Rehabilitation stroke units have now clearly been shown to offer better results than care on general wards although it remains uncertain as to what specific features of a stroke unit are effective. Whether rehabilitation is better provided in hospital or at home after the acute phase of the illness is currently being evaluated. Longer term rehabilitation has been shown to be slightly cheaper and more effective for most patients when provided at home rather than in day hospitals or outpatient departments.

The evidence to support the use of alternative therapies is not presented. There may be a role for treatments such as art and music therapy alongside some of the treatments provided by psychologists. There is also interest being shown in the use of acupuncture and other alternative therapies such as marma therapy. It may be important for some patients to have access to therapies outside the conventional medical model for use when standard treatment has failed and it may therefore be a mistake to subject all of these treatments to formal evaluation.

This chapter serves as an introduction to the sections on the role of specific therapies. Included is a list of questions about rehabilitation that still need addressing.

The priorities for research should therefore be:

1. A study to determine which components of the rehabilitation 'black box' are particularly effective for which subgroups of patients; and trials of increasing the doses of these components to assess whether there is an impact on outcome.

2. A trial of prolonged rehabilitation either given continuously or intermittently to determine whether continued improvement can be achieved or deterioration prevented.

3. A study using position emission tomography to look at changes in brain function in those patients who continue to recover after six months to help understand the mechanisms of neurological recovery.

4. Further studies to determine the most appropriate place to deliver rehabilitation after stroke, comparing hospital, specialist rehabilitation units and home.

5. Evaluation of the relevance of ethnicity and personality on treatment and outcome.

6. Studies of the patterns of recovery and most appropriate forms of rehabilitation for different stroke subtypes

# References

Brocklehurst JC, Andrews K, Richards B, Laycock PJ. How much physical therapy for patients with stroke? Br Med J 1978; 1: 1307-10.

Brown M, Glasenberg M. Mortality factors in patients with acute stroke. JAMA 1973; 224: 1493-5.

Dam M, Tonin P, Cassons S, Erman M, Pizzolato G, Laia V, Battistin L. The effects of long-term rehabilitation therapy on post stroke hemeplegic patients. Stroke 1993; 24: 1186-91.

Dennis M, Langhorne P. So stroke units save lives: where do we go from here? Br Med J 1994; 309: 1273-7.

Depippo KL, Holas MA, Reding MJ, Mandel FS, Lesser ML. Dysphagia therapy following stroke: a controlled trial. Neurology 1994; 44: 1655-60.

Depippo KL, Holas MA, Reding MJ. Validation of the 3oz water swallow test for aspiration following stroke. Arch Neurol 1992; 49: 1259-61.

Effective Health Care: Stroke Rehabilitation. London HMSO, 1992, 2: 1-11.

Gladman JFR, Lincoln for the DOMINO Study Group. Follow-up of a controlled trial of domiciliary stroke rehabilitation (DOMINO Study). Age Ageing 1994; 23: 9-13.

Gladman JFR, Lincoln NB, Barer DH. A randomised controlled trial of domiciliary and hospital-based rehabilitation for stroke patients after discharge from hospital. J Neurol Neurosurg Psychiatry 1993; 56: 960-6.

Jorgensen HS, Nakayama H, Raaschou HO, Larsen K, Hubbe P, Olsen TS. The effect of a stroke unit; reductions in mortality, discharge rate to nursing home, length of hospital stay, and cost. A community based study. Stroke 1995; 26: 1178-82.

Kalra L, Dale P, Crome P. Improving stroke rehabilitation: a controlled study. Stroke 1993; 24: 1463-7.

Keith RA, Cowell KS. Time use of stroke patients in three rehabilitation hospitals. Social Sci Med 1987; 24: 529-33.

Langhorne P, Williams BO, Gilchrist W, Howie K. Do stroke units save lives? Lancet 1993; 342: 395-7.

Langton-Hewer R. Rehabilitation after stroke. Q J Med. 1990; 76: 659-74.

Lewinter M, Mikkelsen S. PatientsÕ experience of rehabilitation after stroke. Disabil Rehab 1995; 17: 3-9.

Lindmark B, Hamrin E. A five year follow-up of stroke survivors: motor function and activities of daily living. Clin Rehab 1995; 9: 1-9.

Nydevik I, Hulter-Asberg K. Sickness impact after stroke. Scand J Prim Health Care 1992; 10: 284-9.

Pound P, Bury M, Gompertz P, Ebrahim S. Stroke patients' views on their admission to hospital. Br Med J 1995; 311: 18-22.

Schuling J, Groenier KH, Meyboom-de-Jong B. Home treatment of patients with cerebrovascular accident [Dutch] Nederlands Tijdschrift voor Geneeskunde 1993; 137: 1918-22.

Tinson DJ. How stroke patients spend their days. An observational study of the treatment regime offered to patients in hospital with movement disorders following stroke. Int Disability Studies 1989; 11: 45-9.

Wade DT, Collen FM, Robb GF, Warlow CP. Physiotherapy intervention late after stroke and mobility. Br Med J 1992; 304: 609-13.

Wade DT, Langton Hewer R, Skilbeck CE, Bainton D, Burns-Cox C. Controlled trial of a home care service for acute stroke patients. Lancet 1985; I: 323-6.

Wolfe CDA, Taub NA, Woodrow J, Richardson E, Warburton FG, Burney PGJ. Pattern of acute stroke care in three districts in southern England. J Epidemiol Community Health 1993; 47: 139-43.

Young JB, Forster A. The Bradford community stroke trial; results at six months. Br Med J. 1992; 304: 1085-9.

Young JB, Forster A. The Bradford community stroke trial: eight week results. Clin Rehab 1991; 5: 283-92.

# CHAPTER 6

# PHYSIOTHERAPY FOR STROKE

*Tony Rudd, Liza Robinson*

**Chapter outline**

## Introduction

Physiotherapy is regarded by many stroke survivors as the most important form of treatment they received (Pound *et al.* 1994) and patients frequently express the view that if they had only had more, then their level of function would have increased. The level of patient faith in physiotherapy is not matched by scientific evidence of efficacy. A lack of evidence does not of course equate with lack of benefit, but it is understandable that purchasers are reluctant to invest more resources without a clearer link being made between input and outcome (Tyson 1995). If physiotherapy is of benefit, then what is the most effective way for it to be given, how intensively and at what stage after a stroke? Are there certain types of stroke where physiotherapy is of particular importance and what are the best ways of measuring and predicting outcome? Are there pharmacological agents available or likely to become available which might augment the work of the physiotherapist? The need for research is well recognised within the profession (Durward and Baer 1995). There is certainly a lack of consensus amongst physiotherapists in the United Kingdom about the best way to provide therapy. Andrews (1985) surveyed 196 geriatric units and found a wide range of different methods being employed. This section will review the literature about stroke and physiotherapy and highlight areas where research might be possible.

## Basic science research

The close links between some departments of neurology, physiology and physiotherapy have produced some interesting work, creating a better understanding of the basic mechanisms that underlie the impairments seen in stroke. Understanding of some of the mechanisms of spasticity (Lance 1980; Carr *et al.* 1995) have unfortunately not yet led to a breakthrough in management. Given *et al.* (1995) have shown that some of the stiffness that may sometimes be attributed to spasticity is in fact due to immobilisation changes in muscle connective tissue, particularly in slow twitch fibres. Maintaining passive movements in the early stages of paralysis is therefore probably of great importance. It is suggested in this paper that there may be some indication for splinting or casting of the ankle joint in some cases and this may be worthy of further investigation.

Understanding the normal pattern of motor recovery is important for both the planning of treatment and for organising and interpreting research. Partridge *et al.* (1987) described the recovery of 368 patients with hemiplegia and Duncan *et al.* (1992) similarly followed the motor deficits of 104 patients but there has still not been enough research in this area, in particular with reference to stroke subtypes. A number of reports have been published looking at specific areas of motor impairments and recovery, including the effect of facilitation techniques on motor potentials in the paralysed hand (Hummelstein *et al.* 1995), the recovery of and factors limiting walking (Nakamura *et al.* 1988), the influence of sway on stability after stroke and the use of biofeedback in recovery (Shumway-Cook *et al.* 1988) and the effect of hemiplegia on trunk muscle strength (Bohannon *et al.* 1995). The extent to which recovery occurs as a result of neuroplasticity is another area that remains contentious, but if proven to occur, this offers great potential for understanding the scientific basis for physiotherapy.

The whole area of motor control after stroke needs more detailed research. With the development of sensitive techniques to look at brain structure (MRI scanning) and brain function (position emission tomography (PET)), enormous opportunities exist for this. Without an understanding of the pathology, treatment is likely to remain at best haphazard.

## Is it effective?

The Effectiveness Bulletin (1992) describes the important studies that had been done up until then evaluating the efficacy of physiotherapy. The principle studies are those of Sunderland *et al.* (1992) who compared conventional with intensive physiotherapy in 137 patients and demonstrated a small but significant increase in arm function in the intensively treated group. Only 31% of possible patients were recruited to the trial, excluding the mildly and severely affected groups. The trial of Smith DS *et al.* (1992) was similar in design, again comparing intensive therapy with conventional therapy but on this occasion including a no therapy group in a cohort of outpatients. Again small differences in ADL scores were found between the intensively treated group and the no therapy group. Unfortunately the relevance of the trial for general clinical practice is difficult to interpret, because of the exclusion of 90% of the stroke population from the study.

Richards *et al.* (1993), in a randomised controlled pilot study of 27 patients with middle cerebral artery infarction, again compared intensive with conventional therapy. Gait velocity at six weeks after starting treatment was faster in the experimental group, although this difference had disappeared by three and six months. A larger trial was planned. Sivenius *et al.* (1985) selected 95 patients out of a possible 373 for intensive or normal physiotherapy. As in the other studies of similar design, ADL function recovered better in the first three months in the intensively treated group. An intensive programme of gait retraining for 4 weeks in mobile hemiparetic patients failed to produce any significant benefits (Hesse *et al.* 1994). Taking patients who might be expected to be stable over one year after stroke, Wade *et al.* (1992) performed a randomised crossover trial of physiotherapy intervention. Treatment was limited to assessment and the provision of advice but nevertheless an improvement in walking speed resulted. Once treatment was withdrawn the patients again deteriorated. Clearly in these patients therapy had an effect and this study is probably the single most important study performed so far on the effectiveness of stroke physiotherapy. In several of these studies the term conventional therapy is used without further clarification as to precisely what it involved. The whole area of defining terms and techniques in physiotherapy needs to be addressed.

In a follow-up study of 155 patients from the Oxfordshire Community Stroke Study (Davies *et al.* 1989), no difference in recovery of function was observed between the group of patients who received remedial therapy and those who did not. The difficulties of interpreting such data retrospectively is of course great and the results must therefore be read with caution. Another retrospective study (Davidoff 1991) of 139 patients with moderate disability compared those who received no outpatient rehabilitation with those who did. No differences were again observed between the groups. Seitz *et al.* (1987), looking at data from 212 patients, tried to correlate the amount of therapy given with outcome. The greater the time spent in therapy the greater the improvement, although again in an uncontrolled retrospective study this result becomes almost meaningless. Wade *et al.* (1984), looking primarily at what determined how much physiotherapy was given, also failed to demonstrate a specific beneficial effect of therapy.

Indirect evidence for the efficacy of physiotherapy may be the benefits shown for patients admitted to stroke units. Smith ME *et al.* (1982) showed that stroke unit patients received more and earlier physiotherapy and had better outcomes than those treated on general medical wards.

For a treatment which has been used for so long and is now so widely accepted and purchased around the world, the paucity of decent research evidence to justify its use is unacceptable. Properly conducted randomised controlled trials of physiotherapy should be a top priority for stroke research.

## What type?

Bobath (1990) or the motor relearning program of Carr and Shepherd (1989) or a more pragmatic approach? Using modern technology such as biofeedback techniques or staying with traditional low-technology physiotherapy? Early mobilisation in wheelchairs or not? A functional approach where it matters less how you do it and more what you do or concentration on quality in the hope of better long-term function? Using walking aids or not?

These are some of the questions for which there are as yet no answers. There are, however, a lot of strongly held beliefs amongst the physiotherapy fraternity.

Basmajian *et al.* (1975) and Colborne (1993) advocate the use of biofeedback for foot drop and hemiplegic gait and Bogataj (1995) obtained good results with multichannel electrical stimulation therapy in the rehabilitation of gait. Engardt *et al.* (1993, 1994) obtained better results for the recovery of sit to stand when biofeedback was used instead of conventional therapy. In a randomised study of 78 patients, Magnusson (1994) used vibrators attached to calf muscles or galvanic vestibular stimulation and demonstrated improvement in postural recovery compared to normal treatments. However in a meta-analysis of biofeedback compared to conventional therapy (Moreland and Thompson 1994), neither form of therapy was superior to the other.

Basmajian *et al.* (1987) compared Bobath therapy with a behavioural approach and found no differences. Again, Dickstein (1986) compared Bobath therapy with traditional exercise activities and proprioceptive neuromuscular facilitation techniques and found no substantial differences between any of the three therapeutic approaches.

A study is being considered to compare the two most widely used and accepted therapeutic techniques, Carr Shepherd and Bobath. Arising out of the 1994 King's Fund conference, preparation is also being made for a multicentre clinical trial to evaluate the effectiveness of physiotherapy following stroke.

## When should physiotherapy be given?

Examination of the effectiveness of early or delayed rehabilitation is complicated by the enormous variability in natural recovery and the inaccuracy of predictive variables (Tangeman *et al.* 1990). Little work has been done to show whether outcome is affected by early or delayed intervention with stroke, although time to being seen by the physiotherapist has been used as a marker for quality of care in some audit packages for stroke. Only the Wade study (1992) has examined the benefits of very late intervention.

## Assessment of outcome

As with all other aspects of stroke research, having a reliable set of outcome measures that are widely accepted is a key requirement. General outcome measures are described in a separate chapter. Discussion here is limited to those measures specifically developed for use within the physiotherapy profession. In 1994 the King's Fund, funded by The Stroke Association, published the results of a workshop entitled: 'The evaluation of physiotherapy for people with stroke.' Key components of recovery for each of the major stages of rehabilitation were defined. Specific adverse events were identified such as pressure sores, joint contractures and shoulder pain, where the quality of physiotherapy was considered to have an impact on the frequency of occurrence. The measures identified now need to be validated and a few selected key indicators introduced into routine clinical practice.

A number of motor rating scales have been developed for use by physiotherapists (Ashburn 1982; Lincoln and Leadbitter 1979; Fugl-Meyer *et al.* 1975; Keenan *et al.* 1984; Carr *et al.* 1985; Dean and Mackey 1992) and there have been attempts to develop specific rating scales for particular components of the rehabilitation process

(Sunderland *et al.* 1989; Sandin and Smith 1990; Nieuwboer *et al.* 1995; Haas and Crow 1995). The link between some of these scores and functional outcome has been assessed (Bohannon and Walsh 1992; Dean and Mackey 1992; Morgan 1994. As yet no consensus has been reached about the most reliable and applicable measures.

## Pharmacology and physiotherapy

For many years physicians have attempted to treat spasticity with baclofen, dantrolene and benzodiazepines. They are of limited value in reducing muscle tone and have unacceptable side effects in many patients (Losseff and Thompson 1995). Intrathecal baclofen, useful in paraplegia, is of much less benefit after stroke. There is clearly a need for the drug companies to find alternatives for what would be a very lucrative market. Koyama *et al.* (1992) report the benefits of phenol blocking for hip flexor muscle spasticity but this is unlikely to be widely applicable. Perhaps of more interest for the local treatment of spasticity is the relatively recently introduced treatment of local injection with Botulium toxin (Hesse *et al.* 1994). The cost of treatment is high and long-term benefits need evaluation.

A double blind pilot study of eight patients (Crisotomo *et al.* 1988) suggested a single dose of amphetamine assisted motor function when combined with physiotherapy. The definitive study has not materialised. The original observation seems worthy of further evaluation.

## Adverse outcomes

Shoulder pain following a stroke is a major cause of persisting disability (Smith *et al.* 1982). An arm can be rendered almost useless by a painful frozen shoulder. In a prospective study of 110 patients, malalignment of the shoulder occurred in 46% with consequent delay and limitation in restoration of function. Bruton reviewed the subject in 1985 and there was a further prospective study in 1994 (Roy et al.). Of 76 patients, 55 experienced shoulder pain at some stage which was strongly correlated with prolonged hospital stay and poor recovery of arm function. Trials of strapping or the use of cuffs are needed, comparing outcome with improved positioning and handling.

The cause of shoulder hand syndrome is not understood. Braus *et al.* (1994), in a prospective study, identified it in 27% of a cohort of 132 hemiplegic patients. In a non-blinded placebo controlled trial, 31 of the 36 patients responded promptly to the use of low-dose steroids. Shoulder joint biopsies in seven patients showed evidence for trauma as an initiating cause, further indicating the need for improvement in the care of the shoulder. A larger trial repeating the treatment with steroids is needed and a trial of the introduction of a protocol for shoulder care would also be of value.

The role of physiotherapists in the prevention of pressure sores is in identifying at-risk patients and providing guidance on positioning and handling. A similar role may also be important in the prevention of the complication of 'pushing' where the patient overcompensates for the hemiparesis by using the unaffected side to push the trunk across the midline towards the weak side. It is believed that incorrect handling and positioning of patients early in the course of the disease may contribute to 'pushing'. Certainly a patient with the problem presents very considerable problems in rehabilitation, which may be slower and ultimately less successful as a result. This phenomenon needs further research to establish a cause and the most effective ways of prevention and treatment.

Contractures arise from immobilised joints. Many therapists would suggest their development is a sign of inadequate treatment. Again the best ways of preventing and treating are not well defined and need more research. Guidelines for the appropriate use of passive movement and splinting or even casting in plaster of paris need developing.

# Executive summary and priorities for research

Physiotherapy is perceived by the patients, carers and health care professionals as a key component of the care needed after stroke. Failure to recover is sometimes attributed by patients as being due to insufficient physiotherapy. Many of the techniques used do have their basis in scientific fact. The normal patterns of recovery for different stroke subtypes is not well understood and, likewise, the mechanisms by which recovery occurs at a cellular level need more research.

Studies of effectiveness of care have also been disappointing. No well conducted trial has been performed comparing physiotherapy with no physiotherapy and it would probably no longer be acceptable to undertake such a trial. There have been several studies comparing intensive with standard therapy, demonstrating modest benefits for an increased quantity of rehabilitation, and one study of rehabilitation late after stroke, again showing small improvements.

Given the resource implications of providing physiotherapy to all stroke patients and the faith put in it by the patients, a clear priority in stroke research must be trials of effectiveness.

Many different approaches are used in stroke physiotherapy. These need clearer definition and trials need to be performed to evaluate which techniques are most effective for which types of patient. Development of widely acceptable stroke outcome measures for use by physiotherapists is needed and work is in progress to achieve this.

Basic scientific understanding of the mechanisms of spasticity has increased but so far this has not been translated into any significant pharmacological developments.

One of the key roles of physiotherapy is to prevent adverse outcomes, including shoulder pain and subluxation, pressure sores and contractives. The most effective preventive techniques and treatments also need clarification.

*The priorities for research should therefore be:*
1. Definition of the natural history of motor recovery of stroke subtypes.

2. Development of clearer definitions of the techniques currently being employed by physiotherapists.

3. Trials comparing the major physiotherapy techniques to determine which are most effective and under what circumstances.

4. Trials to determine the ideal intensity and duration of physiotherapy following stroke. In particular the role of long-term physiotherapy continuing for months or years after stroke needs to be tested.

5. There is a need for the development of standardised outcome measures for physiotherapy.

6. Research is required to examine, at the level of the neurone, what the mechanism of motor recovery is after stroke and whether physiotherapy can be shown to affect cellular function; how much recovery of function is a consequence of neuroplasticity and how much due to recovery of neuronal function in the ischaemic area.

7. Further basic science research is need to identify mechanisms of spasticity with a view to the development of drugs to effect treatment.

# References

Andrews K. Rehabilitation of the elderly stroke patient in the United Kingdom. Int J Rehab Research 1985; 8: 463-4.

Ashburn A. Assessment of motor function in stroke patients. Physiotherapy 1982; 68: 109-13.

Basmajian JV, Gowland CA, Finlayson MA, Hall AL, Swanson LR, Stratford PW, Trotter JE, Brandstater ME. Stroke treatment: comparison of integrated behavioural-physical therapy vs. traditional physical therapy programs. Arch Phys Med Rehab. 1987; 68: 267-72.

Basmajian JV, Kukulla CG, Narayan MG, Takebe K. Biofeedback treatment of foot-drop after stroke compared with standard rehabilitation technique: effects on voluntary control and strength. Arch Phys Med Rehab 1975; 56: 231-6.

Bobath B. Adult hemiplegia: evaluation and treatment 3rd Edition. London Heinemann, 1990.

Bogataj U, Gros N, Kljajic M, Acimovic R, Malezic M. The rehabilitation of gait in patients with hemiplegia: a comparison between conventional therapy and multichannel functional electrical stimulation therapy. Physical Therapy 1995; 75: 490-502.

Bohannon RW, Cassidy D, Walsh S. Trunk muscle strength is impaired multidirectionally after stroke. Clin Rehab 1995; 9: 47-51.

Bohannon RW, Walsh S. Nature, reliability and predictive value of muscle performance measures with hemiparesis following stroke. Arch Phys Med Rehab 1992; 73: 721-5.

Braus DF, Krauss JK, Strobel J. The shoulder-hand syndrome after stroke; a prospective clinical trial. Annals Neurology 1994; 36: 728-33.

Bruton JD. Shoulder pain in stroke patients with hemiplegia or hemiparesis following a cerebrovascular accident. Physiotherapy 1985; 71: 2-4.

Carr JH, Shepherd RB. A motor learning model for stroke rehabilitation. Physiotherapy 1989; 75: 372-80.

Carr JH, Shepherd RB, Ada L. Spasticity: Research findings and implications for intervention. Physiotherapy 1995; 81: 421-9.

Carr JH, Shepherd RB, Nordholm L, Lynne D. Investigation of a new motor assessment scale for stroke patients. Physical Therapy 1985; 65: 175-80.

Colborne GR, Olney SJ, Griffin MP. Feedback of ankle joint angle and soleus electromyography in the rehabilitation of hemiplegic gait. Arch Phys Med Rehab 1993; 74: 1100-6.

Crisostomo EA, Duncan PW, Propst M Dawson DV, Davis JN. Evidence that amphetamine with physical therapy promotes recovery of motor function in stroke patients. Annals Neurology 1988; 23: 94-7.

Davidoff GN, Keren O, Ring H, Solzi P. Acute stroke patients: long-term effects of rehabilitation and maintainance of gains. Arch Phys Med Rehab 1991; 72: 869-73.

Davies P, Bamford J, Warlow C. Remedial therapy and functional recovery in a total population of first stroke patients. Int Dis Studies 1989; 11: 40-4.

Dean C, Mackey F. Motor assessment scale scores as a measure of rehabilitation outcome following stroke. Australian Physiotherapy 1992; 8: 31-8.

Dickstein R, Hocherman S, Pillar T, Shaham R. Stroke rehabilitation. Three exercise therapy approaches. Physical Therapy 1986; 66: 1233-8.

Duncan PW, Goldstein LB, Matchar D, Divine GW, Feussner J. Measurement of motor recovery after stroke. Stroke 1992; 23: 1084-9.

Durward B, Baer G. Physiotherapy and neurology: Towards research based practice. Physiotherapy 1995; 81: 436-9.

Effective Health Care. Stroke Rehabilitation. Leeds: University of Leeds 1992 (Bulletin No 2).

Engardt M. Rising and sitting down in stroke patients. Auditory feedback and dynamic strength training to enhance symmetrical body weight distribution. Scand J Rehab Med 1994; 31: 1-57.

Engardt M, Ribbe T, Olsson E. Vertical ground reaction force feedback to enhance stroke patients' symmetrical body-weight distribution while rising/sitting down. Scand J Rehab Med 1993; 25: 41-8.

Fugl-Meyer AR, Jaasko L, Leyman I, Olsson S, Steglind S. The post-stroke hemiplegia patient: A method for evaluation of physical performance. Scandinavian J Rehab Med 1975; 7: 13-31.

Given JD, Dewald JPA, Rymer WZ. Joint dependent passive stiffness in paretic and contralateral limbs of spastic patients with hemiparetic stroke. J Neurol Neurosurg Psychiatry 1995; 59: 271-9.

Haas BM, Crow JL. Towards a clinical measurement of spasticity? Physiotherapy 1995; 81: 474-9.

Hesse SA, Jahnke MT, Bertelt CM, Schreiner C, Luecke D, Mauritz K-H. Gait outcome in ambulatory hemiparetic patients after a 4-week comprehensive rehabilitation program and prognostic factors. Stroke 1994; 25: 1999-2004.

Hesse S, Lucke D, Bertelt C, Gregoric M, Mauritz KH. Botulinum toxin treatment for lower extensor limb spasticity in chronic hemiplegic patients. J Neurol Neurosurg Psychiatry 1994; 57: 1321-4.

Hummelscheim H, Hauptmann B, Neumann S. Influence of physiotherapeutic facilitation techniques on motor evoked potentials in centrally paretic hand extensor muscles. Electroencephalography Clinical Neurophysiology 1995; 97: 18-28.

Keenan MA, Perry J, Jordan C. factors affecting balance and ambulation following stroke. Clinical Orthopaedics and Related Research 1984; 182: 165-71.

Koyama H, Murakami K, Suzuki T, Suzaki K. Phenol block for hip flexor muscle spasticity under ultrasonic monitoring. Arch Phys Med Rehab. 1992; 73: 1040-3.

Lance JW. Pathophysiology of spasticity and clinical experience with baclofen. In: Feldman RG, Young RR, Koella WP (eds) Spasticity: disordered motor control, Chicago: Year Book Publishers, 1980.

Lincoln N, Leadbitter D. Assessment of motor function in stroke patients. Physiotherapy 1979; 65: 48-51.

Losseff N, Thompson AJ. The medical management of increased tone. Physiotherapy 1995; 81: 480-4.

Magnusson M, Johansson K, Johansson BB. Sensory stimulation promotes normalization of postural control after stroke. Stroke 1994; 25: 1176-80.

Moreland J, Thompson MA. Efficacy of electromyographic biofeedback compared with conventional physical therapy for upper-extremity function in patients following stroke: a research overvieew and meta-analysis. Physical Therapy 1994; 74: 534-47.

Morgan P. The relationship between sitting balance and mobility outcome in stroke. Australian Physiotherapy 1994; 40: 91-6.

Nakamura R, Handa T, Watanabe S, Morohashi I. Walking cycle after stroke. Tohoku J Exp Med 1988; 154: 241-4.

Nieuwboer A, Feys H, DeWeerdt W, Nuyens G, DeCorte E. Developing a clinical tool to measure sitting balance after stroke: a reliability study. Physiotherapy 1995; 81: 439-45.

Partridge C. Evaluation of physiotherapy for people with stroke: Report of a workshop on appropriate outcomes of physiotherapy for people with stroke. King's Fund Centre London 1994.

Partridge CJ, Johnston M, Edwards S. Recovery from physical disability after stroke: normal patterns as a basis for evaluation. Lancet 1987; I: 373-5.

Pound P, Bury M, Gompertz P, Ebrahim S. View of survivors of stroke on benefits of physiotherapy. Quality in Health Care 1994; 3: 69-74.

Roy CW, Sands M, Hill LD. Shoulder pain in acutely admitted hemiplegics. Clin Rehab 1994; 8: 334-40.

Rusi R. Effectiveness of group physiotherapy on motor function in elderly stroke patients. [Finnish] Hoitotiede 1991; 3: 169-75.

Sandin KJ, Smith BS. The measure of balance in sitting in stroke rehabilitation prognosis. Stroke 1990; 21: 82-6.

Seitz RH, Allred KE, Backus ME, Hoffman JA. Functional changes during acute rehabilitation in patients with stroke. Physical Therapy 1987; 67: 1685-90.

Shumway-Cook A, Anson D, Haller S. Postural sway biofeedback: its effect on reestablishing stance stability in hemiplegic patients. Arch Phys Med Rehab 1988; 69: 395-400.

Sivenius J, Pyorala K, Heinonen OP, Salonen JT, Riekkinen P. The significance of intensity of rehabilitation of stroke - a controlled trial. Stroke 1985; 16: 928-31.

Smith DS, Goldenberg E, Ashburn A, Kinsella G, Sheikh K, Brennan PJ *et al.* Remedial therapy after stroke: a randomised controlled trial. Br Med J 1992; 304: 609-13.

Smith ME, Garraway WM, Smith DL, Akhtar AJ. Therapy impact on functional outcome in a controlled trial of stroke rehabilitation. Arch Phys Med Rehab 1982; 63: 21-4.

Smith RG, Cruikshank JG, Dunbar S, Akhtar AJ. Malalignment of the shoulder after stroke. Br Med J 1982; 284: 1224-6.

Sunderland A, TinsonD, Bradley L, Langton-Hewer R. Arm function after stroke. An evaluation of grip strength as a measure of recovery and a prognostic indicator. J Neurol Neurosurg Psychiatry 1989; 52: 1267-72.

Sunderland A, Tinson DJ, Bradley EL, Fletcher D, Langton-Hewer R, Wade DT. Enhanced physical therapy improves recovery of arm function after stroke. A randomised controlled trial. J Neurol Neurosurg Psychiatry 1992; 55: 530-5.

Tangeman PT, Banaitis DA, Williams AK. Rehabilitation of chronic stroke patients: changes in functional performance. Arch Phys Med 1990; 71: 870-80.

Tyson SF. Stroke rehabilitation: what is the point? Physiotherapy 1995; 81: 430-2.

Wade DT, Collen FM, Robb GF, Warlow CP. Physiotherapy intervention late after stroke and mobility. Br Med J 1992; 304: 609-13.

Wade DT, Skilbeck CE, Langton-Hewer R, Wood VA. Therapy after stroke: amounts, determinants and effects. Int Rehab Med 1984; 6: 105-10.

# CHAPTER 7

# SWALLOWING DISORDERS FOLLOWING STROKE

*Julie Quinn*

**Chapter outline**

# Introduction

In the last decade, there has been an increased interest in the assessment and management of dysphagia following stroke. The main focus of research in this field has been in documenting the pathophysiology of swallowing and of identifying the clinical correlates of oro-pharyngeal dysphagia in the acute phase post stroke. The effects of long-term dysphagia and the efficacy of dysphagia therapy have received less attention.

A variety of swallowing disorders have been documented following stroke. Amongst the physiological disturbances in swallowing, reduced bolus formation and transit, delayed swallow reflex, reduced airway protection and impaired pharyngeal peristalsis, have correlated with aspiration following stroke. These have been found generally to occur in combination rather than as isolated disorders (Veis and Logemann 1985; Robbins and Levine 1988; Gresham 1990). The presence of swallowing problems following stroke clearly has serious implications with regard to morbidity and mortality. Dehydration, malnutrition and aspiration pneumonia are reported to be common consequences of dysphagia. The need for early identification of dysphagia and appropriate management in the acute phase is now recognised as essential.

There currently exists limited agreement over whether the nature of the swallowing disorders differs according to lesion location. Early work indicated that aspiration was limited to brainstem or bilateral lesions. However, more recent studies report that this is not the case. Instead, a high incidence of swallowing disorders has been found, regardless of general site of lesion and lesion location does not necessarily predict the type(s) of disorder(s) exhibited (Veis and Logemann 1985 Horner *et al.* 1988; Horner and Massey 1988; Alberts *et al.* 1992). However, Horner *et al.* (1988) did find that patients with combined cerebral-brainstem strokes with bilateral cranial nerve signs were at greatest risk of aspiration.

# Epidemiology

The incidence and prevalence of swallowing disorders in acute stroke is well documented (Veis and Logemann 1985; Groher and Bukatman 1986; Gordon *et al.* 1987; Barer 1989). Bedside swallowing assessments have estimated that 28-45% of individuals post stroke have a swallowing disorder. Studies performed in later phases of stroke using videofluoroscopy, have shown prevalence rates of 49-65% in both hemispheric and brainstem strokes (Horner *et al.* 1988, 1991). The variation in findings may be due to differences in factors such as the population studied, methods and timing of assessment and lack of consensus opinion over primary outcome measurement.

Despite swallowing problems being common (30%-50%) in the first week following stroke, within a month recovery is noted in the majority of individuals (Barer 1984, 1989; Gordon *et al.* 1987). Wade and Hewer (1987) reported the presence of swallowing problems in 43% of conscious patients one week post-stroke, whereas at three weeks less than 2% had marked difficulties. Kidd *et al.* (1995), using videofluoroscopy, found 42% aspirating at 72 hours but only 8% at three months. It should however be noted that the effects of therapeutic intervention were not controlled for in this hospital sample.

## Implications for speech and language therapy provision

The "dysphagia boom" of the eighties has highlighted a number of ethical and professional issues for speech and language therapists. These include issues related to their role within the multidisciplinary team, the need for specialist postgraduate training in dysphagia management, professional accountability and liability, and increased referral rates for those with acute and chronic dysphagia.

The role of the speech and language therapist in the assessment and management of post-stroke dysphagia has dramatically increased over recent years. Involvement in the management of dysphagia has been shown to place an increased burden on already overstretched speech and language therapy services. The increases in referral rates, and concerns over maintaining existing levels of service for those with communication problems following stroke, have been highlighted by several reports (Edelman 1988; Royal College of Speech and Language Therapists RCSLT 1990, 1992). There are concerns that those with speech and language impairments following stroke are neglected by therapy services.

# Assessment of oro-pharyngeal dysphagia

A multidisciplinary approach to the assessment and management of dysphagia has been widely advocated (Logemann 1983; RCSLT 1990; Park and O'Neill 1994). The role of the speech and language therapist in dysphagia management is well documented (Logemann 1983, 1988; RCSLT 1990; Groher 1993) and will be focused on in this report.

Assessment involves a detailed bedside swallowing evaluation by a dysphagia-trained speech and language therapist. Clinical evaluation is generally based on assessment of: oro-motor and oro-sensory function; protective reflexes; respiratory and phonatory status and trial swallows of different textures and amounts of food and liquid. Observations on level of arousal, cognitive-linguistic status and perceptual ability are also noted.

The use and availability of standardised clinical swallowing assessment is limited. Assessments such as the Rehabilitation Institute of Chicago's Clinical Evaluation of Dysphagia (Cherney *et al.* 1986) and the Paramatta Hospital's Assessment of Dysphagia (Warms *et al.* 1990) are rarely used in Britain. Both assessments require further investigation into their reliability and validity.

The development and availability of instrumental techniques to supplement findings from clinical evaluation have emerged. These include videofluoroscopy (Logemann 1983, 1986), videoendoscopy (Langmore *et al.* 1988; Wilson *et al.* 1992), manometry (Olsson *et al.* 1995), electromyography (Bryant 1991; Perlman *et al.* 1989) and ultrasound (Stone and Shawker 1986; Sonies *et al.* 1988). However, it is videofluoroscopy which is used most widely as a clinical diagnositic tool.

Experimental studies indicate that bedside examinations are unreliable at detecting aspiration. Studies have shown that 40-58% of individuals were silently aspirating but this was not detected by bedside evaluation (Logemann 1983; Splaingard *et al.* 1988). However, in both research and clinical practice, there exists great variability in the type of bedside evaluation carried out. In several studies extremely limited clinical swallowing evaluations were carried out. For example, Barer (1989) rated swallowing function on a three-point scale based on a single observation of the subject's ability to swallow 10ml of water.

It has been advocated that bedside evaluation should be combined with videofluoroscopy in order to examine the pharyngeal phase more objectively and to identify silent aspiration (Linden and Siebens 1983; Horner and Massey 1988). However, in clinical practice, the availability of videofluoroscopy may be limited and it may be inappropriate for many individuals following stroke due to cognitive and language impairments. A survey by Edelman (1988) revealed that of the 71 district health authorities studied, only 12 had routine access to videofluoroscopy and held regular clinics with an established multidisciplinary team. This study is dated and assessment of the current situation is required.

Little agreement exists as to specific clinical correlates of oro-pharyngeal dysphagia and as to which prognostic indicators should be used in the prediction of aspiration from a clinical swallowing evaluation. Wet, hoarse voice post swallow has been shown as a sensitive index of the likelihood of aspiration (Linden and Siebens 1987; Horner *et al.* 1988). Kidd *et al.* (1993) report that loss of pharyngeal sensation shows a significant relation with aspiration. An impaired or absent gag reflex has proved to be of limited prognostic value (Horner *et al.* 1988) and in fact has been shown to be frequently present in healthy elderly people (Davies and Kidd 1994).

Another important question which is yet to be fully addressed is the clinical significance of aspiration and the individual variations in ability to tolerate pulmonary aspiration. Not all individuals who aspirate go on to develop aspiration pneumonia or other pulmonary complications (Croghan *et al.* 1994). Tolerance of aspiration and development of aspiration pneumonia following stroke is likely to be dependent on a multitude of risk factors such as medical condition, premordid respiratory status and physical function.

## Management of oro-pharyngeal dysphagia

The overall aims of dysphagia management following stroke are to: i) minimise the risks of aspiration; ii) maximise levels of nutrition and hydration; iii) increase functional eating/drinking skills; iv) increase the individual's/carer's knowledge of dysphagia and its consequences; v) facilitate adjustment to the psychosocial consequences of long-term dysphagia.

The use of behavioural rather than prosthetic, surgical or pharmacological management of dysphagia, is now explored. Extensive reviews of research into the efficacy of dysphagia management have been completed by Langmore and Miller (1994); Langmore (1995); and Rosenbek (1995). These, together with other authors (Logemann 1987, 1990; Silver *et al.* 1990), have highlighted several flaws in the research methodology in this area. Despite claims that a relatively large percentage of individuals can benefit from a swallowing management programme following stroke (Gresham 1990; Groher 1993; Neumann 1993), research demonstrating the efficacy of behavioural methods for treating those with dysphagia is scarce.

Early research into efficacy of dysphagia management programmes and use of specific techniques was often based on anecdotal accounts of therapeutic successes. Heterogenous groups were used in terms of medical diagnosis and times since onset and there was a lack of standardised assessment approaches and therapy regimes. Other concerns relate to issues of treatment effects versus spontaneous recovery following stroke. Studies have failed to include control groups or to control for environmental, treatment, and subject variables.

However, during this last decade specific dysphagia approaches and techniques have been subjected to closer clinical scrutiny. Technological advances such as videofluoroscopy have provided the opportunity to study swallowing behaviour with greater precision and have enabled more accurate monitoring over time.

The outcome measures used generally fall into two categories: physiological outcomes and functional outcomes. The first include measures of improved swallowing function as the desired outcome and the second use measures such as nutritional status and elimination of aspiration. Traditionally, the emphasis in research and indeed in clinical practice has been on the measurement of changes at the level of impairment i.e. the signs of abnormal swallowing physiology measured at bedside or instrumentally using videofluoroscopy. Primary outcome measures such as the frequency and amount of aspiration, the speed of bolus transit and percentage of bolus swallowed are frequently measured. Little emphasis is given to measuring functional changes such as time taken for the individual to finish a meal or drink a cup of tea. The level of handicap experienced by the individual is rarely considered. This may include refusing to eat in public, depression and fear over choking and loss of enjoyment of eating.

## Specific swallowing therapies

Recently, there has been an increased focus on exploring the efficacy of specific swallowing therapies and of identifying objective criteria for selection of subjects. Decisions regarding selection will be dependent on a number of factors such as level of arousal, cognitive-linguistic status, time post onset of swallowing problem and medical status. Logemann (1991) has identified three main treatment methods for oro-pharyngeal dysphagia, namely compensatory strategies, direct therapy and indirect therapy.

### i) Compensatory strategies

These strategies are aimed at relieving the symptoms of dysphagia. For example, it has been shown that diet consistency modification and controlling bolus size can have a beneficial impact on reducing the incidence of aspiration (Groher 1987). Postural changes in head or body have also been proven to be successful. In a study of individuals with unilateral pharyngeal paresis and reduced pharyngeal clearance following medullary infarcts, Logemann *et al.* (1989) and Logemann and Kahrilas (1990) demonstrated that swallowing efficiency was significantly improved by use of head turning technique. Using videofluoroscopy, a significant reduction in transit time and an increase in the percentage of bolus swallowed were shown. Finally, the chin tuck has been advocated for use in reducing the risks of aspiration (Rasley *et al.* 1993; Welch *et al.* 1993; Shanahan *et al.* 1993). It has been found to be particularly useful with those individuals who have premature leakage of the bolus into the valleculae prior to the swallow reflex being triggered.

### ii) Direct therapy

These strategies aim to change the physiological and anatomical relationships of the structures involved in swallowing. The use of the Mendelsohn Manoeuvre has been well documented on normal populations (Kahrilas *et al.* 1991) and on individuals post stroke. This technique involves a volitional prolongation of laryngeal elevation during midswallow and is recommended for those with inadequate laryngeal elevation during swallow. The effectiveness of the technique was demonstrated in a case study of an individual with long-standing dysphagia secondary to medullary infarct (Logemann and Kahrilas 1990). Using videofluoroscopy, it was found that the upper oesophageal sphincter opening increased, the duration of maximal laryngeal elevation increased and the bolus head transit time reduced. These measurable physiological changes showed an increased function with a greater proportion of bolus being cleared during the swallow.

Thermal stimulation has shown potential as a therapeutic technique by helping to trigger a more brisk swallow in individuals with delayed swallows (Lazzara *et al.* 1986; Rosenbeck *et al.* 1991). The long-term functional gains from thermal stimulation are yet to be proven.

### iii) Indirect therapy

These techniques aim to improve neuromuscular control and are performed without a bolus. Such techniques aim to increase oro-motor and laryngeal function. Despite being widely used in clinical practice, there has been little systematic research into the effectiveness of oro-motor exercise programmes in swallowing rehabilitation. Studies report increased range of motion and strength of oral movements (Jordan 1979; Logemann 1983) but further evaluation of efficacy is required.

# Executive summary and priorities for research

The last 10 years has seen a major change in the role of speech and language therapy after stroke with a significant proportion of the time now spent on swallowing rather than speech.

The prevalence of swallowing disorders is between 28 and 65% in the first week, falling to 2% at three weeks in one study. Development of bedside methods for the assessment of dysphagia and aspiration are still not sufficiently reliable to substitute for videofluoroscopy. The link between aspiration and pulmonary complications is debated.

A number of techniques for the management of dysphagia have been developed over the last decade. Compensatory strategies to modify the diet or posture during swallowing have been shown to be effective at reducing aspiration. Direct therapy to change the physiological and anatomical relationships of the structures involved in swallowing, for example, by thermal stimulation are as yet of unproven efficacy and indirect therapy to improve neuromuscular control has been even less researched.

*The priorities for research are therefore:*

1. A longitudinal study to define the rate and extent of recovery in different stroke groups depending on either site or size of lesion or clinical features. Clinical evaluation, videoflouroscopy and nutritional evaluations are needed. Most studies focus on acute hospital populations and do not continue beyond six months.

2. Evaluation of the effectiveness of general dysphagia programmes and specific therapy techniques. More specific outcome criteria against which to measure the effectiveness of rehabilitative management are recommended. Treatment of long-term dysphagia needs to have a positive influence not only at the level of impairment but at the level of disability and handicap.

3. Further use of single case study experimental design to evaluate which types and intensity of specific therapy techniques or combinations of techniques are most effective in: restoring oral feeding as soon as possible; maximising patient comfort and quality of life; and preventing medical complications such as aspiration pneumonia.

4. Greater focus on investigating those living in the community with long-term dysphagia. The prevalence of long-term dysphagia post stroke needs to be established as does the use of percutaneous endoscopic gastrostomy following stroke.

5. For outcome measures to look at changes not only at the level of impairment but also to include measures of disability and handicap. There have been no studies which have investigated psychosocial adjustment to dysphagia or the psychological reactions to dysphagia (e.g. fear of choking, embarrassment) and these need to be performed.

6. Development and validation of the sensitivity and specificity of bedside evaluation and comparison with results from videofluoroscopy.

# References

Alberts MJ, Horner J, Gray L, Brazer SR. Aspiration after stroke: lesion analysis by brain MRI. Dysphagia 1992; 7: 170-3.

Barer DH. Dysphagia in acute stroke. Br Med J 1987; 295: 1137-8.

Barer DH. Lower cranial nerve motor function in unilateral vascular lesions of the cerebral hemisphere. Br Med J 1984; 289: 1622.

Barer DH. The natural history and functional consequences of dysphagia after hemisphere stroke J Neurol Neurosurg Psych 1989; 52: 236-41

Bryant M. Biofeedback in the treatment of a selected dysphagic patient. Dysphagia 1991; 6: 140-144.

Cherney LR, Cantieri CA, Pannell JJ. RIC Clinical Evaluation of Dysphagia. 1986. Maryland: Aspen Systems Corporation.

Croghan JE, Burke EM, Caplan S, Denman S. Pilot study of 12 month outcomes of nursing home patients with aspiration on videofluroscopy. Dysphagia 1994; 9: 141-6.

Davies AE, Kidd D. Prevalence of the gag reflex and pharyngeal sensation in healthy elderly subjects. Age Ageing 1994; 23: 15 (Abstract).

Edelman GM. Dysphagia survey. College of Speech and Language Therapists' Bulletin, April 1988.

Gordon C, Hewer RL, Wade DT. Dysphagia in acute stroke. Br Med J 1987; 295: 411-4.

Gresham SL. Clinical assessment and management of swallowing difficulties after stroke. Med J Aust 1990; 153: 397-399.

Groher ME. Bolus management and aspiration pneumonia in patients with pseudobulbar dysphagia. Dysphagia 1987; 1: 215-6.

Groher ME. Dysphagia: diagnosis and management. Boston: Butterworths 1993.

Groher ME, Bukatman R. The prevalence of swallowing disorders in two teaching hospitals. Dysphagia 1986; 1: 3-6.

Horner J, Buoyer FG, Alberts MJ, Helms MJ. Dysphagia following brainstem stroke - clinical correlates and outcome. Arch Neurol 1991; 48: 1170- 3.

Horner J, Massey EW. Silent aspiration following stroke. Neurology 1988; 38: 317-9.

Horner J, Massey MD, Riski JE, Lathrop MA, Chase KN. Aspiration following stroke: clinical correlates and outcome. Neurology 1988; 38: 1359-62

Jordan K. Rehabilitation of patients with dysphagia. Ear Nose Throat J 1979;58: 86-87.

Kahrilas PJ, Logemann JA, Drugler C, Flanagan E. Volitional augmentation of upper esophageal sphincter opening during swallowing. Am J Physiol 1991; 260: 26450-6.

Kidd D, Lawson J, Nesbitt R, MacMahon J. Aspiration in acute stroke: a clinical study with videofluoroscopy. Qu J Med 1993; 86: 825-9

Kidd D, Lawson J, Nesbitt R, MacMahon J. The natural history and clinical consequences of aspiration in acute stroke. Qu J Med 1995; 88: 409-13.

Langmore S. Efficacy of behavioural treatment of oropharyngeal dysphagia. Dysphagia 1995; 10: 259-62.

Langmore S, Miller RM. Behavioural treatment for adults with oropharyngeal dysphagia. Arch Phys Med Rehab 1994; 75: 1154 -60.

Langmore S, Schatz K, Olsen N. Fibreoptic endoscopic examination of swallowing safety: a new procedure. Dysphagia 1988; 2: 216-9.

Lazzara G de L, Lazarus C, Logemann JA. Impact of thermal stimulation on the triggering of the swallow reflex. Dysphagia 1986; 1: 73-7.

Linden P, Siebens AA. Dysphagia: predicting laryngeal penetration. Arch Phys Med Rehab 1983; 64: 281-4.

Logemann JA. A manual for videofluoroscopic evaluation of swallowing. San Diego: College Hill 1986.

Logemann JA. Criteria for studies of treatment of oral-pharyngeal dysphagia. Dysphagia 1987; 1: 193-9.

Logemann JA. Dysphagia. Semin Speech Lang. 1990; 11: 157-63.

Logemann JA. Evaluation and treatment of swallowing disorders. San Diego College Hill 1983.

Logemann JA. Swallowing physiology and pathophysiology. Otolaryn Clin N Amer 1988; 21: 613-23.

Logemann JA. The role of the speech and language pathologist in the management of dysphagia. Otolarynol Clin North Am 1988; 21: 783-8.

Logemannn JA. Approaches to the management of disordered swallowing. Clin Gastroenterol. 1991; 5: 269-80.

Logemann JA, Kahrilas PJ. Relearning to swallow after stroke application of manoeuvres and indirect biofeedback: a case study. Neurology 1990;40: 1136-8.

Logemann JA, Kahrilas PJ, Kobara M, Vakil NB. The benefit of head rotation on pharyngoesophageal dysphagia. Arch Phys Med Rehab 1989; 70: 767-71

Neumann S. Swallowing therapy with neurologic patients: results of direct and indirect therapy methods in 66 patients suffering from neurological disorders. Dysphagia 1993; 8: 150-3.

Olsson R, Nilsson H, Ekberg O. Simultaneous videoradiography and pharyngeal solid state manometry (videomanometry) in 25 non-dysphagic volunteers. Dysphagia 1995; 10: 36-41.

Park C, O'Neill. Management of neurological dysphagia. Clinical Rehab 1994; 8: 166-74.

Perlman AL, Luschei ES, DuMond CE. Electrical activity from the superior pharyngeal constrictor during reflexive and non-reflexive tasks. J Speech Hear Res 1989; 32: 749 -54.

Rasley A, Logemann JA, Kahrilas PJ, Rademaker AW, Pauloski BR, Dodds WJ. Prevention of barium aspiration during videofluoroscopic swallowing studies: value of change of posture. Am J Radiol 1993; 160: 1005-9.

Robbins J, Levine RL. Swallowing after unilateral stroke of the cerebral cortex: preliminary experience. Dysphagia 1988; 3: 11-17.

Rosenbek JC. Efficacy in dysphagia. Dysphagia 1995; 10: 263-7.

Rosenbek JC, Robbins J, Fishback B, Levine RL. Effects of thermal application on dysphagia after stroke. J Speech Hear Res 1991; 34: 1257-68.

Royal College of Speech and Language Therapists. Dysphagia working party: position paper on dysphagia 1990.

Royal College of Speech and Language Therapists. Policy Review Forum on Dysphagia: Proceedings 1992.

Shananhan TK, Logemann JA, Rademaker AW, Pauloski BR, Kahrilas PJ. Chin-down posture effect on aspiration in dysphagic patients. Arch Phys Med Rehab 1993; 74: 736-9.

Silver K, DuChane AS, Kuhlemeier K. Response to Kasprisin *et al.* the efficacy of rehabilitative management of dysphagia. Dysphagia 1990; 5: 166-8.

Sonies BC, Parent LJ, Morrish K, Baum BJ. Durational aspects of the oral-pharyngeal phase of swallowing in normal adults. Dysphagia 1988; 3: 1-10.

Splaingard ML, Hutchins B, Salton LD, Chaudhury G. Aspiration in rehabilitation of patients: videofluoroscopy vs bedside clinical assessment. Arch Phys Med Rehab 1988; 69: 637-40.

Stone M, Shawker T. An ultrasound examination of the tongue movements during swallowing. Dysphagia 1986; 1: 78-83.

Veis SL, Logemann JL. Swallowing disorders in persons with cerebrovascular accident. Arch Phys Med Rehab 1985; 66: 372-5.

Wade DT, Hewer RL. Motor loss and swallowing difficulty after stroke: frequency, recovery and prognosis. Acta Neurol Scand 1987; 76: 50-4.

Warms TS, Champion R, Mortensen L. PHAD validation and correlation with the modified barium swallow. Adult Speech Pathology Department, Westmead Hospital, NSW, Australia 1990.

Welch MV, Logemann JA, Rademaker AW, Kahrilas PJ. Changes in pharyngeal dimensions effected by chin-tuck. Arch Phys Med Rehab 1993; 74: 178-81.

Wilson PS, Hoare TJ, Johnson AP. Milk nasendoscopy in the assessment of dysphagia. J Laryngol Otol 1992; 106: 525-7.

# CHAPTER 8

# COMMUNICATION PROBLEMS FOLLOWING STROKE

*Julie Quinn, Heather Campbell*

**Chapter outline**

## Introduction

The nature of communication problems following stroke is well documented (Darley *et al.* 1975; Nicholas *et al.* 1993; Wade *et al.* 1986; Enderby *et al.* 1987). Impairments such as dysphasia, dyspraxia and dysarthria have been found to be possible sequelae of stroke. More recently there has been increased attention on communication problems associated with right cerebral hemisphere strokes. These problems include: difficulties with the interpretation of emotional and linguistic prosody; lexical-semantic comprehension deficits; and problems with discourse and the pragmatics of communication (Myers 1983; Code 1987; Bryan 1989).

The main focus of this chapter however will be on dysphasia following stroke. Dysphasia may present the individual with difficulties in the perception, recognition, comprehension and expression of language through both the verbal and/or written modalities (Royal College of Speech and Language Therapists, 1991). Different approaches to the treatment of dysphasia, efficacy of therapy and factors affecting recovery will be explored.

## Epidemiology

It has been suggested that the incidence and prevalence of speech and language problems are frequently underestimated (Enderby and Phillips 1986). Bonita and Anderson (1983) reported that 37% of stroke survivors had a speech and language disorder. Half of these died, or "recovered" their communication ability by six months. Prevalence rates of between 0.05% (Hopkins 1975; Matsumoto *et al.* 1978) and 0.03% (Bonita and Anderson 1983) have been reported for those with dysphasia or dysarthria following stroke. No epidemiological studies have explored communication disorders following right cerebral hemisphere strokes.

With regard specifically to dysphasia, Wade *et al.* (1986) noted dysphasia in the first week post stroke in a quarter of conscious patients, with 12% of individuals remaining dysphasic at six months.

Results from a survey into dysphasia services in the United Kingdom found that in an average district of 250,000, over 100 referrals will be received for people with dysphasia each year. Forty per cent of districts will receive over 200 referrals per year. It is suggested that there will be an annual national referral to speech and language therapy services in the U.K. of approximately 13,680 new dysphasic stroke cases (MacKenzie *et al.* 1992, 1993). They clearly represent a significant group within the stroke population - one which is often neglected in research and clinical practice.

## The impact of dysphasia on the individual

Language and communication are central to social and psychological functioning. Therefore the loss of language functioning will produce its own unique psychological and social effects for both the individual and the family (Lebrun and Hoops 1976; Brumfitt 1993; Code and Muller 1992). It is believed that those with dysphasia suffer a double isolation from many aspects of human experience. It is reported that they suffer greater levels of social isolation than they would from purely physical disability (Brust *et al.* 1976; Code and Muller 1983; Brumfitt and Clarke 1983).

The emotional consequences of dysphasia and the necessity of considering these aspects in therapeutic intervention have been documented. In a study of chronic non-fluent dysphasics (Herrmann and Wallesch 1989), relatives identified depression, anger and resignation as being the main psychological changes since the stroke. With specific regard to research concerning depression and dysphasia, there is evidence to suggest that depressive changes are common and severe in those with dysphasia (Gainiotti 1972; Starkstein and Robinson 1988). The extent to which depression is due to a secondary reaction to the loss of language and other functional skills is unclear, as is the degree to which depression is linked to neurobiochemical changes resulting from damage to the left hemisphere of the brain.

## Treatment approaches

Since World War II the treatment approaches followed in aphasia therapy can be described in terms of the linguistic or psychological school to which the therapists belong. Howard and Hatfield (1987) identify eight of these schools, of which the most significant for current practice are the stimulation (Schuell 1965), pragmatic (Davis and

Wilcox 1985), neo-classical (Goodglass and Kaplan 1983), neurolinguistic (Poeck *et al.* 1977), and cognitive neuropsychological (Colthart *et al.* 1987) schools. For each of these schools there is a battery of published assessments which reflect the type of treatment to be adopted.

The stimulation school regarded aphasia as a unitary disorder differing only in severity and Schuell's Minnesota Test for the Differential Diagnosis of Aphasia (Schuell 1965) aims to provide a diagnosis and prognosis for all levels of aphasia.

The pragmatic school views aphasia as a functional communication problem and believes that assessment should focus on identifying the aphasic's preserved communication skills as viewed from observation of role-played situations e.g. Functional Communication Profile (Sarno 1969); Communicative Abilities in Daily Living (Holland 1980); Edinburgh Functional Communication Profile (Skinner *et al.* 1984). It follows then that treatment focuses on improving the patient's communicative ability in various personally relevant contexts (e.g. shopping, using the telephone) and enabling the patient to convey information by whatever means, verbal or non-verbal, s/he has available (Promoting Aphasics Communicative Effectiveness, Davis 1980).

Proponents of the neo-classical school diagnosed aphasia syndromes according to localisationist classifications (Boston Diagnostic Aphasia Examination, Goodglass and Kaplan 1980; Western Aphasia Battery, Kertesz 1982). There is a wide variation of treatment approaches which can be grouped loosely under this heading, with a common theme being to capitalise on the aphasic's preserved linguistic skills in order to achieve an improvement (e.g. voluntary control of involuntary utterances, Helm and Barresi 1980; visual action therapy, Helm and Benson 1978; Helm-elicited language rogramme for syntax stimulation, Helm-Estabrooks *et al.* 1981).

The neuro-linguistic school views aphasia as a linguistic disorder and specific treatments are described to treat specific linguistic deficit (Weriger *et al.* 1987).

The cognitive neuropsychological school regards aphasia as a breakdown of information processing in terms of language comprehension and production. A large number of unstandardised tests have been produced by therapists and researchers in this field. These aim to identify at which precise point in the theoretical model of language processing the breakdown occurs.

The Psycholinguistic Assessments of Language Processing in Aphasia (Kay *et al.* 1992) is a comprehensive battery of many of these tests and is widely used by aphasia therapists in this country. Treatments for specific language breakdown tend to be individual as no two patients will share exactly the same profile of deficits and, as such, are described in a large number of single case studies (Jones 1986). However some of these methods have been successfully replicated with similar patients (Le Dorze *et al.* 1991; Byng 1988; Byng *et al.* 1994; Nickels *et al.* 1991).

In clinical practice, speech and language therapists draw on a variety of approaches for assessment and treatment. Decisions on which approach to use are dependent on a large number of factors e.g. the communicative needs of clients, time post onset, the setting in which therapy takes place, the dysphasic's linguistic profile and his/her psychological, cognitive and physical state.

## Aims of speech and language therapy intervention

• To reduce the linguistic impairment and disability through detailed assessment and treatment of specific areas of language breakdown.

• To facilitate the individual's adjustment to the social, psychological and emotional consequences of communication disability.

• To educate carers to maximise the dysphasic's communicative potential within different social situations.

• To support carers in coming to terms with the person's altered communication and possibly social skills and emotional state.

• Where necessary, to develop alternative communication strategies.

Intervention involves a process of continuous assessment of the person's changing communicative skills and evaluation of his/her communicative environment. Rehabilitation may last months or years.

## Efficacy

In a survey of studies examining the efficacy of speech and language therapy for dysphasia, Whurr *et al.* (1992) state that few published prior to 1986 met with the basic requirements of experimental validity and as such their results can only be regarded as inconclusive. A frequently cited study (Lincoln *et al.* 1984) used by clinicians attempting to prove the value of their therapy to the medical profession has been criticised (Howard and Hatfield 1987) as being methodologically flawed, mainly because of patients not receiving the anticipated quantity of therapy.

The difficulty with such studies is that the issues involved are far more complex than the question "Is speech and language therapy effective for dysphasia?" would imply. The reasons for this are that:

• Patients with dysphasia do not form a homogeneous population and there are thus many confounding variables which can affect the results of treatment (e.g. type or severity of dysphasia, the interaction of other medical, social and psychological factors). There is a paucity of studies which attempt to match the subjects in pairs.

• There are ethical considerations in withholding treatment from control groups.

• The therapy in such studies is not described or uniform e.g. in Lincoln *et al.*, there were 32 therapists involved, trained in three different countries and "no particular type of therapy was advocated".

• In many of the published studies there are difficulties in fulfilling the relevant criteria e.g. in Lincoln *et al.*, 75% of patients received less than 18 hours' treatment rather than the 48 hours specified.

• The effect of spontaneous recovery needs to be considered and disagreement about the duration of this phase exists.

• The nature of communication impairment itself is such that its recovery may be influenced by uncontrollable factors such as social support and stimulation and the individual's personality, mood and motivation in both treated and untreated subjects.

• It is impossible to generalise from the results of the existing studies because too few variables are controlled for.

• Speech and language therapy is rarely specified or described in the large-scale group studies.

• The outcome measures used are either based on subjective scales of improvement or on wide-ranging standardised assessments, the sub-tests of which may not relate directly to the type of therapy given or to the behaviour of the dysphasic patient in actual communicative situations.

For a fuller discussion of these issues, see Darley (1972).

## Factors affecting recovery

There are inevitably many variables affecting recovery; not enough is known about their precise nature and how they interact. However, there are published studies which have sought to assess the significance of:

### 1. Type of aphasia
It is difficult to analyse the data on this topic as, depending on their theoretical perspective, not all researchers regard aphasia as being subdivided into various types and thus may classify their subjects differently. Most studies report that "global" dysphasics (i.e. severely affected across all language modalities) have the poorest prognosis, making the least gains in early therapy studies (Wepman 1951; Sarno *et al.* 1970). However, in a more recent study by Shewan and Kertesz (1984), Broca's dysphasics made the most gains as measured on the Language Quotient of the W.A.B but they were closely followed by globals and then Wernicke's, with anomics and conduction aphasics falling some way behind. These results are linked to initial severity.

### 2. Initial severity
Shewan and Kertesz (1984) also found that patients of initial moderate severity made the greatest gains with treatment, followed by the severely affected, then mild.

### 3. Age
Age itself does not seem to be a reliable predictor of language recovery although it was cited as significant in early studies of aphasia in trauma cases, with younger patients doing better. In studies which include aphasia arising from CVAs it was not found to be

of significance (Basso *et al.* 1975; Basso *et al.* 1979). With increasing age, however, an increase is found in complicating factors which might affect outcome and well-designed studies would need to match subjects for age in addition to other variables.

### 4. Time post onset

Using PET scan evidence of cognitive reorganisation following brain injury in aphasics, Demeurisse and Capon (1987) state that if recovery (of verbal expression) is to occur, it needs to take place early on and that the type of reorganisation differs according to the presenting language disorder. This has been borne out from the evidence of many therapy studies (Vignolo 1964), which find that patients whose treatment is initiated early tend to make more progress than those who start later. This tends to indicate that the effects of spontaneous recovery can be capitalised on with early intervention. That is not to say that there is no evidence of improvement past the accepted stage of spontaneous recovery (three months to one year) (Broida 1977; Hagen 1973; Dabul and Hanson 1975). David (1983) suggests that studies are needed where patients are studied at the same length of time post onset and compared according to whether their treatment was started earlier or later.

### 5. Amount of therapy

David (1983), comparing the results of several studies, concludes that 'very intensive therapy' (18 to 25 hours per week) seems to be more effective than a more intermittent regime. In a review of 22 studies, Shewan (1986) found that intensity and duration of therapy varied extensively and depended more on financial considerations rather than other factors. However, where comparisons are made, Smith *et al.* (1972) reported that patients who received 20 to 40 weeks (500-1000 hours) of treatment made greater language gains than a group who received five to ten weeks of treatment (125-250 hours).

### 6. Influence of the therapist

Studies evaluating the effect of treatment delivered by   trained speech and language therapists compared with general stimulation or supervised programmes provided by volunteers have been fraught with methodological problems and their results are inconclusive (Meikle *et al.* 1979; David *et al.* 1982).   One of these showed some evidence that professionally supported volunteers may be as effective as speech therapists. In one trial speech therapists and professionally supported volunteers were compared (David *et al.* 1982). Both groups improved and there was no significant difference in their progress. The trial had a high (38%) drop out rate and a low (but representative) treatment level.

In the Meikle *et al.* study, only 29 subjects were studied, with no controls for time post onset or amount of therapy received. Although the mean gain on the overall Porch Index of Communicative Ability scores was higher in the conventionally treated group than the volunteer group the small number of subjects meant that the difference in scores could not reach statistical significance.

In David *et al.*'s (1982) study, treatment lasted for only 15 weeks and was confounded by effects from spontaneous recovery. Subjects were included who had suffered previous episodes and the aetiology of aphasia was various.

### 7. Place of treatment: hospital vs. community

Most studies of this issue have been large-scale rehabilitation trials where several therapies are involved (e.g. occupational, physiotherapy) and it is not possible to extrapolate speech and language therapy data from the results, particularly where the outcome measures used are of a general nature or insensitive to specific linguistic or functional changes.

## Research design

The problems of using large scale randomised controlled trials (RCTs) have been outlined above. Fitzgibbon (1986) calls for well-designed RCTs in which the definition, operalisation and implementation of treatments are categorised and rated. These categories should then be related to the effects which are located in each RCT. In addition, Whurr *et al.* (1992) recommend the use of studies which conform to the requirements of experimental design in the measurement of disorder, which specify variables to be measured and describe tools employed for measurement of effect, and which provide a complete specification of the treatment programme.

Howard and Hatfield (1987), however, make the point that the requirements of valid RCTs are impossible to meet in clinical practice, due to the difficulty of finding sufficient numbers of patients for whom a particular type of treatment would be appropriate.

It is perhaps for this reason that so many single case studies, mainly based on the cognitive neuropsychological model, have emerged in recent years. The advantages of such studies are:

• They are economical, requiring only one therapist and one patient.

• They can be carried out in the course of normal clinical practice.

• Because inter-subject variables have been eliminated, it becomes easier to specify the nature of the impairment being treated and to give specific details of the therapy.

• Such studies are beneficial to the speech and language therapy profession because they can guide practice.

• They enable clinicians to generate hypotheses about the nature of language breakdown and its recovery.

However, they have their disadvantages as results cannot be assumed to replicate to other aphasics even with similar profiles (see Marshall 1995 for a recent discussion of this issue).

# Executive summary and priorities for research

Although a wide variety of communication problems have been described following stroke, this review concentrates on dysphasia. Up to 37% of stroke survivors have communication problems in the early stage. No prevalence studies have explored communication problems following right hemisphere stroke. Dysphasic patients have been shown to have greater psychopathology than non-dysphasic patients.

There are close academic links between speech and language therapy, linguistics and neuropsychology, providing it with a scientific tradition not seen in physiotherapy and occupational therapy. Treatment approaches reflect this, although there is still a dearth of trials evaluating effectiveness. Major methodological problems have hindered effective research, including a wide variety of clinical pretensions, ethical issues, a lack of standardisation of therapy techniques and the variability in the natural history of recovery. Some studies have attempted to identify the variables affecting recovery and these include the type of aphasia, initial severity, aetiology and age. A few studies have shown that recovery is better if more therapy is provided but so far the evidence is weak. Given the clinical importance of this question to service planners, more research in this area is needed.

Because of the difficulties outlined in performing randomised controlled trials, speech and language therapists have developed single case study methodology and it may be that some of the current dilemmas will begin to be resolved as results from these studies emerge.

The priorities for research and development are therefore:

1. To determine the optimal stage after stroke for speech and language therapy intervention and to assess the intensity and duration of treatment.

2. To develop and select appropriate outcome measures in order to reflect the multifunctional consequences of dysphasia and therefore the diversity of rehabilitation objectives. There is a need to ensure that those with dysphasia are not excluded from research into psychosocial outcome following stroke. Methods of assessment and intervention need to be developed which are not totally dependent on intact language skills to establish emotional and psychological state.

3. Long-term studies on dysphasia outcome which include the effect on carers (see Chapter 14).

4. The development of qualitative research methods in order to obtain the personal perspective of individuals with dysphasia.

5. Continued use of single case study experimental design needs to be replicated in dysphasia efficacy studies using subjects of similar cognitive neuropsychological profiles.

6. Study of the outcome of dysphasia when treated with low levels of therapy compared with high levels.

# References

Basso A, Capitani E, Vignolo LA. Influence of rehabilitation on language skills in aphasia patients: a controlled study. Arch Neurol 1979; 36: 190-6.

Basso A, Faglioni P, Vignolo LA. Etudee controllee de la reeducation du language dans l'aphasie: comparison entree aphasique traites et non-traites. Rev Neurol. 1975; 131: 607-14.

Bonita R, Anderson A. Speech and language disorders after stroke: an epidemiological study. New Zealand Speech Language Therapy J 1983; 38: 2-9.

Broida H. Language therapy effects in long-term aphasia. Arch Phys Med Rehab 1977; 58: 248-53.

Brumfitt SM. Losing your sense of self: what aphasia can do. Aphasiology 1993; 7: 569-71.

Brumfitt SM, Clarke PRF. An application of psychotherapeutic techniques to the management of aphasia. In C. Code and DJ. Muller (eds) Aphasia Therapy. London: Arnold 1983.

Brust JC, Shafer SQ, Richter RW, Bruun B. Aphasia in acute stroke. Stroke 1976; 7: 167-74.

Bryan K. The right hemisphere language battery. London: Whurr Publications 1989.

Byng S, Nickels L, Black M. Replicating therapy for mapping deficits in agrammatism: remapping the deficit. Aphasiology. 1994; 8: 315-41.

Byng S. Sentence processing deficits: theory and therapy. Cognitive Neuropsychology. 1988; 5: 629-76.

Code C. Language, aphasia and the right hemisphere. Chichester: Wiley 1987.

Code C, Muller DJ (eds). Perspectives in aphasia therapy: an overview. Aphasia Therapy. London: Arnold 1983.

Code C, Muller DJ. The Code-Muller Protocols: Assessing perceptions of psychosocial adjustment of aphasia and related disorders. London: Whurr Publications 1992.

College of Speech and Language Therapists. Communicating quality: Professional standards for speech and language therapists. London: CSLT 1991.

Coltheart M, Sarori G, Job R (eds). The cognitive neuropsychology of language. London: Lawrence Erlbaum Associates Ltd 1987.

Dabul B, Hanson WR. The amount of language improvement in adult aphasics related to early and late treatment. Paper presented at the annual convention of the American Speech and Hearing Association 1975.

Darley F, Aronson A, Brown J. Motor Speech Disorders. Philadelphia: WB Saunders 1975.

Darley FL. The efficacy of language rehabilitation in aphasia. J Speech Hear Disord 1972; 37: 3-21.

David R. Researching into the efficacy of aphasia therapy. In: C. Code and DJ Muller (eds) Aphasia Therapy. London: Edward Arnold 1983.

David R, Enderby P, Bainton D. Treatment of acquired aphasia: Speech therapists and volunteers compared. J Neurol Neurosurg Psychiatry 1982; 45: 957-61.

Davis GA. A critical loook at PACE therapy. In: Brookshire RH (ed) Clinical Aphasiology Conference Proceedings. Minneapolis: BRK 1980.

Davis BA, Wilcox MJ. Adult aphasia rehabilitation: applied pragmatics. Windsor: NFER-Nelson 1985.

Demeurisse B, Capon A. Language recovery in aphasic stroke patients. Aphasiology 1987; 1: 301-15.

Enderby P, Philipp R. Speech and language handicap: towards knowing the size of the problem. Br J Dis Comm 1986; 21: 151-65.

Enderby PM, Wood VA, Wade DT, Langton Hewer LE. Aphasia after stroke: a detailed study of recovery in the first three months. Int J Rehab Med 1987; 8: 162-5.

Fitzgibbon CT. In defence of randomised controlled trials, with suggestions about the possible use of meta-analysis. Br J Disorders Communication 1986; 21: 117-24.

Gainiotti G. Emotional behaviour and hemispheric side of lesion. Cortex 1972; 8: 41-5

Goodglass H, Kaplan E. Assessment of aphasia and related disorders. Philadelphia: Lea & Febiger, 1983.

Goodglass H, Kaplan E. The Boston Diagnostic Aphasia Examination. Philadelphia: Lea & Febiger 1980.

Hagen C. Communication abilities in hemiplegia: effect of speech therapy. Arch Phys Med Rehabil. 1973; 54: 454-63.

Helm NA, Barresi B. Voluntary control of involuntary utterances: a treatment approach for severe aphasia. In Brookshire RH (ed) Clinical Aphasiology Conference Proceedings. Minneapolis: BRK 1980.

Helm NA, Benson DF. Visual Action Therapy for global aphasia. Paper presented at Academy of Aphasia, Chicago 1978.

Helm-Estabrooks NA, Fitzpatrick PM, Barresi B. Response of an agrammatic patient to a syntax stimulation program for aphasia. J Speech Hearing Dis 1981; 47: 385-9.

Herrmann M, Wallesch CW. Psychological changes and psychosocialadjustment with chronic and severe non-fluent aphasia. Aphasiology 1989; 3: 513-26.

Holland A. Communicative abilities in daily living. Baltimore: University Park Press 1980.

Hopkins A. The need for speech therapy for dysphasia following stroke. Health Trends 1975; 7: 58-60.

Howard D, Hatfield FM. Aphasia therapy: Historical and contemporary issues. London: Lawrence Erlbaum Associates Ltd 1987.

Jones EV. Building the foundations for sentence production in a fluent dysphasic. British Journal of Disorders of Communication 1986; 21: 63-82.

Kay J, Lesser R, Colthart M. Psycholinguistic Assessments of Language Processing in Aphasia. London: Lawrence Erlbaum Associates Ltd 1992.

Kertesz A. Western Aphasia Battery. New York: Grune & Stratton 1982.

Le Dorze G, Jacob A, Codere L. Aphasia rehabilitation with a case of agrammatism: a partial replication. Aphasiology 1991; 5: 63-85.

Lebrun Y, Hoops R (eds) Recovery in Aphasics. Amsterdam: Swets & Zeitlinger 1976.

Lincoln NB, Mulley GP, Jones AC, McGuirk E, Lendrem W, Mitchell JRA. Effectiveness of speech therapy for aphasic stroke patients: a randomised controlled trial. Lancet 1984; ii: 1197-200.

MacKenzie C, LeMay M, Lendrem W, McGuirk E, Marshall J, Rossiter D. A survey of aphasia services in the United Kingdom. Eur J Disorders Communication 1993; 28: 43-62.

MacKenzie C. The diversity of speech and language therapy services for aphasic adults in the United Kingdom. Disability and Rehabilitation 1992; 14: 146-51.

Marshall J. The mapping hypothesis and aphasia therapy. Aphasiology 1995. In press.

Matsumoto N, Whisnat J, Kierland L, Okasaki H. Natural history of stroke in Rochester Minnesota. 1955-1969. Stroke 1978; 4: 20-9.

Meikle M, Wechsler E, Tupper A, Benenson M, Butler J, Mulhall D, Stern G. Comparative trial of volunteer and professional treatments of dysphasia after stroke. Br Med J 1979; 2: 87-9.

Myers PS Treatment of right hemisphere communication deficits. In: WM Perkins (ed) Language handicaps in adults. New York: Thieme Stratton

Nicholas ML, Helm-Estabrook N, Ward-Lonergan J, Morgan AR. Evolution of severe aphasia in the first two years post onset. Arch Phys Rehabil. 1993; 74: 830-6.

Nickels L, Byng S, Black M. Sentence processing deficits: a replication of therapy. Br J Disorders Communication 1991; 26: 175-201.

Poeck K, HuberW, Kerschensteiner M, Stachowiak FJ, Weniger D. Therapie der aphasien. Nervenartzt 1977; 48: 119-26.

Sarno MT, Silverman M, Sands ES. Speech therapy and language recovery in severe aphasia. J Speech Hear Res 1970; 13: 607-23.

Schuell HM. Differential diagnosis of aphasia with the Minnesota Test. Minneapolis: University of Minneapolis Press 1965.

Schuell HM. Minnesota Test for Differential Diagnosis of Aphasia, Research ed. Minneapolis: University of Minneapolis Press 1965.

Shewan CM. The history and efficacy of aphasia in treatment. In: Chapey R (ed) Language intervention strategies in adult aphasia. Williams & Wilkins 1986.

Shewan CM, Kertesz A (1984) Effects of speech and language treatment on recovery from aphasia. Brain and Language 1984;23: 272-299.

Skinner C, Wirz S, Thompson I, Davidson J. Edinburgh Functional Communication Profile: an observation procedure for the evaluation of disordered communication in elderly patients. London: Winslow Press 1984.

Smith A, Champaux R, Leri J, London R, Muraski A. Diagnosis, intelligence and rehabilitation of chronic aphasics. University of Michigan, Dept of Physical Medicine and Rehabilitation 1972.

Sarno MT. The functional communication profile: manual of directions. Rehabilitation Monograph 1969;42 New York: Institute of Rehabilitation Medicine.

Starkstein SE, Robinson RG (1988) Aphasia and depression. Aphasiology 1988;2:1-20.

Vignolo LA. Evolution of aphasia and language rehabilitation: a retrospective exploratory study. Cortex 1964;1: 344-367.

Wade DT, Langton Hewer LE, David RM, Enderby PM. Aphasia after stroke: natural history and associated deficits. J Neurol Neurosurg Psych. 1986; 49: 11-16.

Wepman JM. Recovery from Aphasia. New York: Ronald Press 1951.

Weriger D, Huber W, Stachowiak FJ. In: D Howard and FM Hatfield Aphasia therapy: Historical and contempory issues. London: Lawrence Erlbaum Associates Ltd 1987.

Whurr R, Lorch MP, Nye C. A meta-analysis of studies carried out between 1946 and 1988 concerned with the efficacy of speech and language therapy treatment for aphasic patients. European Journal of Disorders of Communication. 1992;27: 1-18.

# CHAPTER 9

## OCCUPATIONAL THERAPY FOR STROKE

*Shona MacKay, Tony Rudd*

**Chapter outline**

## Introduction

While it is generally accepted that occupational therapists make a valuable contribution to rehabilitation of stroke patients, the proportion of stroke patients receiving occupational therapy in the UK varies considerably. A study by Smith *et al.* (1982) showed that 97% of patients treated in a stroke unit and 60% of patients treated in a medical unit following a stroke received occupational therapy. In contrast, Wolfe *et al.* (1993) found only 55% of patients under the age of 75 admitted to hospital received inpatient occupational therapy.

Stroke rehabilitation therefore represents a considerable workload for an occupational therapy workforce. In recent years there has been a greater emphasis within the health service on the efficiency and value of services. Despite general agreement on the need for research into the efficacy of occupational therapy and other therapeutic interventions for stroke patients, there are few published studies. In this paper the available evidence on the efficacy of occupational therapy in stroke rehabilitation is considered from two perspectives: (1) type of occupational therapy intervention and (2) aspects of therapy programmes.

## Types of occupational therapy intervention

In stroke rehabilitation the occupational therapist's primary concern is to facilitate patients' continued participation in daily activities, and to assist with adaptation to the major changes imposed by stroke. The term daily activities is used here in its broadest sense, encompassing the whole range of activities a person may perform during the course of his/her daily life, not just self-care skills. The purpose of occupational therapy with stroke patients is to prevent disability and to fulfil the person's needs by achieving optimum function and independence in work, social and domestic environments (Wilcock 1986).

### Activities of daily living

Occupational therapy intervention with stroke patients typically concentrates on evaluation and retraining of personal and domestic activities of daily living skills, sensorimotor abilities, cognitive and perceptual skills, affective and social skills, and vocational skills. Research studies on the outcome of stroke rehabilitation usually focus on the package of therapy rather than specifically on occupational therapy or on particular interventions used. In many studies, activities of daily living (ADL) status is the dependent variable of primary interest, an appropriate focus according to Gresham (1986), who claims that 'independence in ADL will continue to be a suitable hallmark of physical restoration'.

Smith (1989) found that treatment of personal ADL was the main occupational therapy treatment category used in physical and geriatric settings, taking up twice as much time as any other treatment activity. Despite ADL retraining being a central part of occupational therapy practice, no occupational therapy studies of the efficacy of ADL retraining have been published in recent years. Research has instead focused on the development of standardised assessments of ADL, while the evaluation of practice using ADL status as an outcome measure has become the domain of multidisciplinary and medical research. Occupational therapists need to consolidate their expertise in ADL retraining by developing practice based on research rather than tradition and clinical experience. Occupational therapy studies evaluating the effects of timing, intensity, and different approaches to ADL retraining are required.

Independence in ADL is usually measured by the quantity of activities a person can perform, without considering the quality of the movement used in performance of these activities (Eakin 1991). As both occupational therapists and physiotherapists focus on the quality of performance during treatment, use of ADL outcome measures may not be sensitive enough to detect changes in performance following therapy. Wade *et al.* (1985) outlined five main approaches which may be used in the physical restoration of stroke patients: the Bobath approach, the Brunnstrom approach, the Rood approach, proprioceptive neuromuscular facilitation (PNF), and progressive resisted exercise. Although therapists may use different approaches, or combinations of approaches, in different situations these five approaches continue to be used. The motor relearning program (Carr and Shepherd 1982) has become more widely used and may be added to the list. These approaches are based primarily on assumptions about motor control developed from clinical experience and observation, rather than scientific theories (Gordon 1987). Between these approaches there are conflicts over basic philosophy and techniques. However, there is also general consensus that normal movement is the cornerstone of relearning functional tasks.

Several studies have attempted to compare the effectiveness of these approaches. Logigian *et al.* (1983), in a study involving both occupational therapists and physiotherapists, compared a combination of Bobath and Rood approaches with more traditional therapy comprising muscle strengthening and passive movements. No differences were found in outcome between the two groups. As discussed by Ashburn *et al.* (1993), the study contained several methodological flaws and used insensitive outcome measures.

Lord and Hall (1986) compared facilitation techniques with traditional techniques and found no significant difference in outcome. This study was also methodologically flawed in that subject groups were not comparable, and pre and post-intervention data collection methods differed. Similarly, Dickstein *et al.* (1986), in a study comparing the effects of Bobath, PNF and a conventional approach, found no significant differences. Again, methodological problems including non-homogenous subject groups and treatments not being mutually exclusive limited this study.

Further problems with these studies are that they do not provide specific information regarding the content of the treatment regimes, or other aspects of the rehabilitation programme which may influence outcome, or the skills and experience of the staff, all of which are required for replication.

Although the approaches to treatment discussed above originated in physiotherapy and are primarily concerned with restoration of motor function, they are also used in occupational therapy. Occupational therapy is however 'concerned with the co-ordination of motor function with perceptual, cognitive, and emotional functions in order to produce purposeful activity' (Eakin 1991). Physical techniques are just one component of the occupational therapist's repertoire of skills in stroke rehabilitation. Eakin (1991) cautions that if occupational therapists become dependent on physical therapists, the success of occupational therapy intervention may be limited. The complexity and scale of the occupational therapist's role, and the overlap with other professions confounds the difficulties of efficacy studies.

**Cognitive rehabilitation**

In a study of prediction of outcome of rehabilitation of stroke patients, Galski *et al.* (1993) found that deficits in cognition, specifically abstract thinking, judgement, short-term verbal memory, comprehension, and orientation, play an important role in predicting functional status following inpatient rehabilitation. Stroke patients with such cognitive deficits spent more time as inpatients, and had increased referrals for outpatient therapies and home services after discharge. Carter *et al.* (1988) found a positive correlation between the cognitive skills of stroke patients on admission and ADL outcome scores on discharge. These studies indicate the importance of cognitive factors in the rehabilitation of stroke patients and suggest occupational therapy has an important role to play in remediation of cognitive abilities. Davies *et al.* (1989), however, failed to show that cognitive performance affected the recovery of dressing skills during a one-month course of treatment.

Numerous approaches to the treatment of cognitive deficits are identified in the occupational therapy literature, including sensory integration, transfer of training, functional and neurodevelopmental approaches (Siev *et al.* 1986); adaptive functional approach or remedial approach (Niestadt 1988); behavioural approach (Fussey and Giles 1988; Giles and Clark-Wilson 1988); and information processing in a multi-context approach (Toglia 1989). In practice, a combination of approaches tends to be used depending on the patient's impairments and stage of illness, motivational and affective factors, environmental conditions, and perhaps most importantly the therapist's preference based on clinical experience.

There is a lack of studies in the occupational therapy literature which evaluate specific approaches to cognitive rehabilitation to provide objective information to assist therapists in the selection of approaches. The few published studies of cognitive rehabilitation for stroke patients evaluate a 'package' of cognitive rehabilitation, which is a combination of various approaches.

Evaluation of the effectiveness of a cognitive skills remediation programme which addressed visual scanning, visual-spatial orientation, and time judgement for acute stroke patients indicated that patients participating in the programme made greater improvement on the skills addressed than did patients in a control group receiving conventional therapies (Carter *et al.* 1983). It is suggested that incorporating early treatment of cognitive impairments into occupational therapy with stroke patients would be beneficial. The relationship between cognitive abilities and functional performance in activities of daily living has been demonstrated in various studies (Ben-Yishay and Diller 1983; Bernspang *et al.* 1987; Carter *et al.* 1988), with results indicating that patients receiving remediation training in cognitive skills improved significantly in functional ADL skills. For occupational therapists to be able to justify spending therapy time on cognitive remediation activities, further studies of the effectiveness of cognitive rehabilitation in occupational therapy for stroke patients are required, particularly in terms of functional outcome.

## Perceptual rehabilitation

Perceptual performance has been observed clinically to influence the achievement of rehabilitation goals. However, due to a lack of consistency over the definition and management of perception and its components, discussion continues in the occupational therapy literature as to the importance of perceptual deficits as a prognostic indicator of functional ability after stroke (Titus *et al.* 1991; Jongbloed 1986).

Many different assessments of perceptual performance with variable standards of measurement are used by occupational therapists to identify areas for intervention, evaluate function, and predict rehabilitation potential. Information about the correlation of specific perceptual deficits with performance of activities of daily living and the efficacy of different approaches to treatment of perceptual deficits is required for occupational therapists to intervene more effectively, either by improving perceptual performance in order to improve activities of daily living performance or by teaching patients to compensate for deficits (Titus *et al.* 1991).

Two general categories of treatment techniques for perceptual deficits are used by occupational therapists: adaptive and remedial. Adaptive approaches seek to capitalise on a person's strengths in order to promote adaptation to the environment. Therapy concentrates on training in activities of daily living rather than on discrete skills. Outcome studies have shown these approaches to be effective in improving self-care and community skills (Neistadt 1987; Panikoff 1983). These and other outcome studies have not used experimental designs to compare functional training with other treatment modalities. Remedial treatment involves retraining specific perceptual skills, usually with tabletop perceptual activities or specific sensorimotor exercises, to stimulate neuroplasticity processes and generate new performance strategies. The research literature has not unequivocally shown functional improvement following such treatment. Changes in specific perceptual skills, but no resultant improvement in self-care activities, have been found in several experimental studies (Gordon *et al.* 1985; Carter *et al.* 1983; Riddoch and Humphreys 1983). Methodological problems such as small sample sizes, lack of blinding, and training on tasks similar to pre and post-tests render these studies inconclusive. No definitive information about the efficacy of remedial versus adaptive approaches is available because all of the relevant studies have failed to examine several variables which could be significant to outcomes.

Neistadt (1988) identifies a range of variables and recommends consideration of each in research of occupational therapy for adults with perceptual deficits. These variables include: exact definition of perceptual disorder, standardised assessment of ADL status, length and frequency of treatment, type of treatment, therapist's style, stimulus parameters, feedback conditions, and client's attitudes and involvement. Only through further more rigid experimental studies which consider these variables can occupational therapists ensure treatment to clients with perceptual deficits which is both cost-effective and clinically effective.

## Discharge planning and environmental modification

With an increasing workload, occupational therapists are spending more time helping to plan the safe discharge of stroke patients than actually giving therapy. In the United Kingdom occupational therapists have become key players in the assessment of the home environment and the desirability of the provision of equipment to aid independence. Development of close links with social services and housing departments has also provided an essential bridge between hospital and community. There has been little published data on the formal evaluation of such services. Much of the work undertaken is so clearly essential (such as simple descriptions of the environment e.g. will the wheelchair supplied fit through the door?) that research into the benefits of the work seems superfluous.

There is perhaps a place to evaluate alternative ways of obtaining basic information. Development of standardised tools which could be administered by less qualified staff or even friends or relatives could be tried and if successful could save significant resources. Large sums are spent on the provision of equipment, from stair rails, cutlery, walking aids and foot splints to adapted motor vehicles. An excellent series of articles published in the British Medical Journal between January and April 1988 reviewed 'Everyday Aids and Appliances' and there have been occasional articles since then updating aspects of the subject.

Little information is available based on research evidence as to precisely which pieces of equipment are best, and how and when they should be prescribed. Ankle and foot orthoses were the subject of a study by Lehmann *et al.* (1987) who demonstrated that wearing a splint increased gait speed and pattern in seven patients seen 3-13 years after their stroke. A study is currently being performed to evaluate the effect of the early provision of wheelchairs to stroke patients compared to conventional management where wheelchairs are withheld until it is clear that one will be required long-term.

George *et al.* (1988) did, however, know the importance of monitoring the use of appliances and providing continuing support and education. Of 140 people studied, 92 possessed a walking stick but only four objectively required one. Sixty one of these people used the stick and in 43 the equipment was faulty. Fifteen per cent of hearing aids, reading spectacles and dentures were faulty and up to half the aids were not used.

There is, therefore, a need for more research to be performed on the most effective types of aids and appliances and the most effective way of encouraging their use.

The use of rehabilitation apartments to guide discharge planning has been evaluated (Ardron and Finneston 1990) although not specifically for stroke patients. They were not shown to be of particular value in a group of elderly patients with a range of chronic diseases but would be worthy of a further trial, particularly in stroke patients with perceptual disorders.

## Executive summary and priorities for research

The provision of occupational therapy services around the United Kingdom varies considerably as does the style of practice. Many services concentrate primarily on assessment of activities of daily living and adaptations to the environment. Some are sufficiently well resourced to provide therapy. There is a paucity of research examining the role of occupational therapy after stroke.

The main areas of occupational therapy intervention for stroke patients are ADL retraining, sensorimotor abilities, cognitive and perceptual skills, and discharge planning. While a small amount of research in each of these areas has been published, insufficient evidence exists for the profession to scientifically justify current practice in rehabilitation for stroke patients. Rather, occupational therapists tend to rely on custom, clinical experience, intuition, and expert opinion to guide their intervention. While each of these factors has a role to play in clinical practice, a more comprehensive research base is also required.

As with physiotherapy, occupational therapy has evolved different styles of practice. These have not been the subject of much comparison and clearly this does need further work.

Development of outcome measures for use by occupational therapists both clinically and for research purposes is needed. More studies are required to more clearly define the links between cognitive abilities and functional performance in activities of daily living particularly in patients with major perceptual deficits.

*The priorities for research are therefore:*

1. The development of clearly defined definitions and descriptions of what occupational therapists are currently doing.

2. A trial to study the effects of timing, intensity and different approaches to ADL training.

3. A trial to evaluate the effectiveness of cognitive and perceptual skills remediation programs using functional performance actions measures.

4. Development of outcome measures for use in routine clinical practice.

5. A trial of late occupational therapy to reduce handicap.

6. Comparative studies of adaptive and remedial treatment techniques.

7. Evaluation of alternatives to occupational therapists performing home assessments.

8. Trials of equipment type and timing.

# References

Ardron ME, Finneston A. Use of rehabilitation apartments for elderly patients. Age Ageing 1990; 19: 195-8.

Ashburn A, Partridge C, De Souza L. Physiotherapy in the rehabilitation of stroke: a review. Clin Rehab 1993; 7: 337-45.

Ben-Yishay Y, Diller L. Cognitive remediation. In: Rosenthal M, Griffith E, Bond MB, Miller JD (eds). Remediation of the Head Injured Adult 1983; Philadelphia: FA Davies.

Bernspang B, Asplund K, Eriksson S, Fugl-Meyer A. Motor and perceptual impairments in acute stroke patients: effects on self-care ability. Stroke 1987; 18: 1081-6.

Carr J, Shepherd R. A Motor Relearning Program for Stroke. London; 1992: Heinemann.

Carter LT, Howard BE, O'Neil WA. Effectiveness of cognitive skill remediation in acute stroke patients. Am J Occup Therapy 1983; 37: 320-6.

Carter LT, Oliveira DO, Duponte J, Lynch SV. The relationship of cognitive skills performance to activities of daily living in stroke patients. Am J Occup Therapy 1988; 42: 449-55.

Davies ADM, Gargaro P, Dodd A, Smith C. Mental status and occupational therapy outcome in teaching dressing skills to the disabled elderly. Clin Rehab 1989; 3: 293-8.

Dickstein R, Hocherman S, Pillar T, Sharham R. Stroke rehabilitation: three exercise therapy approaches. Physical Therapy 1986; 66: 1233-8.

Eakin P. The outcome of therapy in stroke rehabilitation: do we know what we are doing? Br J Occup Therapy 1991; 54: 305-7.

Fussey I, Giles GM (eds). Rehabilitation of the severely brain injured Adult: A practical approach 1988; London: Croom Helm.

Galski T, Bruno R, Zorowitz R, Walker J. Predicting length of stay, and aftercare in the rehabilitation of stroke patients: the dominant role of higher order cognition. Stroke 1993; 24: 1794-800.

George J, Binns VE, Clayden AD, Mulley GP. Aids and adaptations for the elderly at home: underprovided, underused and undermaintained. Br Med J 1988; 296: 1365-6.

Giles GM, Clark-Wilson J. The use of behavioural techniques in functional skills training after severe brain injury. Am J Occup Therapy 1988; 42: 658-65.

Gordon J. Assumptions underlying physical therapy intervention: theoretical and historical perspectives. In: Carr J *et al.* (eds). Movement Science Foundation for Physical Therapy in Rehabilitation 1987; London: Heinemann 1-30.

Gordon WA, Ruckdelshel H, Egelko S, Diller L, Scotzin S, Lieberman A, Ragnarsson K. Perceptual remediation in patients with right brain damage. A comprehensive program. Int Rehab Med 1985; 66: 353-9.

Gresham GE. Stroke outcome research. Stroke 1986; 17: 358-60.

Jongbloed L. Prediction of function after stroke: a critical review. Stroke 1986; 17: 765-76.

Lehmann JF, Condon SM, Price R, de Lateur BJ. Gait abnormalities in hemiplegia: their correction by ankle-foot orthoses. Arch Phys Med Rehab 1987; 68: 763-71.

Logigian M, Samuels M, Falconer J. Clinical exercise trial for stroke patients. Arch Phys Med Rehab 1983; 64: 364-7.

Lord J, Hall K. Neuro-muscular re-education versus traditional programs for stroke patients. Arch Phys Med Rehab 1986; 67: 88-91.

Neistadt ME. Occupational therapy for adults with perceptual deficits. Am J Occup Therapy 1988; 42: 434-40.

Neistadt ME. An occuaptional therapy program for adults with developmental disabilities. Am J Occup Therapy 1987; 7: 433-8.

Panikoff LB. Recovery trends of functional skills in the head injured adult. Am J Occup Therapy 1983; 54: 305-7.

Riddoch MJ, Humphreys GW. The effect of cueing on unilateral neglect. Neuropsychologia 1983; 21: 581-99.

Siev E, Freishtat B, Zoltan B. Perceptual and cognitive dysfunction in the adult stroke patient 1986; Thorofare NJ: Slack.

Smith S. How occupational therapy staff spend their work time. Br J Occup Therapy 1989; 52: 82-7.

Smith ME, Garraway WM, Smith DL, Akhtar AJ. Therapy impact on functional outcome in a controlled trial of stroke rehabilitation. Arch Phys Med Rehab 1982; 63: 21-4.

Titus M, Gall N, Yerxa E, Roberson T, Mack W. Correlation of perceptual performance and activities of daily living in stroke patients. Am J Occup Therapy 1991; 45: 410-8.

Toglia JP. Visual perception of objects: an approach to assessment and intervention. Am J Occup Therapy 1989; 43: 587-95.

Wade DT, Langton-Hewer R, Skilbeck CE, David RM. Stroke: A critical approach to diagnosis, treatment and management 1985: London: Chapman Hall.

Wilcock AA. Occupational therapy approaches to stroke 1986; London: Churchill Livingstone.

Wolfe CDA, Taub NA, Woodrow J, Richardson E, Warburton FG, Burney P. Patterns of acute stroke care in three disticts of southern England. J Epid Community Health 1993; 47: 144-8.

# CHAPTER 10

# THE ROLE OF THE NURSE IN STROKE

*Penny Irwin*

**Chapter outline**

## Introduction

Whilst the medical literature indicates the value of the nursing contribution to the management and care of patients with a stroke (Wade 1987; Barer 1990), reviews of the nursing literature demonstrate that nursing research related specifically to stroke has not been extensive, although there is evidence that it has increased and become more rigorous in recent years (Myco 1984; O'Connor 1993; Waters 1994).

## Nursing research specific to stroke

Myco (1984) found the nursing literature in stroke descriptive, uncritical and concentrated in the weekly journals. O'Connor (1993), in a later review of stroke in the English language journals from 1966, categorised the 312 contributions according to subject matter and type of article (Table 1):

**Table 1**

| Category | Case study | Research | Descriptive | TOTAL |
|---|---|---|---|---|
| Provision of care | | | 7 | 7 |
| Assessment | | 3 | 12 | 15 |
| Direct care | 64 | 12 | 112 | 188 |
| Evaluation | | 3 | 4 | 7 |
| Principles of rehabilitation | 4 | 2 | 83 | 89 |
| Stroke unit nursing | | 2 | 4 | 6 |
| **TOTAL** | 68 (22%) | 22 (7%) | 222 (71%) | 312 |

It was notable that only 7% of articles were designated as research. The author found that topics which fall outside the domain of other professionals and which could be addressed by nurses were not covered in any detail in the literature reviewed. Such topics include continence care, sleep and rest promotion, and counselling (including sexual counselling), as they relate to stroke patients.

Since 1990, nursing research in Britain has focused on defining the state of nursing in stroke care and identifying the underlying issues rather than testing the effectiveness of specific interventions. The methods employed have tended to be surveys of opinions of nurses as to their perceived role in stroke care (Gibbon 1991; Gibbon 1994), action research (Gibbon and Little 1995), and observational studies in rehabilitation (Waters 1994). In the last few years, particularly in the USA, qualitative research by nurses with stroke carers (Rosenthal *et al* 1993; Williams 1994; Enterlante and Kern 1995; Robinson-Smith 1995) has produced important information to inform more sensitive service provision as well as future research.

This review of nursing research relating to stroke will cover the literature concerning the nursing role followed by the research related to the different phases of stroke care.

## The nursing role

The nursing literature identifies the nursing role in stroke as the maintenance of hygiene, in particular maintaining the integrity of skin, bowels and bladder; the organisation and co-ordination of care on a 24-hour day-to-day basis; the continuation of therapy; and patient/carer education, support and counselling (Myco 1994; O'Connor 1993; Waters 1994). Whilst this fits easily into the pattern of care in the acute stage of stroke, there are difficulties with nurses having a defined role when it comes to rehabilitation. This review will predominantly focus on the British nursing research with some reference to literature from abroad where this is thought helpful to inform the debate.

### 1. Acute phase

This section would be incomplete without some acknowledgement of the nursing research into the broad domains of nursing which are relevant to stroke patients, although the studies concerned may not have specifically addressed stroke. This includes research into the organisation of care; preventing the complications of bed-rest, such as pressure sores; and the management of incontinence.

### a) The organisation of nursing to give individualised care

Qualitative research of stroke patients' views of their admission to hospital demonstrates the importance to patients' well-being of being treated and valued as an individual by the professionals caring for them (Pound *et al* 1995). This highlights the importance of the organisation and co-ordination of nursing to ensure an individualised approach to care.

The introduction of individualised care planning into British nursing in the 1970s in the form of the nursing process was possibly not as well thought out as it might have been (Gibbon *et al* 1995) but it became a part of the movement to develop an individualised, patient-centred approach to patient care. Systems of nursing organisation to promote the patient's individuality followed, and include (along an increasing continuum) systems such as patient allocation, team nursing, primary nursing (the named nurse) and case management. Whether the benefits of primary nursing over task allocation (Macdonald 1988; Pearson 1987) are realised in practice has depended on the nature of implementation (Wright 1990). It has taken longer to introduce into areas where a culture of organisational routine predominates over the needs of individual patients (Waters 1994), with implications for the quality of care and the experiences of patients.

### b) Co-ordinated care and integrated care pathways

In recent years, with there being a greater emphasis on patient-centred care and a multidisciplinary team approach to care, interest has grown in integrated care pathways as a means of ensuring the consistency of care for a specified condition during a hospital admission. Care pathways are essentially multidisciplinary care plans agreed in advance. All those involved in the care of a patient with a particular condition examine the processes of care and agree the sequence and timing of interventions by each discipline. The process of defining the pathway helps clarify the shared processes of care and the most effective means of achieving the goals. Benefits resulting from this process include enhanced understanding of the roles of other care-givers and a rationalisation of care processes (Sovie 1995; Rossiter and Thompson 1995; Ebener *et al* 1996). Variances from the pathway (whether in the delivery of care or in the achievement of goals) are documented, identifying where possible the reasons. The variances should be followed up by regular review (approximately each month) so that appropriate action can be taken to remedy faults in the systems of care.

Critical pathways have their roots in the industrial quality improvement techniques to minimise variation in the production process. In health care in the USA, critical care pathways (or integrated care pathways) are part of the wider framework of case management to ensure cost-effective care within their prospective payment health systems (Zander 1988; Ebener *et al* 1996). The routine cases are therefore admitted under the agreement that they use the routine care pathway. In case management, the more complex cases are actively managed by nurse specialists in conjunction with an identified physician, with a case manager and physician who together supervise the entire patient stay whichever department is involved, and ensure appropriate discharge and follow up at home (Sovie 1995). In the UK, care pathways have been implemented without a formalised system of case management, although interest is growing in it despite the weak evidence to support it (Hale 1995).

There has as yet been little systematic research to evaluate the effectiveness of pathways in medical specialties in the UK. What literature there is in Britain tends to be descriptive (Rossiter *et al* 1995; Morris and Mylotte 1995; Johnson 1994; 1995). There is concern that because some medical conditions such as stroke have such a variable course that pathways have a limited use. However, as many centres have now adopted care pathways for stroke patients, some form of evaluation to compare them with centres which have not done so would be appropriate. In the USA, Odderson and McKenna (1993) evaluated the introduction of a pathway for the management of acute non-haemorrhagic stroke and concluded that outcomes for patients during the first year of the pathway demonstrated a reduction in length of stay, costs and complications. Such benefits have also been shown in other studies introducing a more integrated approach to the management of stroke where care pathways were not used. It could be that the success or otherwise has something to do with more effective co-ordination of the multidisciplinary team. There is therefore a need to evaluate the effectiveness of care pathways for stroke in the context of the different patterns of care in the UK.

## c) Preventing complications

In the acute phase of stroke, the care to prevent complications includes patient positioning to prevent contractures, pressure sore prevention, continence management and the management of dysphagia.

### i) Patient positioning

The care after stroke to prevent the onset of spasticity and contractures by careful patient positioning was reviewed by Carr and Kenney (1992). In the extensive literature on the subject they identified a consensus among authors' recommendations for most aspects of positioning. The recommendations they reviewed were based on theories of neurophysiology from a wide range of disciplines. The areas covered included all aspects of positioning. There was general agreement for protraction of the shoulder when lying on the affected side, alignment of the spine, avoidance of external rotation of the hip, extension of the fingers on the affected side and avoidance of pressure against the soles of the feet. Recommendations conflicted regarding elbow flexion/extension and the positioning of the unaffected limbs. These areas therefore, and any changes to the theories underpinning these practices, could be areas for future research.

### ii) Pressure sore prevention

The Effective Health Care Bulletin on prevention and treatment of pressure sores (Cullum *et al* 1995) indicates that most of the equipment available for the prevention and treatment of pressure sores has not been reliably evaluated and that research evidence on clinical or cost-effectiveness grounds is insufficient to guide equipment choice. What evidence there is suggests that large celled alternating pressure mattresses should be used for patients at high risk of developing pressure sores. Risk assessment scales in use are criticised in the bulletin on grounds of the ad hoc way in which they were conceived and developed, and their consequent predictive validity is questioned. Nonetheless it is considered that the use of such scales ensures a consistent structured assessment of all patients and that, as indicators of risk, such scales can help in the rational allocation of equipment to those most at risk. The bulletin highlights the need for more randomised controlled trials and economic analysis of different intervention strategies.

*iii) Continence management*

Research into continence management in general has been long-standing and strategies for its management well documented (Norton 1986). Continence advisors ensure research-based practice is part of these strategies in both hospitals and community. Nursing research into incontinence specifically in stroke is not common. An American study by Owen *et al* (1995) in a sample of 42 stroke patients attempted to identify the characteristics of patients with persistent incontinence following a rehabilitation and bladder management programme. The conclusion of the study was that more research was required to determine the effects of cognitive deficits on the ability of patients to achieve continence with a standard bladder management programme. In the social integration literature, a long-term follow up of stroke patients in a district in Britain (Greveson *et al* 1991) found that incontinence was poorly managed in the community with an inflexible response to need resulting in 'rationing' of incontinence pads and no assistance with laundry problems. Given the social taboos surrounding incontinence and its profound effect on psychosocial function, the effectiveness of incontinence management services to meet the needs of stroke patients and the appropriateness of the interventions used would seem to be an area which would benefit from evaluative research.

*iv) The management of dysphagia*

Nursing literature in this area tends to rely heavily on the research and advice of other professions, such as speech therapy, medicine and dietetics (Negus 1994; Beadle 1995) and commends the importance of a multidisciplinary approach to care. The possible risks of aspiration, and the secondary effect of reduced nutrition on strength and energy required for later rehabilitation are highlighted to emphasise the important role of the nurse in strategies for management of both these problems.

## 2. The rehabilitation phase

During rehabilitation the therapy professions have a pre-determined role by nature of their expertise, whilst the contribution of nursing in this process remains more diffuse. Some authors have pointed to the potential maintenance role for nurses in rehabilitation, indicating a process where nurses can enable patients to practise what they learn with the therapists, and ensure therapy becomes a 24-hour process instead of one based on sessions (Henderson 1980; Mayer 1991; Waters 1986). However, research in this area shows that the daily reality of the work of nurses, and their attitudes to rehabilitation, do not always reach this ideal.

Gibbon's (1991) survey of the attitudes of medical ward nurses to stroke rehabilitation was followed up with an action research project (Gibbon and Little 1995) which included an education programme to improve the nurses' knowledge and understanding of their role and the patients' care. The aim of the study was to improve stroke care on a medical ward, to encourage interdisciplinary collaboration, to introduce objective measures of patients' progress and to evaluate the effectiveness of revised nursing process documentation. The authors claimed the project achieved most of its aims, although the changes in nursing knowledge and attitudes were not significant and the effects of the changes on patients were not systematically evaluated. Whilst the methods of action research serve to introduce change in a measured way, the small sample sizes and lack of controls make generalisability of the findings difficult. The value of this particular study is what it unearthed about some of the influences on the quality of care, such as the cultural and structural difficulties associated with therapy being delivered away from the ward, and the issues surrounding team working when there is not an identifiable team approach such as exists in stroke units. It demonstrated the importance of introducing systems such as multidisciplinary meetings and good documentation to improve multidisciplinary communication in these circumstances.

In a non-participant observation study, Waters (1994) studied the styles of staff/patient interaction during dressing in the early morning on two wards in a rehabilitation unit for elderly people. Early morning dressing was chosen as an example of service delivery to illustrate how institutional practices determine patients' experiences and their rehabilitation. In this study patients were woken at 0600am by the night nurses and dressed in a routine way which was appropriate to their rehabilitation in only 39% (12/31) of cases. There was no regard given to the dressing practice undertaken with the occupational therapist (working office hours), who had devised individual dressing plans tailored to the patient's specific disabilities, because the night nurses had no contact with the occupational therapist. While the sample size is small, this study illustrates some of the potential mechanisms barring effective multidisciplinary communication and the direct effects this has on the quality of care and the rehabilitation process. The researcher points out that the setting for her study was not unusual and that routine care as recognised consistently for 30 years by nursing research in elderly care wards is nursing's default mechanism in the absence of other guidance or an alternative model of care. She called for better educational preparation for rehabilitation nursing.

Little nursing research exists comparing nursing approaches to rehabilitation. What there is tends to be American or Scandinavian. In an American nursing study comparing the neurodevelopmental approach (based on restoring bilateral function and use of the affected side) with so-called traditional techniques (emphasising the use of the unaffected side), Salter *et al* (1991) found no difference in outcome between two groups of (37 and 43) similar patients when initial differences were taken into account. The researchers reported that their findings contradicted previous studies on this topic which they claim had small samples. They identified a need for further research with larger samples to compare the neurodevelopmental with the traditional techniques of rehabilitation.

## Patient and carer education

Research into the educational needs of stroke patients and their carers has received little attention from British nurse researchers. McLean *et al* (1991), in a small interview study of 20 stroke survivors and their informal carers following discharge from hospital, showed they required more information. In the American nursing literature, research into the educational needs of patients and carers has received increasing attention. A study by Kernich *et al* in 1988 tried to demonstrate the effectiveness of a stroke family support and education programme, but the study suffered from poor design and sample selection. However, Vanetzian *et al* (1995) used adult learning theory to identify the importance of four categories of educational wants of family care-givers. These were: assisting the adult with disabilities; maintaining their own well-being; maintaining family well-being; and understanding health and human resources. Men and women's responses varied in accordance with their prior learning as adult learning theories suggest. The researchers concluded that the differences in the prior experiences of care-givers have implications for the planning of education programmes. In terms of nursing research in Britain, this study demonstrates that carer education should be more closely informed and evaluated by well-tested adult learning theories.

## Carer support

The needs expressed by carers in recent qualitative American studies of the effects of stroke on the wives of stroke victims (Rosenthal 1993; Enterlante and Kerne 1995; Robinson-Smith G 1995) demonstrate the added responsibilities undertaken by the carer for areas of life with which they were unfamiliar, on top of their responsibility for caring for the stroke patient. In view of the well-documented effects of carer strain in quality of life and social re-integration, this would be an important area for research to develop better information for carer education and counselling programmes.

## Community nursing

Gibbon (1994) surveyed the views of district nurses on their contribution to the care and management of stroke patients in the community. He found that:

a) Nursing need was assessed in terms of bowel management, personal hygiene and catheter care needs. Once the needs were identified they were often undertaken by nursing auxiliaries, now care assistants under Social Services.

b) The measurement of patients' progress was not to any objective scale.

c) The frequency of visits was determined by patients' dependency or the inability of the carer to cope.

d) District nurses in this study did not see rehabilitation as part of their role and had received little education about it in their specialist district nurse training. They saw hospital admission for acute stroke or rehabilitation as a positive event - both for treatment and to see the consultant for reassurance.

Gibbon concluded that in England district nurses do not perceive that they have a role until the patient chronicity reaches a point where they and their carer can no longer cope with their hygiene and continence needs. Research identifying the importance of social support for patient outcome both in the short-term (Glass *et al* 1993) and the long-term (Greveson *et al* 1991) highlights potential areas for development of the nursing role in the community to include greater support and education of the family. This could include a more proactive rehabilitative role to re-integrate the patient into their community, as identified in the research by Young and Forster (1995), where a nursing support service encouraged activities outside the home such as visits to the pub, supermarket or local stroke support group.

## Nurse education for rehabilitation

Research to evaluate the effectiveness of basic nurse education in rehabilitation is currently being commissioned by the English National Board for Nursing, Midwifery and Health Visiting. Given the time frame of completion within six months this will require the in-put from one of the few university nursing departments with an interest in rehabilitation nursing (such as Liverpool, Manchester, King's College London or Southampton). There are two post-basic education courses in rehabilitation nursing validated by the English National Board - the ENB 913 (Care and Rehabilitation of Physically Disabled People), run at six centres in England, consisting of 20 days either in a block or on a day release basis; and the A67 (Care and Management of Clients requiring Rehabilitation) run at one centre (Kings College London), lasting 24 weeks over one year. A course in stroke nursing is currently in the process of curriculum planning (personal communication Professor Fentem).

# Executive summary and priorities for research

The nursing literature relating to stroke is not extensive and much of it is not of good quality. Nursing research has focused on the process of care rather than the effectiveness of outcome. The role of the nurse and nursing techniques in stroke care are not defined and their effectiveness has not been assessed. Generally, nursing research in the field of stroke should be encouraged, along with the evaluation of training methods in the care of stroke patients. The role of the nurse as part of the multidisciplinary team and in the rehabilitation process should be investigated.

*The priorities for research are:*

1. Provision of support for training of nurses in research methodologies applicable to stroke.

2. Evaluation of methods of training nurses, both in the care of stroke patients and in the provision of information and support to carers.

3. Evaluation of the role of the nurse in the rehabilitation process in primary care.

4. Evaluation of the use of critical care pathways in the management of stroke.

5. Evaluation of research into the management of patient positioning after a stroke.

6. Evaluation of pressure sore prevention and treatment interventions.

7. Development of effective services for the management of incontinence.

8. Evaluation of systems to improve multidisciplinary communication in the management of stroke patients.

# References

Barer DH. Stroke rehabilitation: panacea or placebo. Geriatr Med 1990: 20: 45-9 (part 1).

Beadle L. The management of dysphagia in stroke. Nurs Stand 1995; 9: 37-9.

Carr EK, Kenney FD. Positioning of the stroke patient: a review of the literature. Int J Nurs Stud 1994; 29: 355-69.

Cullum N, Deeks J, Fletcher A, Long A, Mouneimne H, Sheldon T, Song F The prevention and treatment of pressure sores: how effective are pressure-relieving interventions and risk assessment for the prevention and treatment of pressure sores? Eff Health Care Bull 1995; 2: ISBN: 0965-0288.

Ebener MK, Baugh K, Formetta NM. Proving that less is more: Linking resources to outcomes. J Nurs Care Quality 1996; 10: 1-9.

Enterlante TM, Kern JM. Wives reported role changes following a husband's stroke: a pilot study. Rehab Nurs 1995; 20: 155-60.

Gibbon B. A reassessment of nurses' attitudes towards stroke patients in general medical wards. J Adv Nurs 1991; 16: 1336-42.

Gibbon B. Stroke nursing care and management in the community: a survey of district nurses' perceived contribution in one health district in England. J Adv Nurs 1994; 20: 469-76.

Gibbon B, Little V. Improving stroke care through action research. J Clin Nurs 1995; 4: 93-100.

Glass TA, Matchar DB, Belyea M, Feussner JR. The impact of social support on outcome in first stroke. Stroke 1993; 24: 64-70.

Greveson GC, Gray CS, French JM, James OFW. Long-term outcome for patients and carers following hospital admission for stroke. Age Ageing 1991: 20: 337-44.

Hale C. Case management and managed care. Nursing Standard 1995; 9: 33-5.

Henderson VA. Preserving the essence of nursing in a technological age. J Adv Nurs 1980; 5: 245-60.

Johnson S. Patient focused care without the upheaval. Nurs Standard 1994; 1: 20-2.

Johnson S. Pathways to the heart of care quality. Nurs Management 1995; 1: 26-7.

Kernich CA, Robb G. Development of a stroke family support and education program. J Neurosci Nurs 1988; 20: 193-7.

Mayer A. Rehabilitation round the clock. Nurs Times 1991; 67: 65-8.

Macdonald M. Primary nursing: is it worth is? J Adv Nurs 1988; 13: 797-806.

McLean J Roper-Hall A, Mayer P, Main A. Service needs of stroke survivors and their informal carers. J Adv Nurs 1991; 16: 559-64.

Morris E, Mylotte A. The management of childhood asthma through care pathways. Nurs Times 1995; 91: 36-7.

Myco F. Stroke and its rehabilitation: the perceived role of the nurse in medical and nursing literature. J Adv Nurs 1984; 9: 429-39.

Negus E. Stroke-induced dysphagia in hospital: the nutritional perspective. Br J Nurs 1994; 3:263-269.

Norton C. Nursing for continence. 1986 Beaconsfield Publishers.

O'Connor SF. Nursing and rehabilitation: the interventions of nurses in stroke patient care. J Clin Nurs 1993; 2: 29-34.

Odderson IR, McKenna BS. A model for management of patients with stroke during the acute phase: Outcome and economic implications. Stroke 1993; 24: 1823-7.

Owen DC, Getz PA, Bulla S. A comparison of characteristics of patients with completed stroke: those who achieve continence and those who do not. Rehab Nurs 1995; 20: 197-203.

Pearson A. Primary nursing 1987. Groom Helm.

Pound P, Bury M, Gompertz P, Ebrahim S. Stroke patients' views on their admission to hospital. BMJ 1995; 311: 18-22.

Robinson-Smith G, Mahoney C. Coping and marital equilibrium after stroke. J Neurosci Nurs 1995; 27(2): 83-9.

Rosenthal SG, Pituch MJ, Greninger LO, Metress ES. Perceived needs of wives of stroke patients. Rehab Nurs; 1993; 18: 148-53, 167.

Rossiter D, Thompson AJ. Introduction of integrated care pathways for patients with multiple sclerosis in an inpatient neurorehabilitation setting. Disabil Rehab 1995; 17: 443-8.

Salter J, Camp Y, Pierce LL, Mion LC. Rehabilitation nursing approaches to cerebrovascular accident: a comparison of two approaches. Rehab Nurs 1993; 16: 62-6.

Sovie MD. Tailoring hospitals for managed care and integrated health systems. Nurs Economics 1995; 13: 72-80, 83.

Vanetzian E, Corrigan BA. A comparison of the educational wants of family caregivers of patients with stroke. Rehab Nurs 1995; 20: 149-54.

Wade DT. Who looks after stroke patients? Br J Hosp Med 1987; March: 200-4.

Waters K. Role recognition. Senior Nurse 1986; 9: 15-6.

Waters K. Getting dressed in the early morning: styles of staff/patient interaction on rehabilitation hospital wards for elderly people. J Adv Nurs 1994; 19: 239-48.

Williams A. What bothers caregivers of stroke victims? J Neurosci Nurs 1994; 26: 155-61.

Wright SG. My patient - my nurse: the practice of primary nursing. 1990; Scutari.

Young J, Forster A. A randomised trial of nurse-led community stroke support. Paper at Stroke Association Research Conference 1995; 15/9/95.

Zander K. Nursing case management: Strategic management of cost and quality outcomes. J Nurs Admin 1988; 18: 23-30.

# CHAPTER 11

# PSYCHOLOGICAL ASPECTS OF STROKE

*Shuli Reich*

**Chapter outline**

# Introduction

Currently, in Britain, there are few clinical psychologists involved in working with stroke patients, whether in hospital or in the community. Although the young 'physically disabled' represent a well established client group for clinical psychologists, the primary fields of work within this speciality usually involve patients with head injury, and young chronically sick patients such as those with multiple sclerosis and other neurodegenerative disorders.

Clinical posts dedicated to working with physically disabled elderly patients, in contrast to the elderly mentally ill, are also very few in number. The majority of patients with stroke are over 65 years of age and it is possible that both areas of work suffer from a similar ageist stereotype, namely, that elderly people are on a slope of inevitable physical decline such that clinical services have little to offer.

Stroke, however, is a life-threatening illness and constitutes a major life event for patients as well as for their families and carers. Although one-third of patients die within the first six months after the event, and approximately one-third of survivors recover to their former level of physical function, there are many patients who will recover a proportion of their function but remain moderately or severely disabled for the rest of their lives. Their quality of life may be reduced dramatically and they constitute a significant burden for their carers and community services.

A further characteristic of the management of stroke disease, particularly in Britain, has been the tendency to conceptualise the illness and its rehabilitation in primarily physical terms. The aetiology of stroke is undoubtedly physical, as are many of the sequelae such as hemiplegia, dysphagia and even coma. Personality disorders and behavioural disturbances were thought to occur relatively infrequently. Furthermore, cognitive impairments, such as disorders of memory, visual perception, thinking, and problem solving, have until recently been considered to be subtle problems which recover spontaneously by three to six months post onset and which contribute little to the process of physical recovery or the final quality of life.

In contrast, impairments of speech and language such as expressive and receptive dysphasia have attracted considerable attention, with the result that the provision of early and even community follow-up speech therapy for stroke is considered essential.

Thus, it is possible that for a number of different and inappropriate reasons, recruitment of psychology services to the assessment, management and rehabilitation of patients with stroke has been a low priority.

## Current clinical practices

A number of recent studies have reported better outcomes for patients managed on stroke units compared to general medical wards (Langhorne *et al.* 1993). One of the factors that has been thought to contribute towards these effects has been the coherence and integrated working of the multi-disciplinary team on stroke units relative to the more fragmented therapy offered on general medical wards. However, despite the apparent efficiency of stroke units, the multidisciplinary team may encounter a number of obstacles to the management and treatment of patients.

Occupational therapists and physiotherapists in Britain are largely untrained in, and ignorant of, the cognitive disorders that may accompany and even underpin the disabilities and handicaps which they are treating. Repeated occupational therapy practice and training sessions to improve, for instance, a dressing dyspraxia may fail or achieve only limited success. Similarly, patients may be able to accomplish assisted transfers with the help of one person but fail to achieve independent transfers despite persistent training and encouragement by physiotherapists. Therapists may be further impeded and frustrated in their efforts when these patients appear to have minimal motor and sensory impairments. Patients may themselves become frustrated by the lack of progress and may also be sensitive to the failure to consistently achieve therapeutic goals or targets. Before long, a cycle of negative expectations and underachievement may become established whereby patients and therapists experience repeated failures and the rehabilitation process becomes inefficient. Neuropsychological assessment of these patients may reveal a number of cognitive impairments such as disorders of short-term memory, object recognition, distance perception or sequencing. Repeated practice with tasks such as dressing or transfers may be insufficient to overcome these difficulties and rehabilitation may be terminated on the grounds of patients having 'motivational' problems. Although direct rehabilitation of these cognitive impairments has been poorly evaluated, it is critical for these problems to be accurately identified in order for realistic and achievable goals to be set and reviewed.

There is a great need for psychological services to be recruited to the assessment and management of cognitive dysfunction in the early stages after stroke and for enhancement of the effectiveness of the multidisciplinary team.

The last 10 to 15 years has heralded a number of new clinical and research advances in relation to the psychological sequelae of stroke. Primary amongst these are the investigation of mood disorders, cognitive rehabilitation and, more recently, perceptions of patients and carers regarding the impact of stroke on their lives.

## Mood disorders

Until the mid 1980s, mood disorders and particularly clinical depression were considered to be understandable responses to the traumatic and disabling effects of stroke. A further assumption was that these disorders recovered spontaneously after several months and did not merit, or were not amenable to, antidepressant treatment. Since then, a range of studies have indicated that depressed mood, and more frequently depressive symptoms, are highly prevalent after stroke and occur in 20% to 60% of patients. Unfortunately, there has been a striking lack of consensus regarding the classification, aetiology, prevalence and duration of these disorders.

In groups of patients with moderate to severe disabilities who were resident in deprived inner-city areas and who were initially hospitalised for their stroke, the prevalence of minor and major depression was high (about 50%) and frequently persisted for one year or more if untreated (Robinson *et al.* 1987). Other studies that have focused on patients of high socio-economic status, resident in relatively prosperous rural areas and only about 40% of whom were admitted to hospital, have reported a lower incidence of depressive symptoms (20%) which fell to even lower levels (11%) after six months (Sharpe *et al.* 1990; House *et al.* 1991). Robinson *et al.* argued further that in addition to the reactive or functional aetiology of depressed mood, there was an association between depression and site of cerebral lesion. Patients with left anterior cortical or subcortical lesions or right posterior cortical lesions were at greater risk of becoming depressed than patients with lesions of similar volume but in different areas of the brain. These studies, as with many other investigations in this area suffer from a number of methodological flaws. In general, small cohorts of patients have been investigated and the criteria for the diagnosis of clinical depression (whether major or minor) have been frequently violated or ignored. In addition, groups of patients with different demographic characteristics have been used in the various studies, combined with diverse and often inadequate criteria for identifying depressed mood. Longitudinal studies have also often failed to follow up the original patient cohort due to high attrition rates, instead recruiting new patients for follow up at the six and 12-month assessment periods.

Mood disorders such as anxiety or depression are notoriously hard to detect in medically ill patients and patients with physical disability, with the result that they are consistently under-diagnosed (Schubert *et al.* 1992a). Somatic symptoms are prevalent in patients with and without concurrent illness and may therefore lead to type 1 errors in diagnosis. In addition, physically ill patients commonly experience somatic symptoms, withdrawal, fatigue and lethargy without evidence of depressed mood (type 2 error).

In spite of the methodological issues cited above, several converging pieces of evidence have emerged from the literature. Depressive symptoms after stroke seem to occur more frequently than in age and sex-matched control patients (Eastwood *et al.* 1989). It is also possible that the prevalence rates for these symptoms are higher than in patients after other disabling illnesses, although the preliminary evidence is based on very small samples (Folstein *et al.* 1977).

In addition, it is likely that once depression has occurred after stroke, additional risk factors for its maintenance include low socio-economic status, pre-existing social and financial difficulties, poor social support and pre-morbid depressed mood (Morris *et al.* 1992; Astrom *et al.* 1993)). There is also a suggestion that depressed mood in stroke inpatients may lead to a slower recovery of physical function and longer length of stay and be a poor prognostic indicator for discharge ADL (Henley *et al.* 1985; Anderson 1992; Schubert *et al.* 1992b). Depressed mood after stroke may not only have a short-term but also a long-term impact on survival. Mortality rates examined 10 years after stroke were higher for patients who were depressed than for those who had not exhibited depression (Morris *et al.* 1993). However, in general, these studies have used small cohorts of selected patients and need to be replicated with larger samples and with appropriate diagnostic criteria.

There are three additional and important qualifications to the above studies. Firstly, some have argued that in view of the inappropriate diagnostic criteria, patients with emotional lability have mistakenly been identified as having symptoms of depression (House *et al.* 1989; Sharpe *et al.* 1990). However, although this may be the case, emotional lability is currently identified on the basis of a scale containing three questions. The sensitivity and specificity of this scale remains to be determined. Secondly, few of these studies have employed age-specific criteria for identifying mood disorder despite the fact that the majority of patients with stroke are over 65. Katona (1994) has suggested that the presentation of depressed mood in people over 65 may differ from that in younger cohorts and may therefore be missed or misclassified if inappropriate screening and diagnostic instruments are used. Finally, in all these studies, patients with a significant degree of dysphasia were excluded from the investigations as they were unable to adequately complete or provide answers to the questions regarding mood. Reliable methods for the assessment of mood in dysphasic patients need to be developed and validated.

## Treatment of mood disorders

The effect of antidepressant medication on depressed mood after stroke has attracted remarkably little attention in the literature. Depression after stroke is commonly under-diagnosed and under-treated (Wade *et al.* 1987) even when psychiatric liaison services are provided (Ramasubbu and Kennedy 1994). Lipsey *et al.* (1984) conducted a double blind placebo controlled trial of nortriptyline in 34 elderly patients. The drug was found to be significantly more effective than placebo in reducing symptoms of depression after an average of six weeks of treatment. Antidepressant medication has also been found to be helpful in reducing physical symptoms after stroke. Reding *et al.* (1986) reported a beneficial effect of tradozone hydrochloride relative to a placebo group. Patients were treated on average 44 days after stroke, for an average of 32 days in the treatment group and 25 days in the placebo group. Six patients from the drug and six from the placebo group were dropped from the study because of sedating and perceived side-effects in the two groups respectively. Thus although there was a trend towards greater improvement of Barthel scores in the treated relative to the placebo group, the small numbers of patients in the trial make it difficult to draw any definitive conclusions.

Recently, the selective serotonin reuptake inhibitors (SSRI) and reversible selective inhibitors of monoamineoxidase (RIMA) have been increasingly favoured for use with elderly patients as preliminary evidence suggests that they have a better side-effect profile than the monoamine oxidase inhibitors (MAOI) and tricyclic groups of drugs (Katona 1994). Others have examined the efficacy and tolerability of fluoxetine in elderly depressed patients (Altamura *et al.* 1989). In their double blind study, fluoxetine was compared with amytriptyline in 28 elderly inpatients. After five weeks of treatment both groups of subjects improved equally in terms of reduction of depressive symptoms, but the drop-out rate was significantly higher in the amytriptyline group due to orthostatic hypotension, drowsiness and other anti-cholinergic side-effects.

Hutchinson *et al.* (1991) conducted a double blind randomised study of paroxetine versus amytriptyline in 101 elderly depressed patients. Although the two patient groups demonstrated equivalent and significant improvements in mood after six weeks of treatment, those taking paroxetine experienced significantly fewer adverse side-effects than patients taking amytriptyline.

To date, there has been only one large-scale investigation of the efficacy and tolerability of SSRIs in elderly depressed stroke patients. Andersen *et al.* (1994) conducted a six-week double blind placebo controlled trial of citalopram in 66 patients with depressed mood after stroke. Patients were included in the trial on average 12 weeks post onset although with a wide variation around this time, by which time the majority (74%) had been discharged home. The six-week outcome of patients with citalopram was significantly better than the placebo group on two measures of depressed mood. Interestingly, this effect was entirely the product of patients who had been entered into the study at seven weeks post onset. Patients treated earlier after stroke failed to demonstrate significant improvements of mood with placebo or drug. Thus, patients who became depressed after several weeks post onset appeared to have benefited more than patients who became depressed early after stroke. However, the small numbers in this study make it difficult to draw any firm conclusions. In addition, the authors did not follow up the patients to determine the long-term effects of a short treatment intervention. They also did not investigate the potential effects of depressed mood on recovery of physical or cognitive functions.

There is a great need for further studies in this area using larger cohorts of patients with longitudinal measures. Clearly, more information is also required about the normal rates of recovery of cognitive and physical function in non-depressed stroke patients.

A few studies have also reported beneficial effects of antidepressant medication on emotional lability following brain injury (Sloan *et al.* 1992; Seliger *et al.* 1992). However, stroke patients represented only a proportion of the small number of subjects used in each study. In addition, the patients were reported in the form of series of short single case studies, and no control groups were included for comparison.

## Cognitive impairment

### Assessment

A number of medical and physical factors have been examined to determine prognostic indices for outcome measures such as discharge functional ability (ADL), length of stay and discharge status. Although anecdotal evidence suggested that certain cognitive factors such as visual neglect may complicate the recovery of functions such as dressing and walking independently, there has been little interest in the literature regarding these questions.

Until recently, the literature indicated that visual neglect and other cognitive factors were highly prevalent in the first few days and weeks after stroke, but that they recovered spontaneously and were almost non-existent by three months post onset (Hier *et al.* 1983). However, a few studies have reported that deficits of higher cognitive function, such as learning and delayed recall of new information, may persist beyond three or even six months after the stroke (Wade *et al.* 1986) and that the presence of these and other cognitive deficits within the first few days after the stroke may be associated with a poor outcome in terms of physical function at discharge or after six months (Novack *et al.* 1987; Fullerton *et al.* 1988; Galski *et al.* 1993). In some cases, cognitive impairments were strongly associated with the presence of lower initial ADL scores and higher levels of physical disability. Certain of these impairments, however, were also associated with ADL on discharge independently of ADL on admission and therefore constituted useful prognostic indices of functional outcome (Reich *et al.* in preparation). Nevertheless, these studies are few in number and contain relatively small samples of subjects. Further longitudinal investigations are also required to determine whether cognitive and perceptual disorders on admission actually impede and delay recovery of physical function. However, these impairments are hard to identify without detailed cognitive or neuropsychological assessment. It could be argued that, in the absence of adequate knowledge about cognitive dysfunction, the multidisciplinary team may 'continue in a round of unsuccessful rehabilitation programmes that end up frustrating both patient and provider' (Gresham 1986).

## Cognitive rehabilitation

The vast majority of studies in the field of neuropsychological rehabilitation have been conducted with patients suffering from head injury. In particular, behavioural and other training techniques have been employed to improve and assist the residual and often persistent effects of disorders of attention, short-term memory, new learning and high-level reasoning. Although the results have in general indicated beneficial effects of rehabilitation, few of these approaches have been attempted with stroke patients.

The most significant area in which cognitive rehabilitation has been addressed to the needs of stroke patients is in the field of visual perceptual disorders, particularly in the context of visual neglect.

In the 1970s and 1980s Diller and his colleagues at New York University's Institute of Rehabilitation Medicine published a number of studies concerning the cognitive rehabilitation of visual neglect and other perceptual impairments underlying spatial dysfunction in groups of stroke patients (Weinberg *et al.* 1977; Weinberg *et al.* 1979; Gordon *et al.* 1985). Using a number of visual scanning training techniques, rehabilitation was associated with a beneficial effect on specific impairments such as reading, writing and arithmetic relative to control subjects who received equivalent time with standard occupational therapy. Furthermore, the effects of training generalised to other tasks not employed in the training sessions. However, training failed to generalise to more complex tasks or to tasks which differed dramatically from those addressed in training. In addition, the subjects used were exclusively patients with right hemisphere stroke disease. Subsequently, a number of studies have attempted to replicate and extend the range of this type of rehabilitation but failed to obtain significant generalisation effects (Lincoln *et al.* 1985). The possible reasons for these failures are discussed in detail by Calvanio *et al.* (1993). In essence, their thesis is that the lack of success was due to a number of methodological and conceptual flaws including the failure to incorporate task specific features into the impairment training programme. If tasks that depend on the number of integrated cognitive functions are grossly dissimilar to the functions addressed in rehabilitation, the results of training seem to be less likely to be beneficial.

There are almost no studies, apart from the individual case reports, that have assessed rehabilitation training of perceptual functions using task-specific training, in contrast to impairment training in controlled laboratory conditions. Although the results of these investigations have been promising in demonstrating beneficial effects for tasks such as wheelchair transfers (Stanton *et al.* 1983), the findings need to be replicated with larger samples of subjects and adequate controls. The effects of concurrent spontaneous recovery also need to be disentangled from the gains obtained in rehabilitation, or at least controlled for by providing cognitive training after physical performance has plateaued. A number of studies have examined the role of biofeedback training to facilitate recovery of paretic limbs. However, a meta-analysis of the results obtained from eight studies was inconclusive and failed to obtain consistent effects (Glanz *et al.* 1995).

Other cognitive rehabilitation approaches have been used to improve functioning in the context of disorders of memory and learning. However these rehabilitation techniques have been implemented almost exclusively with head-injured patients. Although the results of these interventions have been variable, repetition and practice per se have proved of little or no value (Wilson 1989).

Apart from one or two isolated case studies, no research has been conducted with stroke patients. Some have suggested that group support may be of assistance in remediating memory disorders. Others have argued that although these groups may be beneficial in reducing anxiety and depression, there is little evidence to suggest that they lead to improvements in memory performance (D'Esposito *et al.* 1995).

Other disorders of cognitive function after stroke, such as thinking or problem solving, have not been addressed in rehabilitation, despite their detrimental effects on everyday living.

Since stroke patients differ widely in terms of their pre-morbid skills, intellectual function, and site and size of lesion, as well as in their range of impairments, disabilities and handicaps, it is also important to be able to identify the characteristics of patients most likely to benefit from cognitive rehabilitation. Neither single case studies nor small poorly defined cohorts of patients with mixed aetiologies studied at different times post onset address these questions.

Finally, behavioural approaches derived from learning theory have been commonly applied to the rehabilitation of patients with cognitive disorders after acquired brain damage (Giles and Fussey 1988). In order to modify behaviour, a functional analysis needs to be conducted of: a) its antecedents or settings, b) the frequency and duration of behaviour, and c) its consequences (Goldstein 1993). For example, an analysis of the performance of transfers from wheelchair to plinth may reveal that these are accomplished successfully in the context of the controlled conditions of the physiotherapy gym but occur rarely in the setting of the hospital ward. A systematic analysis of the different environmental settings may identify a number of factors that distinguish the two situations. Staff in the gym may subtly prompt behaviour of a complex task that patients with disorders of sequencing are unable to accomplish unaided. The patterning of the floor may differ in the two situations creating varying levels of difficulty for patients with an impairment of distance perception. There may also be fewer distracting stimuli in the form of other patients or staff in the gym relative to the ward, rendering the two contexts unequal. Finally, patients may have developed trust and confidence in one or two physiotherapists which they have difficulty in generalising to different members of staff such as nurses. Once these difficulties have been identified, the transition between the two environments may be graded in smaller, more achievable steps. Other behavioural techniques such as reducing the size of goals, modelling, cueing and backward training may be applied to facilitate the process of learning. The selective use of reinforcements such as praise or a cup of tea may also improve the rate of learning in rehabilitation particularly when tasks are an effort or do not appear to have immediate relevance for patients' real life goals.

Although behavioural analysis and training have been developed and evaluated in the context of animal models of brain damage, they have clear relevance for the rehabilitation of adults with acquired brain injury (Oakley 1983). The literature is replete with anecdotal and single case reports of improvement in function as a result of the application of these approaches to patients with head injury or stroke.

However, they remain to be systematically investigated and evaluated by means of randomised controlled double blind studies and in the context of larger cohorts of stroke patients.

## Patients' and carers' perceptions of illness

A number of recent studies have examined the perceptions of stroke patients and carers regarding their illness, treatment in hospital and follow-up care. Although in general most patients are satisfied with their treatment and rehabilitation in hospital, the studies have identified a number of areas in which patients felt their care was inadequate. In some cases, patients and carers felt they had insufficient information and support about the stroke in terms of the cognitive, social and psychological sequelae, particularly after discharge (Lewinter and Mikkelsen 1995). Carers were uncertain as to how to relate to the patient and were disturbed by the patient's personality change and the patient 'not being himself' (Carnwath and Johnson 1987; Wilkinson *et al.* in preparation).

In other studies, carers and relatives felt that they were left alone to deal with the patient in terms of his or her psychosocial needs and thought that more advice and family counselling after discharge from hospital would have been helpful. Although carers' stress in looking after their relatives with dementia has been found to be more strongly related to the mental rather than the physical disabilities of patients, relatively little research has been conducted with stroke patients. There is some indication however that the stress experienced by carers is unrelated to the patients' physical disability and strongly associated with depression, increasing irritability or behavioural problems in the patient (Carnwath and Johnson 1987; Anderson *et al.* 1995).

Patients with a residual mental and/or physical disability may experience a loss of role, mastery and control, particularly if they were formerly the dominant member of the family (Anderson 1992). Carers frequently report a lack of advice and help offered to patients and themselves while in hospital or after discharge, particularly with regard to the impact of stroke on the patients' family.

Counselling and/or short-term family therapy is often requested and may be helpful in enabling successful adjustment to the effects of stroke (Langton Hewer 1990) and in preventing the emergence of maladaptive responses, but these services are rarely provided or evaluated. Stroke patients, particularly in cases of high pre-morbid IQ or middle to high socio-economic status, may feel stigmatised by even minimal disability and handicap and may withdraw from their former social network (Anderson 1992; Labi *et al.* 1980). Although, in general, a good social network is one of the factors associated with better physical outcome and quality of life, recent research has suggested that maladaptive responses such as overprotectiveness by close relatives may develop (Thompson and Sobolew-Shubin 1993). In these cases, patients may fail to thrive emotionally and may not maintain the level of physical independence that they achieved in the hospital setting.

Depressed mood after stroke may be misinterpreted by family or friends and attributed to increased eccentricity or even deliberate non-compliance, particularly if the patient is elderly. Externally directed frustration, anger and hostility may occur independently of depressive symptoms and may lead to an increase in long-term physical disability as well as increased tension and stress amongst family members or friends (McFarlane *et al.* 1987). In the absence of adequate information, guidance and treatment, coping strategies may flounder with a consequent reduction in quality of life for all parties.

## Counselling and psychotherapy

Few systematic psychotherapeutic interventions have been attempted with stroke patients and their families. Short-term focused cognitive behaviour therapy has been demonstrated to be effective with adults suffering from primary depression, particularly when used in conjunction with antidepressant medication. Patients with head injury have also been successfully treated for depression with cognitive behaviour therapy and other psychotherapeutic interventions. The majority of reports in the literature with regard to stroke patients refer to single case studies.

Although the results have in general demonstrated decreases in severity of depressive symptoms, it is difficult to draw any general conclusions from these studies, particularly as no control subjects were employed. Larger-scale double blind placebo controlled investigations with standardised appropriate screening and diagnostic instruments urgently need to be conducted.

It is likely that, as with adults with primary mood disorders, counselling per se or attempts to improve the quality of social relationships may be less effective in facilitating the emergence of appropriate coping strategies and in reducing depressive symptomatology than structured in-depth psychotherapeutic approaches such as cognitive behaviour therapy. It is also important for psychotherapy and antidepressant medication not to be considered as mutually exclusive options. Combined cognitive behaviour therapy and antidepressant medication has been found to have been more effective in adults with primary depression than either treatment alone (Blackburn *et al.* 1981). Stroke patients who are depressed in the early stages of their illness may be ineligible for psychotherapeutic interventions because of medical illness, weakness, fatigue, loss of insight and severe cognitive disorders such as short-term memory loss. At this stage, antidepressant medication may be the most effective line of intervention. As patients improve, and are discharged to their own homes, they are obliged to confront the real impact of their disabilities and handicaps on everyday living. It is possible that this is the most appropriate time to involve psychotherapeutic services. However, these suggestions are at present untested and need to be investigated.

## Perceptions of illness and adjustment

Extensive research has been conducted to examine patterns of responses and coping after a major life event. A number of distinct responses occurring sequentially have been identified during the bereavement period after loss or death of a partner (Parkes 1972). Initially, denial occurs often followed by anger and depression. All of these reactions are thought to occur in the normal process of loss and grieving before a successful adjustment to the trauma is achieved.

This period of adjustment and adaptation varies in time as a function of the nature of the loss and its significance for the individual, although much research remains to be done in this area. Maladaptive responses, occasionally leading to extended and unremitting periods of depression may occur and are characterised by the individual remaining fixed at a particular stage e.g. anger. The mechanisms underlying successful adjustments by patients and their carers to a life-threatening illness such as stroke are as yet minimally researched or understood.

In general, patients and carers are left to their own devices to come to terms to the traumatic and long-term impact of stroke despite high risks of stress and depression.

Some have suggested, in a cross sectional study of stroke and orthopaedic patients, that patients with an internal locus of control (i.e. regarding themselves as being able to influence the course and progress of their illness) have a better prognosis in terms of functional outcome than patients with similar initial levels of disability who identify chance factors or other people such as doctors as determining their recovery (Partridge and Johnston 1989). Others have argued that a successful search for the cause and meaning of a stroke is significantly associated with better psychological adjustment (Thompson 1991). Patients with more severe (disabling) strokes were in general found to be more poorly adjusted than patients with lower levels of disability. However, when the effect of disability was controlled, patients and carers were better adjusted 'if they reported finding meaning in the experience, if they did not ask themselves "why me?", if they did not hold themselves responsible and if they had identified a cause of the stroke' (Thompson and Sobolew-Shubin 1993). However, both studies used a cross-sectional design and it is unclear whether different styles of coping are more adaptive at different stages in recovery after stroke. It also remains to be determined whether successful adjustment leads to the search for appropriate causes of stroke and a reduction in the tendency to blame oneself for, or feel victimised, by the stroke or vice-versa.

Others have suggested that pre-morbid dispositional styles such as optimism (Sheier and Carver 1985) or type A behaviour patterns (Shima *et al.* 1994) may determine the interpretation of one's situation and adjustment in patients.

Finally, no longitudinal information is available as to whether successful adjustment reactions by patients and carers may serve as a buffer against the long-term sequelae of stroke by reducing stress and improving functional outcome. Specific short-term interventions such as increased information or assistance in the development of appropriate cognitive coping strategies may also be helpful in reducing stress and in facilitating adaptive adjustment responses.

# Cultural determinants of illness perception

Significant cultural variations exist in the interpretation of a meaning attributed to illness, particularly to psychiatric symptoms (Littlewood and Lipsedge 1981). Psychotic symptoms may be considered relatively 'normal' behaviour patterns within certain cultures. Even when these symptoms are regarded as abnormal or deviant, the cause and frequently the remedies for the illness may be sought outside the realms of orthodox Western medicine. Even within Western society, different cultures may interpret and react to illnesses in a number of ways. Mediterranean cultures appeared to react to pain and illness in a more overt and distressed manner than people from the USA or Britain (Zborowski 1952). In addition, religious individuals from any of these cultures may react to illness and disease processes as though they were preordained, or delivered as a punishment for previous wrong-doings. These beliefs may lead to feelings of guilt, soul searching and a passive, fatalistic attitude to rehabilitation and long-term outcome.

Elderly people from different cultures may also be treated differently by their families in the event of serious or life-threatening illnesses than younger adults. Patients with moderate and even minimal disability may be confined to bed and rendered increasingly dependent by their anxious and overprotective families.

Although all these reactions may be identified informally amongst patients and carers on stroke units of inner-city hospitals, there have been no systematic investigations of the effects of these belief systems on the morbidity or mortality rates of patients after stroke.

Furthermore, it is not clear to what extent the attitudes and practices of health professionals are able to modify these beliefs, particularly when they conflict with those of patients and their families. Health promotion programmes which attempt to encourage patients to change their lifestyles and reduce risk factors for further strokes (such as smoking and alcohol consumption) may also meet with considerable resistance and limited success.

# Executive summary and priorities for research

There are few clinical psychologists involved in working with stroke patients, whether in hospital or in the community in the United Kingdom. A further characteristic of the management of stroke disease, particularly in Britain, has been the tendency to conceptualise the illness and its rehabilitation in primarily physical terms. Recruitment of psychology services to the assessment, management and rehabilitation of patients with stroke can be considered to have been a low priority.

There is a need to train members of the multidisciplinary team managing stroke patients with regard to psychological aspects of stroke disease and counselling.

The last 10 to 15 years has heralded a number of new clinical and research advances in relation to the psychological sequelae of stroke. Primary amongst these are the investigation of mood disorders, cognitive rehabilitation and perceptions of patients and carers regarding the impact of stroke on their lives.

Studies of mood disorders have been hampered by small numbers, and a lack of case-definition and failure to control for differences between groups studied. It would, however, appear that depressive symptoms are more common after stroke than in age and sex-matched controls. The effect of depression on outcome is unclear. The effect of antidepressant medication on depressed mood after stroke has attracted remarkably little attention and remains unclear. There is, therefore, a great need for further studies in this area.

The effect of various cognitive factors on the natural history and outcome of stroke is not known. There have been few studies assessing the effectiveness of neuropsychological rehabilitation. Few systematic psychotherapeutic interventions have been attempted with stroke patients and their families.

This chapter identifies an important gap in the provision of psychology services, and has reviewed the literature regarding the existing research on psychological aspects of stroke disease. There are a number of serious shortcomings associated with a range of these investigations as well as several unanswered questions. In view of these factors a few particularly important areas need to be addressed. These are summarised in order of priority in each of the two sections.

**Service provision**

An increase in psychology resources is required in order to identify and manage disorders of mood and cognition and potentially to increase the cost-effectiveness of the rehabilitation team. A crucial component of these posts would include multidisciplinary staff training with regard to psychological aspects of stroke disease and counselling.

Psychology resources are also needed in the community to facilitate patients' and carers' adjustments to the longer-term social and psychological impact of stroke, and to provide cognitive and behavioural psychotherapy.

The priorities for research are therefore:

1. A longitudinal study to determine the incidence, prevalence and natural history of cognitive and mood disorders following stroke and their effects on recovery and long-term outcome of physical function.

2. Further trials of antidepressants, particularly the new SSRI drugs in post-stroke depression. The effects of this intervention on the recovery of physical and cognitive function in addition to mood needs to be evaluated.

3. Investigation of the effect of pre-morbid personality and ethnicity on interpretation of, and reactions to, stroke by patients and carers.

# References

Altamura AC, Percudani M, Guercetti G, Invernizzi G. Efficacy and tolerability of fluoxetine in the elderly: a double blind study versus amitriptyline. Int Clin Psychopharm 1989; 4: 103-6.

Andersen G, Vestergaard K, Lauritzen L. Effective treatment of post stroke depression with the selective serotonin reuptake inhibitor citalopram. Stroke 1994; 25: 1099-104.

Anderson CS, Linto J, Stewart-Wynne EG. A population based assessment of the impact and burden of caregiving for long-term stroke survivors. Stroke 1995; 26: 843-9.

Anderson R. The aftermath of stroke, the experience of patients and their families. Cambridge University Press 1992.

Astrom M, Adolfsson R, Asplund K. Major depression in stroke patients: A three year longitudinal study. Stroke 1993; 24: 976-82.

Blackburn IM, Bishop S, Glen IM, Whalley LJ, Christie JE. The efficacy of cognitive therapy in depression: a treatment trial using cognitive therapy and pharmacotherapy, each alone and in combination. Br J Psychiat 1981; 139: 181-9.

Calvanio R, Levine D, Petrone P. Elements of cognitive rehabilitation after right hemisphere stroke. Behav Neurol 1993; II (1) 25-57.

Carnwath TCM, Johnson DAW. Psychiatric morbidity among spouses of patients with stroke. BMJ 1987; 294: 409-11.

D'Esposito MD, Alexander MP. The clinical profiles, recovery and rehabilitation of memory disorders. Neurorehab 1995; 5: 141-59.

Eastwood MR, Rifat SL, Nobbs H, Ruderman J. Mood disorder following cerebrovascular accident. Br J Psychiat 1989; 154: 195-200.

Folstein MF, Maiberger R, McHugh PR. Mood disorder as a specific complication of stroke. J Neurol Neurosurg Psychiat 1977; 40: 1018-20.

Fullerton KJ, Mackenzie G, Stout RW. Prognostic indices in stroke. QJ Med 1988; 66: 147-62.

Galski T, Bruno RL, Zorowitz R, Walker J. Predicting length of stay, functional outcome and after care in the rehabilitation of stroke patients: the dominant role of higher-order cognition. Stroke 1993; 24: 1794-800.

Giles GM, Fussey I. Models of brain injury rehabilitation: from theory to practice. In: LI Fussey and GM Giles (eds). Rehabilitation of the severely brain injured adult; a practical approach. Croom Helm, London 1988; 69-101.

Glanz M, Klawansky S, Stason W, Berkey C, Shah N, Phan H, Chalmers TC. Biofeedback therapy in post stroke rehabilitation: A meta-analysis of the randomised controlled trials. Arch Phys Med Rehab 1995; 76: 508-15.

Goldstein L. Behaviour problems. In: R Greenwood, MP Barnes, TM McMillan and CD Ward (eds). Neurolo Rehab 1993; 389-401.

Gordon WA, Hibbard MR, Egelko S *et al*. Perceptual remediation in patients with right brain damage: a comprehensive programme. Arch Phys Med Rehab 1985; 66: 353-9.

Gresham GE. The rehabilitation of the stroke survivor. In: JM Barnett, JP Mohr, BM Stein and FM Yatzu (eds). Stroke: patho-physiology, diagnoses and management. 1986; 1259-74. New York, Churchill Livingstone.

Henley S, Petit S, Todd-Pokropek A, Tupper A. Who goes home? Predictive factors in stroke recovery. J Neurol Neurosurg Psychiatr 1985; 48: 1-6.

Hier DB, Mondlock J, Caplan LR. Recovery of behavioural abnormalities after right hemisphere stroke. Neurology 1983; 33: 345-50.

House A, Dennis M, Molyneux A, Warlow C, Hawton K. Emotionalism after stroke. BMJ 1989; 298: 991-4.

House A, Dennis M, Mogridge L, Warlow C, Hawton K, Jones L. Mood disorders in the year after first stroke. Br J Psychiat 1991; 158: 83-92.

Hutchinson DR, Tong S, Moon CAL *et al*. A double blind study in general practice to compare the efficacy and tolerability of paroxetine and amitriptyline in depressed elderly patients. Br J Clin Res 1991; 2: 43-7.

Katona CLE. Depression in old age. John Wiley and Sons, 1994.

Labi MLC, Phillips TF, Gresham GE. Psychosocial disability in physically restored long-term survivors. Arch Phys Med Rehab 1980; 61: 561-5.

Langhorne, P. Williams BO, Gilchrist, W, Howie K. Do stroke units save lives. Lancet 1993; 342: 395-7.

Langton Hewer R. Rehabilitation after stroke. Q J Med 1990; 76: 659-74.

Lewinter M, Mikkelsen S. Patients' experience of rehabilitation. Disabil Rehab 1995; 17: 3-9.

Lincoln NB, Whiting SE, Cockburn J, Bhavani G. An evaluation of perceptual retraining. Int Rehab Med 1985; 7: 99-110.

Lipsey JR, Robinson RG, Pearlson GD *et al*. Nortriptyline treatment of post stroke depression: a double-blind study. Lancet 1984; 1: 297-300.

Littlewood R, Lipsedge M. Aliens and alienists: ethnic minorities and psychiatry. London: Penguin, 1981.

McFarlane AC, Hobbin ER, Kneebone CS. The determinants of illness behaviour in stroke patients. Psychiat Med 1987; 5: 133-41.

Morris PLP, Robinson AG, Andrzejewski P, Samuels J, Price TR. Association of depression with ten year post stroke mortality. Am J Psychiat 1993; 150: 124-9.

Morris PLP, Robinson RG, Raphael B, Samuels J, Molloy P. The relationship between risk factors for affective disorder and post stroke depression in hospitalised stroke patients. Aust NZ J Psychiatry 1992; 26: 208-17.

Novack TA, Haban G, Graham K, Satterfield WT. Predictions of stroke rehabilitation from psychologic screening. Arch Phys Med Rehab 1987; 68: 729-34.

Oakley DA. Learning capacity outside neocortex in animals and man: implications for therapy after brain injury. In G. Davey (Ed). Animal models of human behaviour: conceptual, evolutionary and neurobiological perspectives. John Wiley, Chichester. 1983; 247-66.

Parkes CM. Bereavement: Studies of grief in adult life. 1972. New York. Int. Univ. Press.

Partridge C, Johnston M. Perceived control of recovery from physical disability: measurement and prediction. Br J Clin Psychol 1989; 28: 53-9.

Ramasubbu R, Kennedy SH. Factors complicating the diagnosis of depression in cerebrovascular disease, Part 1 - phenomenological and nosological issues. Can J Psychiatry 1994; 39: 596-600.

Reding MJ, Orto, LA, Winter SW, Fortuna IM, Di Ponte P, McDowell FH. Antidepressant therapy after stroke: a double-blind trial. Arch Neurol 1986; 43: 763-5.

Robinson RG, Bolduc PLR, Price TR. Two year longitudinal study of post stroke mood disorders: diagnosis and outcome at one and two years. Stroke 1987; 18: 837-43.

Robinson RG, Kubos KL, Starr LB, Rao K, Price TR. Mood disorders in stroke patients. Brain 1984; 107: 81-93.

Scheier MF, Carver, CS. Optimism, coping and health: assessment and implications of generalized outcome expectancies. Health Psychol 1985; 4: 219-47.

Schubert DSP, Burns R, Paras W, Siason E. Increase of medical hospital length of stay by depression in stroke and amputation patients: a pilot study. Psychother Psychosomat 1992b; 57: 61-6.

Schubert DSP, Taylor C, Lee S, Mentari A, Tamaklo W. Detection of depression in the stroke patient. Psychosomatics 1992a; 33: 290-4.

Seliger GM, Hornstein A, Flax J, Herbert J, Schroeder K. Fluoxetine improves emotional incontinence. Brain Injury 1992; 6: 267-70.

Sharpe M, Hawton K, House A, Molyneux A, Sandercock P, Bamford J, Warlow C. Mood disorders in long-term survivors of stroke: associations with brain lesion location and volume. Psychol Med 1990; 20: 815-28.

Shima S, Kitagawa Y, Kitamura T, Fujinawa A, Watanabe Y. Post stroke depression. Gen Hosp Psychiatr 1994; 16: 286-9.

Sloan RL, Brown KW, Pentland B. Fluoxetine as a treatment for emotional lability after brain surgery. Brain Injury 1992; 6: 315-9.

Stanton KM, Pepping M, Brockway JA, Bliss L, Frankel D, Waggener S. Wheelchair transfer training for right cerebral dysfunctions: an interdisciplinary approach. Arch Phys Med Rehab 1983; 64: 276-80.

Thompson SC. The search for meaning following a stroke. Basic Applied Soc Psychol 1991; 12: 81-96.

Thompson SC, Sobolew-Shubin A. Over-protective relationships: A non-supportive side of social networks. Basic Applied Soc Psychol 1993. 14: 363-83.

Wade DT, Legh-Smith J, Hewer RA. Depressed mood after stroke. A community study of its frequency. Br J Psychiatr 1987; 151: 200-5.

Wade DT, Parker V, Langton-Hewer R. Memory disturbance after stroke: Frequency and associated losses. Int Rehab Med 1986; 8: 60-4.

Weinberg J, Diller L, Gordon WA *et al.* Training sensory awareness and spatial organisation in people with right brain damage. Arch Phys Med Rehab 1979; 60: 460-77.

Weinberg J, Diller L, Gordon WA *et al.* Visual scanning training effect on reading related tasks in acquired right-brain damage. Arch Phys Med Rehab 1977; 58: 470-86.

Wilson B. Models of cognitive rehabilitation. In: R L Wood and P Eames (eds) Models of brain injury rehabilitation. John Hopkins University Press; 1989; 117-41.

Zborowski M. Cultural Components in responses to pain. J Soc Issues 1952; 8: 16-30.

# CHAPTER 12

# THE ROLE OF THE PRIMARY HEALTH CARE TEAM IN STROKE

*Frances Bunn*

**Chapter outline**

## Introduction

It is only in more recent years that there has been an exploration of the role of the general practitioner and other members of the primary health care team in the prevention of stroke and the care of stroke patients. Indeed there is still little information on stroke and the primary health care team and this may be because an average general practitioner (GP) sees only four new stroke patients a year. Most of the work that has been done concentrates on primary prevention of stroke and cardiovascular disease.

Although there has been little research, the role of primary care is an important one in stroke care, both in prevention and management, particularly in ensuring co-ordination of care for patients.

There seems to be a general consensus that prevention in primary care is desirable. A report by the Royal College of General Practitioners in 1981 into prevention of arterial disease in general practice said: 'About half of all strokes in people under 70 are probably preventable by the application of existing knowledge.' It recommended that everyone should have their blood pressure measured at least once every five years, that smoking behaviour should be recorded and that patients should have weight and height measured as a useful and visible indicator of increased lipid concentration. Bennet *et al.* (1989) found that of the sample of people they looked at in south Birmingham, nearly half the population screened in primary care were seriously overweight, a quarter had serum cholesterol levels sufficiently high to warrant some intervention and one-third smoked.

Despite such evidence of risk, it still appears to be an area neglected in primary care. A study by Wolfe *et al.* (1993) followed up patients three months after their stroke. It found that only 70% of survivors had seen their GP. Those patients not admitted to hospital were unlikely to be referred by the primary health care team for rehabilitation. A study by Fleming and Lawrence (1981) looked at recorded information about preventive measures in 38 practices. They found that of men in their 40s, 47% had no record of their blood pressure having been taken during the previous 10 years, and information about smoking habits was available in only 23% of records. Wallace *et al.* (1987) looked at whether GPs were doing enough to promote healthy lifestyles; of the smokers in their study, they found that 27% had definitely, and 13% probably, received advice on smoking. They concluded that patients are concerned about their lifestyles, that most would welcome relevant counselling, and that doctors should become more concerned with prevention of this kind.

Calnan *et al.* (1994) looked at the involvement of the primary health care team in coronary heart disease prevention. They sent questionnaires to a sample of practices to both the GPs and the practice nurses. In total 94% of GPs who replied reported that they were involved in assessing lifestyle risk factors in the routine consultation and most were commonly involved in blood pressure testing and inquiring about smoking status. Eighty six per cent of the surgeries had well-person clinics, which were usually run by the practice nurses. Of the practice nurses who replied, 98% stated that they routinely asked about smoking, 97.3% asked about weight, 97.4% asked about blood pressure and 86.5% asked about cholesterol. District nurses and health visitors appeared to be little involved in preventive care. Although such a study is useful, only 64% of GPs and 71% of practice nurses replied. It might also be reasonable to assume that those who replied were in fact more involved in preventive care. Also, the study relies on self-reporting by the health care professionals involved.

## The role of the general practitioner

A study by Mant *et al.* (1985) undertook a three-year follow up of patients with raised blood pressure identified at health checks in general practice. All records of blood pressure, weight and smoking habits in the medical record were abstracted for the three years after the initial health check. Those patients with an initial diastolic blood pressure of 105 mmHg or above and most of the patients with an initial pressure of 90-104 mmHg had at least one further measurement of their blood pressure. Follow up of smoking habits and of weight was less complete, with only half the smokers having any documented follow-up of these risk factors. They found only a modest decrease of blood pressure in their sample group and this could not be attributed to the health checks because of an absence of a control group. They say that their results 'emphasise the need to develop formal protocols for dietary and anti-smoking interventions and to evaluate formally the effectiveness of health checks'. Fotherby *et al.* (1992) sent a postal questionnaire to GPs to look at the way they managed hypertension in elderly patients.

They conclude that 'the variation among GPs in the criteria for the measurement, diagnosis and treatment of hypertension in elderly patients emphasises the need for clear management guidelines in this age group'. It would seem then that there is a lack of clarity about the way GPs should be monitoring and treating raised blood pressure, despite there being no doubt of the importance of this intervention. Fleming and Lawrence (1981) write that 'since 90% of patients attend over a five-year period, there is great scope for screening for hypertension on an opportunistic basis; screening all men in their 40s would seem to be a goal which all practices could reach'.

It would seem that case-finding of patients by general practitioners can be effective. Shaper *et al.* (1986) devised a strategy for identifying men at high risk of acute myocardial infarction or sudden ischaemic death. Their risk score looked at cigarette smoking, mean blood pressure, recall of ischaemic heart disease or diabetes mellitus, history of parental death from heart trouble, and the presence of angina. The top fifth of the score distribution identified 53% of men who experienced major ischaemic heart disease over the next five years. Coppola *et al.* (1995) devised a scoring system, for use in general practice, to identify men at high risk of stroke. Subjects were randomly selected. A simple scoring system derived from logistic regression, using age, systolic blood pressure, current cigarette consumption, and evidence of anginal chest pain was able to predict more than 80% of all strokes occurring within five years in the top fifth of score distribution. The combination of smoking and hypertension, while much less sensitive than the scoring system, was a better indicator of risk than any single risk factor, all of whose predictive values were poor. They conclude that 'this scoring system could be used in general practice to identify men at high risk of stroke who would benefit from further intervention'. Effective identification of high-risk individuals requires assessment of the combined effects of multiple risk factors. It would seem then that there is evidence that risk factor screening can be done effectively in general practice, although at present it is often not being done with any consistency or thoroughness.

## The role of the practice nurse

There is an increasing emphasis in the literature on the role of the practice nurse in primary prevention. A study by Fullard *et al.* (1987) looked at promoting prevention in primary care by the use of a facilitator and the practice nurses. It was a controlled trial of a low-technology, low-cost approach; patients were recruited to the trial when they visited their GP. They say that 'during the study the increase between intervention and control practices in blood pressure recording was doubled and in the recording of smoking habit it was quadrupled, and there was a five-fold increase in the recording of weight'. They calculated that using their method of prevention should only cost a practice £10 a week although an accurate assessment of doctors' time was not made. They concluded that 'the results of this study show that ascertaining the major risk factors for cardiovascular disease in primary care may be substantially improved by an opportunistic, systematic approach using practice nurses'.

Sanders *et al.* (1989) undertook a randomised controlled trial of the value of anti-smoking advice by nurses in general practice. General practitioners see the majority of smokers on their practice lists at least once a year and are expected by their patients to take an active interest in behaviour that affects health, including smoking (Wallace *et al.* 1984). Also, advice from general practitioners has been shown to be effective in helping patients to stop smoking (Russell *et al.* 1979; Richmond *et al.* 1986). However, in accordance with the growing interest in the role of the nurse in prevention, Sanders and colleagues looked at the efficacy of anti-smoking advice when given by practice nurses. Smokers were asked to make an appointment with the practice nurse. Only 26% did so. Of those who did attend they found that 'in terms of the number of smokers reporting non-smoking at both one month and one year, and the number of smokers who claimed sustained cessation for one year, the intervention group performed significantly better than the control group'. Owing to the problem of poor attendance, which has also been found by others (Pill *et al.* 1988), the authors came to the conclusion that 'it is possible that the most appropriate role for the practice nurse is not in giving initial advice to stop - which may be best done opportunistically by the general practitioner - but in the provision of longer-term support and follow up which may be necessary to achieve sustained cessation'.

A study in south Birmingham by Bennet and colleagues (1989) looked at a district approach to the prevention of heart disease. They used practice nurses to provide health checks in GPs' surgeries, combined with direct access to secondary care. If appropriate, patients were offered further intervention such as stress management or smoking cessation groups. They were also referred to the GP if it was necessary. They found that they achieved a significant decrease in blood pressure and serum cholesterol levels and that a substantial number of smokers had ceased smoking since attending the smoking cessation groups. The OXCHECK study (1994) also looked at the effectiveness of health checks conducted by nurses in primary care. A randomised controlled study was undertaken to assess the effectiveness of health checks by nurses in reducing risk factors for cardiovascular disease in patients from general practice. It was found that the intervention by the nurses did lower cholesterol and blood pressure but did not decrease the number of people smoking. The conclusion was that general health checks by nurses are ineffective in helping smokers to stop smoking, but they help patients to modify their diet and total cholesterol concentration.

It would seem then that there is mixed evidence for the benefits of the role of the nurse in primary prevention. However, all of the studies mentioned did find some beneficial effect, although the evidence about smoking does not seem to be conclusive. Indeed, nurses themselves have expressed a lack of confidence in the effectiveness of their role in this area (Sanders *et al.* 1986). It would seem then that there is a role for the practice nurse in the prevention of stroke. However, Calnan *et al.* (1994) do have some reservations about the way prevention is organised in general practice. They say: 'This division of activities appears to be less a result of organised teamwork and deployment of skills and expertise to a clearly defined management protocol, and more a product of the general practitioner contract and management arrangements which tended to encourage an approach to general practice health promotion revolving around the role of the practice nurse...this also hindered the development of a broader team-based approach to planning and delivery of health promotion in relation to the needs of the practice population.'

There is also the issue of whether practice nurses are qualified to fulfil this role. Cant *et al.* (1993) found that practice nurses often felt that they had not had enough training and particularly wanted training in smoking and diabetes control. Calnan and Williams (1993) also found that GPs were less enthusiastic about the benefits of clinics because they felt clinics attracted the worried rather than those most at risk.

# Implications of screening

The benefits of screening are still not clear as outlined in Chapter 1. There are some negative implications of comprehensive screening programmes, for example the increase in workload and the increase in expense. The OXCHECK study looked into the prevalence of risk factors for heart disease and the implications of screening in primary care (1991). Of the 2205 patients in the study, it was found that overall almost three-quarters needed specific advice or follow up; 15% needed only follow up for hyperlipidaemia or hypertension; 9% needed advice on smoking only; and 35% needed follow up advice on a combination of risk factors. This study found that there were definite implications for the workload of a practice if screening is done: 'If the entire adult population of a practice is offered health checks systematically, the acceptance rate is lower and the follow up workload is higher than previously understood. Not only are there the implications of the cost of the initial tests but also the follow up.' The authors say: 'Health checks are only the beginning of a successful preventive programme - the challenge is to provide effective intervention and follow-up.' Also, as seen in the research, uptake is a problem and it may be that those most in need of such programmes are not reached by them. Waller *et al.* (1990) found that attenders at health checks were more likely to be women, married, non-smokers and of higher social class than patients who did not respond to the invitation. Indeed the likelihood of acceptance of an invitation to attend was inversely related to the patient's cardiovascular risk for all factors measured except age. As indicated in Chapter 2, the targeting of health promotion to different groups of the population has not been evaluated. At United Medical and Dental Schools of Guy's and St Thomas' a group is currently assessing the prevalence of risk factors in different ethnic groups and their attitudes towards strategies for risk factor reduction.

## Executive summary and priorities for research

Primary care potentially has a pivotal role in the prevention and management of stroke. Research efforts involving GPs have virtually exclusively been in the area of prevention. Although an average general practitioner will only see four new stroke patients a year, stroke is the major cause of adult disability and requires co-ordinated management.

In the 1990s it would appear that most general practices are involved in cardiovascular risk reduction programmes as part of *The Health of the Nation* strategy, but, as outlined in Chapter 2, the evidence to support such activity for stroke is not strong. It is also clear that general practices are not centrally involved in the management of stroke patients after their stroke.

The effectiveness of detection and management of hypertension in reducing the risk of stroke has been discussed in Chapter 2 and it would appear there is a continuing need to audit this in primary care and develop strategies to improve access to care and compliance with treatment.

Scores to predict cardiovascular and cerebrovascular risk have been developed which might be of use in prompting early treatment, thereby reducing the chances of having a stroke. There would not appear to be a consistent use of such an approach in general practice at the present moment. Although efforts have been made to identify risk factors, no research has really addressed how patients use this information and whether in fact risk is reduced.

The role of the practice nurse has expanded over the years but the effectiveness of this role is still to be determined. The training needs for this role require clarification. The increased workload that has been generated by practice nurse clinics cannot currently be considered cost-effective.

The role of the primary health care team in the management of stroke has not been researched and audits of stroke care not undertaken. In view of the small numbers of incident cases seen by GPs and the consequent difficulty that doctors have in maintaining a sufficient knowledge base, the role of primary health care in secondary prevention and rehabilitation needs careful evaluation. There are opportunities for effective secondary prevention in primary care but whether these are being taken up is not known.

Increasingly, the health service is looking at the interface between the hospital and primary care and at multisectoral collaboration with social services. To improve the effectiveness of primary care in stroke prevention and care, the following research and service priorities are suggested:

1. The assessment of different strategies for reducing risk factors in different groups of a practice population.

2. The audit of secondary prevention in primary care and the evaluation of different ways of delivering an effective secondary prevention service, with particular reference to anticoagulation.

3. An assessment of the role and training needs of practice nurses and health visitors in stroke prevention programmes.

4. An assessment of the role and training needs of GPs in respect to the management of stroke patients.

# References

Bennet P, Blackall M, Clapham M, Little S, Player and Williams S. South Birmingham coronary prevention project: a district approach to the prevention of heart disease. Community Med 1989; 11: 90-6.

Calnan M, Cant S, Williams S, Killoran A. Involvement of the primary health care team in coronary heart disease prevention. Brit J Gen Pract 1994; 44: 224-8.

Calnan M, Williams S. Coronary heart disease prevention: the role of the general practitioner. Family Pract 1993; 10(2): 137-51.

Cant S, Killoran A, Calnan M. The role of the community nurse in coronary heart disease prevention, based in general practice. Final report to HEA. Canterbury, University of Kent, 1993, Centre for Health Services Studies.

Coppola WGT, Whincup PH, Papacosta O, Walker M, Ebrahim S. Scoring system to identify men at high risk of stroke: a strategy for general practice. Br J Gen Pract 1995; 45: 185-9.

Fleming DM, Lawrence STA. An evaluation of recorded information about preventative measures in 38 practices. J R Coll Gen Pract, 1981; 31: 615-20.

Fotherby MD, Harper GD, Potter JF. General practitioners' management of hypertension in elderly patients. BMJ 1992; 305: 750-2.

Fullard E, Fowler G, Gray M. Promoting prevention in primary care: controlled trial of low technology, low cost approach. BMJ 1987; 294: 1080-2.

Mant D, McKinlay C, Fuller A, Randall T, Fullard E, Muir J. Three year follow-up of patients with raised blood pressure identified at health checks in general practice. BMJ 1989; 298: 1360-2.

OXCHECK Study Group. Prevalence of risk factors for heart disease in OXCHECK trial: implication for screening in primary care. BMJ 1991; 302: 1057-60.

OXCHECK Study Group. Effectiveness of health checks conducted by nurses in primary care: results of the OXCHECK study after one year. BMJ 1994; 308: 308-12.

Pill R, French J, Harding K, Stott N. Invitaton to attend a health check in a general practice setting; comparison of attenders and non-attenders. J R Coll Gen Pract 1988; 38: 53-6.

Richmond RL, Austin A, Webster IW. Three year evaluation of a programme by general practitioners to help patients to stop smoking. BMJ 1986; 292: 803-6.

Royal College of General Practitioners. Prevention of arterial disease in general practice. 1981. London: Royal college of General Practitioner's.

Russell MAH, Wilson C, Taylor C, Baker CD. Effect of general practitioners' advice against smoking. BMJ 1979; 2: 231-5.

Sanders DJ, Fowler G, Mant, Fuller A, Jones, Marzillier J. Randomized controlled trial of anti-smoking advice by nurses in general practice. J R Coll Gen Pract 1989; 39: 273-6.

Sanders DJ, Stone V, Fowler G, Marzillier J. Practice nurses and anti-smoking education. BMJ 1986; 292: 381-3.

Shaper AG, Plcock SJ, Philips AN, Walker M. Identifying men at high risk of heart attacks: strategy for use in general practice. BMJ 1986; 293: 474-9.

SHEP Cooperative Research Group. Prevention of stroke by antihypertensive drug treatment in older persons with isolated systolic hypertension. JAMA, 1991; 265: 24, 3255-64.

Wallace PG, Brennan PJ, Haines AP. Are general practitioners doing enough to promote health life style? Findings of the Medical Research Council's general practice research framework study on life style and health. BMJ, 1987; 294: 940-2.

Wallace PG, Haines AP. General practitioners and health promotion: what patients think. BMJ 1984; 289: 534-6.

Waller D, Agass M, Mant D, Coulter A, Fuller A, Jones L. Health checks in general practice: another example of inverse care? BMJ, 1990; 300: 1115-8.

Wolfe CDA, Taub NA, Woodrow J, Richardson E, Warburton FG, Burney PGJ. Patterns of acute stroke care in three districts of southern England. J Epidemiol Community Health 1993; 47: 144-8.

# CHAPTER 13

# LONGER-TERM CARE

*Peter Wilkinson*

**Chapter outline**

## Introduction

Two areas of stroke that have received little attention in the UK are the longer-term morbidity and quality of life of survivors. This information is required before decisions can be made about service provision. Most of the studies that have been done have followed a group of hospital patients for several years (Greveson *et al.* 1991). A small amount of long-term outcome work has been reported for a UK community-based group (Weddell and Beresford 1979). The Oxford Community Stroke Project (OCSP) has reported on long-term survival but not yet on disability (Dennis *et al.* 1993). The distinction between whether the study population is community-based or not is important as not all stroke patients are admitted to hospital.

## Long-term outcome of stroke

### South London follow up study

In 1989 a stroke register was established in South East London (Wolfe *et al.* 1993). Over the subsequent 12 months 291 local residents aged under 75 who suffered their first-ever stroke were registered. The survivors of this group have recently been reviewed. The fieldwork was carried out during 1994/95 and has provided information on the longer-term outcome of stroke. The objectives were to determine the survival rate of the cohort and to assess the levels of impairment, disability and handicap as well as the quality of life of the survivors plus the services that they had received.

The patients were assessed at between 4.3 and 5.5 years since their stroke with the mean duration being 4.9 years. At the long-term follow up, 123 (42%) of the original cohort were known to be alive. Fourteen were lost. Of the 106 interviewed survivors, 94 lived in private accommodation. The most disabled patients were only likely to be living in private accommodation if they had an identified carer.

One-third of the interviewed surviving group were severely or moderately disabled, one-third mildly disabled and one-third functionally independent. Two-fifths of the survivors were more disabled at five years than they had been at three months.

The subjects were sometimes uncertain whether the therapy services they had received had been whilst at home or when they were in hospital. With this in mind two-fifths reported receiving physiotherapy, one in seven had received speech therapy and one in 17 occupational therapy for their stroke.

Of the non-therapy services, chiropody and district nursing were the most likely to have been provided. Very few people had received any respite care. Nearly three-quarters had an aid or appliance and over half had had an adaptation to their home. Three-quarters of the subjects were on treatments aimed at preventing further vascular events. The patients' scores on several quality of life scales were related to their degree of disability.

### Where are stroke patients living in the long term?
In the St Thomas' study, of the 123 people alive at the long-term follow up, 107 (87%) were living in private accommodation, nine (7%) were permanently in a nursing home or hospital and one person was in sheltered accommodation with a paid, live-in carer. The remainder were either in hospital at the time of the interview or their type of accommodation was unknown. This compares with 10% of the patients in Weddell and Beresford's (1979) community-based study living in a nursing home or hospital four years after their stroke. That study included people of all ages, but may have missed mild cases of stroke. A further hospital-based study found that three years after their stroke, approximately one-fifth of survivors were not living at home (Greveson *et al.* 1991).

### Long-term impairment and disability
Although the contributing factors to the long-term disability of stroke patients will include the changes of ageing and comorbidities, the overall burden of disease is likely to be stroke-related.

Clinically, 103 of the interviewed patients in the St Thomas' study were fully conscious, and two were somnolent, at the long-term follow up. One person was in a persistent vegetative state and is not included in the following clinical details. Fifty nine (56%) had weakness or paralysis of the hand or arm together with paralysis or weakness of the leg of the same side. Thirty seven (35%) had a speech disturbance resulting from the stroke, but 24 could be completely understood. Eleven patients (10%) had difficulty swallowing as a consequence of the stroke. Three patients (2.9%) were permanently catheterised.

Of the 96 patients who completed the Hospital Anxiety and Depression Scale (Zigmond and Snaith 1983), 22 (23%) had scores suggesting they were depressed and 13 (14%) had borderline scores. Eighteen (19%) of patients had scores suggesting they were anxious and 12 (13%) had borderline scores. The results suggest that the high levels of depression found in other studies at one year (Wade, Legh-Smith and Hewer 1987) and at three years (Greveson *et al.* 1991) after stroke continue in the longer term.

In the St Thomas' study, 36 (34%) of the 106 interviewed patients were functionally independent as assessed by their activities of daily living and 39 (37%) were mildly disabled. This is very similar to the findings of Greveson *et al.* (1991) in a hospital-based cohort three years after their stroke. In the Framingham study, Gresham *et al.* (1979) used a different rating index but found similarly that 32% of stroke patients were dependent in their activities of daily living. The majority of the patients assessed by Gresham *et al.* (1979) had suffered their stroke more than 20 months previously.

Although only approximately one-third of the patients were functionally independent as assessed by their Barthel Index, nearly nine out of ten patients were living in private accommodation. The findings of the St Thomas' study were that 21 (22%) of the 94 people living at home were moderately or severely disabled and that 37 (39%) were mildly disabled. As well as providing an overall score for disability, the Barthel Index gives an idea of the problems the patients and their carers deal with. As has been found in other studies (Wade and Langton-Hewer 1987), the activity of daily living that most patients in the St Thomas' cohort who were at home needed help with was bathing (49%), followed by climbing stairs (44%) and dressing (38%). This gives some insight into the type of support that carers and the support services are providing to stroke patients to maintain them in their own homes. This high level of disability implies that the stroke survivors will require a great deal of help and support from health and from social services as well as from the voluntary sector.

*Handicap*

The long-term consequences of the impairments and disabilities of stroke may manifest themselves as handicap. Ebrahim (1990) suggested that increasing a patient's quality of life, through rehabilitation, may be equated with reducing handicap. The WHO (1980) definition of handicap relates it to the fulfilment of a role that is normal for that individual. This may include such areas as employment and social interaction.

Greveson *et al.* (1991) found that approximately 40% of the patients at home regularly walked outside for over 15 minutes, and 60% regularly took part in social occasions. In the St Thomas' study, 13% of those who were moderately or severely disabled had been on a social outing in the last three months compared with 46% of mildly disabled people and 67% of people who were functionally independent.

Many different factors may contribute to a patient's quality of life. This has resulted in several different approaches to its assessment, often using new measures rather than those already available. A wide range of different measures were used in the current study. These were aimed at assessing impairment, disability and handicap as well as the subjects' own assessment of their general health. The overall picture suggested that four to five years after their stroke the patients' scores on the various quality of life scales were related to their residual disability.

## *Utilisation of services*

In the St Thomas' study, the 94 interviewed people living at home were receiving a wide range of services at the time of the interview. Sixteen (17%) were attending a day centre at least once a week. Fifteen (16%) people had a local authority home help, and three a private home help, at least weekly. Eight (9%) people had at least weekly contact with a district nurse. The service being received regularly by most people was chiropody. Twenty one (22%) people had NHS chiropody, and three had it privately, at least every three months. The services which had been most frequently ever used by the 106 interviewed survivors since the stroke were chiropody, both NHS and private, (30%), district nurses (29%), day centres (24%), local authority home helps (22%) and meals on wheels (16%). These are similar to the findings of other studies at one year, based on a community register of people of all ages (Legh-Smith *et al.* 1986) and at four years (Weddell and Beresford 1979) after the patients had their strokes. In the St Thomas' study, 38% of the subjects reported receiving physiotherapy whilst at home. The weakness of these studies is that it is not possible to compare with non-stroke patients and therefore whether stroke patients are actually utilising more services remains unclear.

The table shows the main services ever received since their stroke by 94 subjects living in private accommodation by their Barthel Index score and disability category at the interview.

| Service | Barthel score and disability category at five years | | | |
|---|---|---|---|---|
| | 0-9 Severe | 10-14 Moderate | 15-19 Mild | 20 Independent |
| Number in each Barthel category | 8 | 13 | 37 | 36 |
| Respite care | 3 | 2 | 0 | 0 |
| Day hospital | 4 | 1 | 4 | 1 |
| Meals on wheels | 0 | 4 | 7 | 3 |
| Local authority home help | 2 | 3 | 9 | 6 |
| Day/luncheon centre | 4 | 5 | 11 | 2 |
| District nurse | 4 | 6 | 9 | 6 |

Combining information from the Barthel scores with the service provision provides a basis for estimating the needs of these patients. For example, half the 94 interviewed patients at home needed help with bathing, but only 25 patients reported ever having seen a district nurse.

Respite care is provided only for the most disabled patients but only five out of twenty one people living at home with a Barthel score less than fourteen had actually received it. The day centre appeared to be used by more mildly disabled patients and the day hospital by more severely disabled patients. The district nurses had contact with all categories of disability, though what they actually did for each group is likely to have varied greatly.

There are many factors which determine the level of service provision required by a stroke patient. Legh-Smith *et al.* (1986) found that the level of disability and the presence or absence of a carer influenced the level of service provision. The presence of a carer would be expected to influence different services in different ways. For example, the carer may provide the meals and do the cleaning and shopping for a very disabled patient who therefore does not require those services from elsewhere. However, because the patient is at home and not in an institution the patient and carer may require nursing help with bathing. A mildly disabled patient without a carer may require meals on wheels and a home help to allow them to stay in their own home.

Clark and Opit (1994) used data from the OPCS disability surveys to estimate the level of services received by people aged over 65 years who had suffered a stroke. They estimated the percentages of stroke patients receiving various services by living conditions and by the intensity of support required. For example, they estimated that 11% of people living alone who needed no or little care received meals on wheels compared with 3% of those who lived with others. This increased to 25% for people living alone with long-interval care needs and 40% for those with short or critical-interval care needs. The percentages for the same groups who lived with others were 3% and 5% respectively. For respite care the percentages were 1%, 9% and 19% for patients living with others who needed little or no care, long-interval care, or short or critical-interval care respectively.

In the St Thomas' study, nearly all of the most disabled people had had an adaptation of some sort for their home. Half of the interviewed cohort had had an adaptation. The most frequent adaptations were grab rails in the bathroom or toilet. The most disabled patients were also much more likely to have an aid or appliance than those who had a mild disability or were functionally independent. Nearly three quarters of the cohort had an aid or appliance. This was usually to help with mobility. Although not directly comparable, Weddell and Beresford (1979) found that four years after their stroke 52% of patients were using aids or adaptations.

A recent study of severely disabled people living on low incomes (Phillips 1995) used data from the Independent Living Fund. The latter is a charitable trust which provides direct financial aid to people meeting certain financial and physical dependency criteria. The average age of the 231 people with a diagnosis of stroke was 70 years and 15% lived alone. Forty eight per cent of the people received care from district nurses, 28% from the voluntary sector and 41% had a local authority home help. Forty two per cent received help from private agencies. The average total number of formal hours of care for each stroke patient was 6.8 hours per week. Of this, 2.5 hours was provided by private agencies, 2.7 hours by district nurses and 1.1 hours by local authority home helps. It was a surprising finding that the private agencies were used so frequently by this group of low-income people. Half of the stroke patients were receiving no formal care from district nurses or local authority home helps. This emphasises the important part informal carers play in filling in the gaps provided by the formal services.

*Who is providing the care?*

As highlighted above, informal carers are providing a great deal of support to stroke patients. Greveson *et al.* (1991) assessed the carers of ex-hospital patients who had suffered their stroke at least three years earlier. The median age of the 44 carers interviewed was 62 years with a range of 29 to 83 years. Of these, 84% lived with the patient and 69% were female. Most of the carers were the patients' spouses (66%) or their children (20%). Using the Nottingham Health Profile, it was found that carers had more problems with emotional reaction, sleep and social isolation than expected from age and sex-matched norms. Using the Caregiver Strain Index, it was found that 13 of 44 carers had evidence of marked strain. The Caregiver Strain Index (Robinson 1983) is made up of 13 separate statements about caring. The individual questions could be used to identify particular problems that carers face. In the community-based study at St Thomas', the patients identified 50 carers, 36 of whom completed the Caregiver Strain Index. The three statements that over half the carers agreed with were related to the changes in the patient, upsetting patient behaviour and changes to personal plans.

## Executive summary and priorities for research

The longer-term outcome of stroke is not well defined and it has been difficult to assess as age and concurrent illnesses also affect outcome assessment. Studies have measured resultant disability but paid little attention to quality of life or the carer perspective. Without adequate assessment of the needs of stroke survivors in the longer term, appropriate services cannot be provided.

Although there are limited data on longer-term outcomes, they have all been part of research projects. The resources required and feasibility of regularly assessing these stroke patients in a defined population has not been estimated.

In a survey in south London, the vast majority of stroke survivors, years after their stroke, lived in private accommodation, and the most disabled were only likely to be in private accommodation if they had an identified carer. One-third of survivors were severely or moderately disabled and two-fifths of survivors were more disabled than they had been at three months after their stroke. Respite care was received by only a few people. Nearly 75% had an adaptation to the environment and 75% were prescribed treatments aimed at preventing further vascular events. Twenty three per cent were depressed and a further 14% had borderline depression scores. The assessment of quality of life suggested that the patients' scores on the various scales were related to their residual disability.

Data from the Independent Living Fund suggests that half of all stroke patients are receiving no formal care from district nurses or local authority home helps. This emphasises the important part informal carers play in filling the gaps in formal service provision.

The priorities for research and service provision are considered below.

1. The assessment of outcome, and need for services, in the longer term is required using stroke register populations. Prospectively collected data on acute care and rehabilitation should enable an assessment of the importance of these interventions on outcome.

2. The longer-term outcome by subtype of stroke requires clarification.

3. The development of appropriate outcome tools which quantify disability, quality of life and the effect on families and carers is required which can be used by health care professionals in the service rather than research setting.

4. The development of a minimum data set is required for use in routine clinical practice for the purpose of longer-term follow up.

5. The development and evaluation of multisectoral collaborative services are required.

6. The evaluation of the most clinically and cost-effective ways of providing respite care is required.

# References

Clark I, Opit L. The prevalence of stroke in those at home and the need for care. J Public Health Med 1994; 16: 93-6.

Dennis M, Burn J, Sandercock P, Bamford J, Wade D, Warlow C. Long-term survival after first-ever stroke: The Oxford Community Stroke Project. Stroke 1993; 24: 796-800.

Ebrahim S. Clinical epidemiology of stroke. 1990 Oxford University Press.

Gresham G, Phillips T, Wolf P, McNamara P, Kannel W, Dawbes T. Epidemiologic profile of long-term stroke disability: The Framingham Study. Arch Phys Med Rehab 1979; 60: 487-91.

Greveson G, Gray C, French J, James O. Long-term outcome for patients and carers following hospital admission for stroke. Age Ageing 1991; 20: 337-44.

Legh-Smith J, Wade D, Langton-Hewer R. Services for stroke patients one year after stroke. J Epidemiol Community Health 1986; 40: 161-5.

Phillips VL. Community care for severely disabled people on low incomes. BMJ 1995; 311: 1121-3

Robinson B. Validation of a caregiver strain index. J Gerontol 1983; 38: 344-8.

Wade D, Langton Hewer R. Functional abilities after stroke: measurement, natural history and prognosis. J Neurol Neurosurg and Psychiatry 1987; 50: 177-82.

Wade D, Legh-Smith J, Hewer R. Depressed mood after stroke: A community study of its frequency. Br J Psychiatry 1987; 151: 200-5.

Weddell J, Beresford S. Planning for stroke patients: a four year descriptive study of home and hospital care. HMSO 1979, London.

Wolfe C, Taub N, Woodrow J, Richardson E, Warburton F, Burney P. Does the incidence, severity, or case fatality of stroke vary in southern England? J Epidemiol Community Health 1993; 47: 139-43.

World Health Organisation. The International Classification of Impairments, Disabilities and Handicaps. 1980 WHO, Geneva.

Zigmond A, Snaith R. The Hospital Anxiety and Depression Scale. Acta Psychiat Scand 1983; 67: 361-70.

# CHAPTER 14

# THE NEEDS OF FAMILIES AND CARERS OF STROKE PATIENTS

*Frances Bunn*

**Chapter outline**

# Introduction

Traditionally, the medical emphasis of stroke care has been on short-term inpatient care with early rehabilitation, generally while the patient is still in hospital (Evans et al. 1992). Part of the hospital culture is of cure rather than long-term care. The longer-term needs of stroke sufferers and their carers have tended to be neglected (Power 1989). Recently there has been an increasing emphasis on the care of stroke patients in the community, with shorter stays in hospital. However it needs to be remembered that in the community much care is undertaken by the family and other informal carers (Briggs 1985; Bonney 1984). Of those stroke patients living at home, that is not in an institution, as many as 79% may live with a carer (Legh-Smith *et al.* 1986). "In practice, informal care has become the cornerstone of policies for health care in the United Kingdom" (Anderson 1988). Brocklehurst *et al.* (1981) found that the largest group of carers were women aged less than 60, with over one-quarter of them having responsibility for other people. In all cases more than half of the chief carers were the patients' spouses. Wade *et al.* (1986) found that the main carer for stroke patients was a spouse for 85%, a son or daughter for 8%, a brother or sister for 4% and a more distant relative or a friend for 2%. Anderson (1992) looked at whom stroke patients identified as the person who helped them most when they were at home; 32% said it was their spouse, 39% a child, 9% a friend, 6% a sibling, and 6% someone else.

# Problems for informal carers

There is no shortage of literature highlighting the sort of problems that stroke sufferers and their carers are likely to face. Wade *et al.* (1986), in a longitudinal study of a community sample of 302 patients in the Bristol area, found significant depression in 11-13% of carers over the first two years after stroke. Carnwath and Johnson (1987) found 39% of spouses of stroke patients were depressed compared with 12% of the control group. Depression in carers may also affect the stroke sufferers themselves, as they may receive less than optimal care if their carer is depressed (Evans *et al.* 1991). Increased levels of anxiety in carers may also be a consequence of stroke, with one study finding increased anxiety to be the most commonly reported change in caregivers after caring for stroke survivors for six months (Wade *et al.* 1986).

The physical and cognitive changes brought about by stroke have been shown to have a substantial effect on the family, influencing marital relations (Williams 1986), family members' health (Brocklehurst *et al.* 1981) and social functioning (Robinson *et al.* 1985). Williams (1994), in a small study of carers of stroke sufferers, found that irritability and demanding behaviour were cited by carers as particular problems. This contrasts with Alzheimer's where carers cite wandering and violent behaviour as the major problems. Findings such as these highlight the need to look at carers of stroke patients specifically and not just at the needs of carers in general. Brocklehurst (1981) found that deterioration in the chief carer's health was common during the first year and Mumma (1986), in a study of losses as a result of stroke, found that a majority of spouses who were carers reported one or more health problems. Enterlante and Kern (1995), in a small pilot study (sample size 10) that looked at wives, reported role changes following a husband's stroke. They found that wives' responsibilities increased after their husbands' stroke and that the wives were more unhappy with their marriages after the stroke.

As well as the documented adverse effects on physical health and well-being, informal carers may face social and financial worries. Loss of social life may affect three-quarters of carers and have adverse financial effects on over half (Holbrook 1982). One study found that 14% of those who had been employed at the time of the stroke subsequently had to give up work (Brocklehurst *et al.* 1981). In a small study of 20 carers of stroke patients, Periard and Ames (1993) found that it was the changes to established patterns of daily life that caused much carer strain; they say "many lifestyle changes were perceived as being precipitated by either actual physical confinement or lack of sufficient blocks of time to engage in activities such as personal care, leisure, and church or community participation". As well as the detrimental effects on the carers' physical and mental well-being, caregiver-related problems can have a collective effect on the stroke sufferer's rehabilitation outcome (Evans *et al.* 1991).

It would seem then that there are many studies which show anxiety, depression and other problems in carers. Yet as Anderson (1987) points out: 'We should study more the quality of life and suffering of carers and not just whether they have clinical indicators of stress. In this broader perspective the importance for the carer's life of the physical aspects of the patient's disability and the effectiveness of the statutory services might become clearer.'

**249**

## Statutory service provision for informal carers

It is difficult to make generalisations about the provision of services for stroke patients and their carers because of the variation that exists from one area of the country to another. Provision of services after discharge from hospital can be poor and indeed patients may feel abandoned once away from the hospital situation (McLean *et al.* 1991). National Health Service provision includes day hospitals, respite care, district nurses, community psychiatric services and nursing homes. Social service provision includes meals on wheels, home helps, occupational therapy assessments and provision of aids, social workers and residential and sheltered housing. To what extent stroke patients and their informal carers receive these services will be discussed further. There is now new legislation to oblige local authorities to assess carers' needs.

In a sample of 436 stroke patients from the Frenchay health district, Legh-Smith *et al.* (1986) found that 38% of those at home were visited by one or more community services, the major ones being district nurse, home help and meals on wheels. Day centres were also used by 42 patients. However, 57 (19%) disabled patients were being looked after at home without any outside help, and patients with carers were much less likely to receive help from the community services. This may indicate that services are refused by carers, that they are not provided for carers, or that the services provided are not those required by the carers. In a follow up five years after stroke of 106 surviving patients, Wilkinson found that 29% were receiving or had at some time in the last five years received a district nurse, 16% meals on wheels, and 22% home help. At the time of interview of the 96 patients in private accommodation, seven were receiving meals on wheels weekly, 15 council home help, eight district nurse services and 16 were visiting a day centre at least once a week (Chapter 13).

McLean *et al.* (1991), in a pilot study of 20 stroke patients and their carers, found that the services most appreciated by the carers were those of the district nurse and the home help, although they did find a variation in satisfaction with these services. Indeed one study found only 25% of carers felt that professionals understood their problems (Nolan and Grant 1989). Various studies have looked at the caseloads of district nurses and the percentage of stroke patients they see as part of their overall workload. Estimates have varied from 11% (Kratz 1978), to 6% (Poulton 1981) to 12% (Hudson and Hawthorn 1989). A strong association has been found between needing help with bathing and seeing the district nurse (McLean *et al.* 1991) and much of this bathing may be done by auxiliary nursing staff (Gibbon 1994). However, more recent policy has seen district nurses moving away from helping patients bath and wash, with care workers employed by social services now often performing this function. It might therefore be reasonable to assume that stroke patients may now make up less of the district nurse caseload than previously thought. Gibbon (1994), in a study of district nurses' perceived role in stroke care, found that district nurses generally became involved in the care of stroke patients when the patient or the carer was no longer able to cope. District nurses spend little time on advice giving and counselling (Ross 1985).

Carers have been found to place great value on respite care (McLean *et al.* 1991, Nolan and Grant 1989). However, studies have found that stroke sufferers may receive little respite care. Jones and Vetter (1985) found, in a sample of 267 carers of elderly dependants, that less than half reported having a break of a few days away from the dependant within the past year. Wilkinson found that only 5% of his sample had received respite care within the previous five years. Lack of sufficient regular respite has also been found to be a problem by others (Nolan and Grant 1989). Neither the Nolan and Grant study or the Maclean *et al.* study had randomised samples.

Although many stroke sufferers are cared for at home, increasing numbers of disabled elderly stroke survivors are being discharged from hospital to private nursing homes. Gladman *et al.* (1991) found that most of the patients in their study who went to nursing homes were severely disabled on discharge from hospital and the Barthel scores of the survivors showed no significant change after four months. They also identified high levels of emotional distress and loneliness using the Nottingham Health Profile.

## Voluntary and non-statutory provision of services for carers

The main voluntary sector provider of services for stroke patients and their carers is The Stroke Association. It is a charitable organisation concerned solely with stroke. It provides a nationwide advisory service from CHSA House in London which deals with over 16,500 calls per year. It produces a range of publications and cassettes to help patients and their carers to understand stroke and its effects and it makes welfare grants to help in cases of financial need. The Stroke Association also has 32 information centres throughout England and Wales which provide advice and information and supply all Stroke Association literature and cassettes (in Scotland the charity remains under the old name of Chest, Heart and Stroke Association and is separate from England and Wales). The need for information for patients and carers is cited by various studies, as is dissatisfaction with the often poor provision of such information. Richardson *et al.* (personal correspondence) found that of 158 GPs and health workers in the Lewisham area, 75% had heard of The Stroke Association but that only 33% of their departments/wards/surgeries carried Stroke Association literature. As the level of knowledge and awareness of The Stroke Association among GPs and health service workers is high in comparison to that of patients (75% to 46%) it would seem that the information is not being disseminated from general practices and hospital wards. Wilkinson, in a five-year follow up, found that only 9% of his sample had received help from The Stroke Association in the previous five years. Considering the general dissatisfaction with the provision of information, it may be that The Stroke Association needs to look at its facilities for disseminating information.

The Stroke Association also provides support for dysphasic patients and their families. There can be many problems associated with dysphasia (Williams and Freer 1986). The Stroke Association has approximately 4000 trained volunteers who complement the work of speech and language therapists. These Dysphasic Support volunteers will visit people in their own homes to help them with communication. They also organise group meetings where interests can be shared and hobbies revived. A study looking at the first 63 such Dysphasic Support schemes, involving 5880 patients, reported that improvements in speech and general confidence were observed in the majority of patients (Eaton Griffith and Pepys 1991). A small study found that patients attending group meetings showed little definite improvement in speech and that the benefits of the club seemed to be largely social (McDonald 1983). A further study in Leeds did find benefits from the Dysphasic Support service, with improved Frenchay Activities Index scores in those who participated in the scheme compared to the control group (Geddes and Chamberlain 1994). The authors concluded that users of the service are more likely to make a better social and functional recovery. They also found that twice as many carers of users of the service had more free time for themselves compared to the control group. The utilisation and value of groups for stroke patients and their carers will be looked at further later.

The Stroke Association also provides family support services (SFSS). There are 43 family support organisers in England and Wales. They visit people at home and provide information, literature and emotional support for stroke patients and their carers/families. They aim to visit hospital wards regularly to make contact with people who have had a stroke and work closely with hospital staff. In the community, referrals generally come from health professionals, social workers and home helps. A recent evaluation of this service has been done in Lewisham. Of 158 GPs and health service workers questioned, only 33% were aware that there was a stroke family support service organiser in Lewisham and only 15% had ever referred a patient to the SFSS. Only one person seen by the SFSS in this study was a community referral. However, 92% of the sample saw this service as being valuable to stroke patients, which would seem to indicate a willingness to use this service. The generally favourable opinion of such a service but somewhat poorer uptake would seem to indicate a need for publicising the service more, especially in the community. Those patients who had been contacted by the SFSS were generally happy with the service and the majority would recommend it (Richardson *et al.* 1995, Personal Communication).

The Stroke Association also helps set up local stroke clubs (over 500 in England and Wales) and provides advice and support for these. Stroke clubs provide support for patients with all types of disability and help to combat feelings of isolation. Different clubs have different activities - some offer therapy, others are just social, but all are friendly and helpful.

Crossroads is another voluntary organisation that offers support to carers. It has approximately 250 branches across the country, and offers respite to carers. The amount of support offered and the waiting list may vary from one area of the country to another. Assessing the effectiveness of some voluntary services is difficult because of the variation from one area of the country to another.

## Needs of informal carers

It is not only the provision of help with personal care and activities of daily living that stroke sufferers and their families require. A need has been shown for more personal support for carers, more information about stroke, and the provision of counselling for stroke patients and their families (Wade *et al.* 1986; McLean *et al.* 1991). Wade *et al.* (1986) conclude that "increased personal support such as that given by stroke support groups may be more important than extra physical support in reducing depression in the carers". It has also been found that regression in self-care activities can be seen in stroke patients when they are discharged home to the primary carer (Andrews and Stewart 1979). This has been blamed on a lack of preparation of carers and a lack of confidence (Anderson 1992), leading to overprotection of the stroke sufferer by family members (Garraway *et al.* 1980; Brocklehurst *et al.* 1981)

American research has shown benefits from the use of support groups, such as the provision of information and the contact they provide with others in a similar situation (Bishop 1986; Kanan *et al.* 1985). Many of these studies have concentrated on groups for carers of patients with Alzheimer's, such as that by Kanan *et al.* (1985). However, little research into self-help groups has been undertaken in Britain (Anderson 1988). Langford (1987) says that "a small group approach allows patients to come together, share experiences, and provide each other with support". Some studies have been performed to look at the effect of groups on stroke patients and their families. However, the numbers in the studies has often been small and there has been no control group. Printz-Fedderson (1990), an American researcher, looked at the group process effect on caregiver burden. She analysed responses from 21 patients in the control group and 17 in the experimental group. The experimental group, however, was drawn from the mailing list of a stroke club and this would obviously bias the sample. The hypothesis was that there would be less caregiver burden in those caregivers who participated in a stroke club than those who did not. She did not however find any significant difference between the groups, although users of the group cited its importance as a source of emotional support and friendship. Pasquarello (1990), in another American study, looked at the use of a stroke recovery group for inpatients. She reported a favourable response to the group from the families of stroke sufferers. However, this group was not well evaluated as all patients could participate in the group and there was no control.

There is some evidence that those who join groups tend to be more educated, female, elderly and 'socially competent' (Brauskaerts 1987). Those families most in need of the support of groups are unlikely to participate (Evans and Baldwin 1989). These authors found that persons with signs of depression seldom participate. However, it was practical problems such as a lack of transport that were the most important factors in preventing families attending support groups. Anderson (1988) found that only 8% of patients in his study of stroke sufferers in the Greenwich area reported that they had received help from a church or voluntary group in the first nine months after their stroke. Only about 3% of patients from his sample of 176 reported that they had been to the local stroke club, although about 11% were aware that the group existed. Of those who had not been to the club, 44% thought that it was a good idea, but only 33% thought that they would go, with a further 4% being uncertain. Those over 75 years of age were less likely to think that they would go, as were more disabled patients. Fifteen per cent of the carers of the stroke sufferers reported that they had been to a social or group meeting for the relatives or friends of stroke patients; and a third of supporters who did not already attend such a group thought they would go if a group was available. It might therefore be inferred that although self-help groups can be of great benefit to many stroke sufferers and their families, they are not necessarily the answer for everyone. It would also seem that there needs to be more work done on the benefits of groups for stroke patients, with special reference made to making such groups relevant to all stroke patients regardless of age, sex or disability.

The educational needs of stroke patients and their carers have also been looked at as an area of importance; although this interest has been emphasised more in the American nursing literature than in the British nursing press. Clark and Rakowski (1983) point out that "family members may be responsible for interpreting the needs of the stroke patient, functioning as liaisons with the healthcare team, and assuming responsibility for caregiver tasks that include the management of health problems". Caregivers may want information on the type of impairment, type of treatment and type of resources available, as well as wanting to know about the sort of emotional responses to expect (Hirst and Metcalf 1986). Education can also be important as families can play a part in the prevention of recurrence (Goldberg and Berger 1988). Evans *et al.* (1988) conducted a randomised controlled study of intervention with families of stroke patients. They looked at the benefits of counselling and education after stroke; they had a sample size of 188, with 63 patients in the control group, 61 in the group receiving counselling and 64 receiving education. They found that counselling and education significantly improved caregiver knowledge, family problem solving, communications, and global family functioning, though counselling was more effective than education alone and resulted in better patient adjustment at one year.

Vanetzian and Corrigan (1995) feel that nurses are in an ideal position to educate carers of stroke patients, but also that the teaching should continue after discharge from hospital. Kernich and Robb (1988) looked at the development of a stroke family support and education program in an American hospital. Families filled out evaluation forms about the group and a favourable response was recorded. Again however, the programme was not properly evaluated and so it is difficult to draw conclusions from this work. Braithwaite and McGown (1993), in an Australian study, observed that carers who are seen as emotionally unstable may not be given information because the medical and nursing staff doubt their capacity to absorb information. In their study though, they found that so called emotionally unstable carers were as capable of learning about stroke as those who were emotionally stable. They do point out though that carers may be more responsive to learning when the initial shock has worn off. This would seem to indicate the importance of education for the carers even after discharge from hospital. It has been pointed out that it is important to remember that adults with different experiential backgrounds have learning needs that may differ from the goals of the educator (Brookfield 1986).

# Executive summary and priorities for research

In recent years there has been an increasing, but unproven, emphasis on the need for stroke services managed in the community. The strategists and health service planners have not considered the considerable proportion of care undertaken by carers and families. As a result of the pressures, carers suffer from depression and anxiety, and family tensions and financial problems are common. Four main areas of concern to carers can be identified through the literature. Carers want information, skills training, emotional support and regular respite. However, these have been highlighted as areas of major deficiency in informal carers' interactions with professionals. Carers frequently mentioned a failure of agencies to supply promised aids or services, a general lack of information and advice, and the provision of irrelevant help. These points obviously have great implications for the type of help offered to carers. The nursing literature does suggest the importance of nurses in information giving and counselling; the support of informal carers must be seen as a legitimate and important focus for nursing interventions. Yet the literature also highlights the fact that on the whole this has not been happening. The literature also cites the benefits of intervention such as support groups for patients and their carers. However, it has also been shown that these may only benefit certain people and there is a lack of proper evaluation of such groups.

The following priorities for research are suggested:

1. The assessment of the need and value of providing information and education for carers and families.

2. The assessment of emotional support and respite care.

3. The evaluation of The Stroke Association Family Support Service and of nurse visitor schemes.

4. The evaluation of the cost of stroke on carers. This should include emotional, financial and physical aspects.

5. Studies on how to improve collaboration between health and social services.

# References

Anderson R. The unremitting burden on carers. BMJ 1987; 294: 73-74.

Anderson R. The contribution of informal care to the management of stroke. Int Disabil Stud 1988; 10: 107-12.

Anderson R. The aftermath of stroke: The experience of patients and their families. 1992; Cambridge University Press, Cambridge.

Andrews K, Stewart G. Stroke recovery: He can but does he? Rheumat Rehab 1979; 18: 43-8.

Bishop DS, Epstein NB, Keitner GI. Stroke: morale, family functioning, health status, and functional capacity. Arch Phys Med Rehab 1986; 67: 85-7

Bonney S, Who cares in Southwark? Association of Carers; 1984 Rochester.

Braithwaite V, McGown A. Caregivers emotional well-being and their capacity to learn about stroke. J Adv Nurs 1993; 18: 195-202.

Brauskaerts J. Self-help and chronic illness. Report of a WHO meeting in Leuwen, Belgium, January 1987.

Briggs. Who cares? Association of Carers. 1985 Rochester.

Brocklehurst JC, Morris P, Andrews K, Richards B, Laycock P. Social effects of stroke. Soc Sci Med 1981; 15:35-9

Brookfield S. Understanding and facilitating adult learning. San Francisco: Jossey-Bass 1986.

Carnworth, Johnson D. Psychiatric morbidity among spouses of patients with stroke. BMJ 1987; 294: 409-11.

Clark NM, Rakowski W. Family caregivers of older adults: Improving helping skills. Gerontologist 1983; 23: 637-42.

Eaton Griffith V, Pepys E. Pioneering scheme helps stroke patients to speak again. Care Elderly 1991; 3: 74-8.

Enterlante T, Kern J. Wives reported role changes following a husbands stroke: A pilot study. Rehab Nurs 1995; 20: 155-60.

Evans RL, Baldwin D. Factors affecting decision to participate in caregiver support groups. Arch Phys Med Rehab 1989; 70-87.

Evans RL, Bishop DS, Haselkorn JK. Factors predicting satisfactory home care after stroke. Arch Phys Med Rehab 1991; 72: 144-7.

Evans R, Hendricks R, Haselkorn J, Bishop D, Baldwin D. The family's role in stroke rehabilitation. Am J Physical Med Rehab 1992; 71: 144-7.

Evans RL, Matlock AL, Bishop DS, Stranahan S, Pederson CK. Family intervention after stroke: Does counselling or education help? Stroke 1988; 19: 1243-9.

Garraway WM, Akhtar AK, Prescott RJ, Hockey L. Management of acute stroke in the elderly: preliminary results of a controlled trial. BMJ 1980; 280: 1040-3.

Geddes ML, Chamberlain MA. Improving social outcome after stroke: an evaluation of the volunteer stroke scheme. Clinical Rehab 1994; 8: 116-26.

Gladman J, Albazzaz M, Barer D. A survey of survivors of acute stroke discharged from hospital to private nursing homes in Nottingham. Health Trends 1991; 23: 158-60.

Goldberg G, Berger G. Secondary prevention in stroke: A primary rehabilitation concern. Arch Phys Med Rehab 1988; 69: 32-40.

Hirst SP, Metcalf BJ. Learning needs of caregivers. J Gerontol Nurs 1986; 12: 24-8.

Holbrook M. Stroke: social and emotional outcome: J Royal College of Physicians of London 1982; 16: 100-4.

Hudson M, Hawthorn P. Stroke patients at home: Who cares? NT 1989; 85: 48-50.

Jones, Vetter N. Formal and informal support received by carers of elderly dependants. BMJ 1985; 291: 643-5.

Kanan J, Kempt B., Staples FR *et al.* Decreasing the burden in families caring for a relative with a dementing illness: A controlled study. J Am Geriatr Soc 1985; 33: 664-70.

Kernich KA, Robb G. Development of a stroke family support and education program. J Neurosci Nurs 1988; 3: 193-7.

Kratz CR. Care of the long-term sick in the community. Churchill Livingstone, Edinburgh, 1978.

Langford R. Chronic Illness: a small group approach. Rehab Nurs 1987; 12: 179-87.

Legh-Smith J, Wade D, Langton-Hewer R. Services for stroke patients one year after stroke. J Epidemiol Community Health 1986; 40: 161-5.

McDonald P. A study of the changes in functional communicative abilities of patients following involvement with a volunteer CVA scheme. Proceedings of XIX Congress of International Association of Logopaedics and Phoniatrics. Edinburgh. Folio Phoniatrica 1983; 35: 1014-9.

McLean J, Roper-Hall A, Mayer P, Main A. Service needs of stroke survivors and their informal carers: a pilot study. J Adv Nurs 1991: 16; 559-64.

Mumma CM. Perceived losses following stroke: Rehab Nurs 1986; 11: 19-24.

Nolan MR, Grant G. Addressing the needs of informal carers: a neglected area of nursing practice. J Adv Nurs 1989; 14: 950-61.

Pasquarello MA. Developing, implementing and evaluating a stroke recovery group. Rehab Nurs 1991; 15: 26-9.

Periard M, Ames B. Lifestyle changes and coping patterns among caregivers of stroke survivors. Public Health Nurs 1993; 10: 252-6.

Power P. Working with families: An intervention model for rehabilitation nurses. Rehab Nurs 1989; 14: 73-5.

Printz-Fedderson V. Group process effect on caregiver burden. J Neurosci Nurs 1990; 22: 164-8.

Richardson E, Warburton F, Rudd A, Wolfe C. Evaluation of Stroke Association family support services in an inner London district. Personal Communication.

Robinson R, Bolduc GA, Kubos K. Social functioning assessment in stroke patients. Arch Phys Med Rehab 1985; 66: 496-500.

Ross F. A challenging district. Nurs Mirror 1985; 160: 35-7.

Stockwell F. The unpopular patient. Royal College of Nursing. London 1972.

Vanetzian E, Corrigan B. A comparison of the educational wants of family caregivers of patients with stroke. Rehab Nurs 1995; 20: 149-54.

Wade D, Legh-Smith J, Langton-Hewer R. Effects of living with and looking after survivors of a stroke. BMJ 1986; 293: 418-20.

Williams A. What bothers caregivers of stroke victims? J Neurosci Nurs 1994; 26: 155-61.

Williams SE, Freer CA. Aphasia: Its effect on marital relationships. Arch Phys Med Rehab 1986; 67: 250-2.

Wilkinson P. Personal communication.

World Health Organisation, Pan-European Consensus Conference, Helsingborg, 1995.

# CHAPTER 15

## OUTCOME MEASUREMENT IN STROKE PATIENTS

*Nada Stojcevic, Peter Wilkinson, Charles Wolfe*

**Chapter outline**

## Introduction

The early use of the term outcome referred mainly to the technical result of a diagnostic procedure or treatment episode. However, this clinical approach was found to be inappropriate for many health service activities. The initial broader population-based approaches were concerned with different components of the quality of health care, and the most influential contribution has been that of Donabedian (1980). He separated three aspects of quality of care, namely the structural characteristics of the service, the process of care, and the outcome of the care.

Donabedian's formal definition of outcome was:

**'A change in a patient's current and future health status that can be attributed to antecedent health care'.**

Recently, however, there has been a growing interest in the measurement of outcomes of health care. The National Health Service reforms have brought many changes. Health care professionals wish to ensure that their patients receive optimal services and managers need to make informed choices about resource allocation. Health commissioners and public health physicians want to purchase the most effective services for their population. This has resulted in numerous attempts to measure the outcome of health care.

Outcome can be defined as the overall long-term impact of health interventions both on the population as a whole and on individuals in particular. For an individual patient outcomes range from impact on performance of everyday tasks to social functioning or general quality of life. What is included in 'outcomes' depends on how broadly or narrowly health and the objectives of health care are defined. Moreover, prior factors external to the health care system have a crucial bearing on health outcome. Age, sex and patient's history are the most obvious, but there are other factors such as socio-economic status of an individual, and broader ones such as the proportion of the gross national product spent on health care, general social expenditure, and the quality of social services. There are many difficulties when it comes to the practical issue of measuring outcomes. It is rarely possible to measure outcome directly, and therefore indirect measures are used. The most widely used indices include mortality rates, morbidity measures, routinely collected statistics on health service use, and health status measurements (Bowling 1991).

## Outcome for whom?

Another issue that needs to be addressed is from whose perspective is outcome being measured? Measures can be used by the users of the service and their families, the primary health care team, the hospital team, purchasers, other agencies and the voluntary sector. Within each of these groups there is a heterogeneity of opinion on outcome; eg, in the hospital team, medical, rehabilitation (occupational, speech and physiotherapy), nursing and social worker perceptions on outcome have to be considered. Long (1995) developed an approach looking at the possible process/outcome measures that could be used by various groups involved with the stroke services (Table 1). This GRID approach does tease out the issues, but one could argue that a multidisciplinary team should work together with common objectives and tools to measure these objectives, although this is not often achieved in practice.

## Outcome of stroke

As long ago as 1987, a review of outcome measures in stroke rehabilitation research criticised the lack of use of broader measures. The authors highlighted the limitations of measuring physical recovery and self-care, and suggested that subjective measures of health status and quality of life should be included in assessments (Seale and Davies 1987). Increasing a patient's quality of life is an important target of rehabilitation. Ebrahim (1990) suggested that this may be equated with reducing handicap and that assessments of quality of life and of handicap for stroke patients may be more relevant than changes in impairment or disability.

This framework for measurements of outcome is the World Health Organisation's classification of impairments, disabilities and handicaps. The fundamental concept behind it is a definition of a disease in terms of its consequences. Thus, any illness can be considered at four levels (planes of experience): pathology, impairment, disability and handicap (WHO 1980).

Table 1: Long (1995)

| Defining group | User/ carer | Primary care team | Hospital team | Commissioner |
|---|---|---|---|---|
| Reasons for interest | At risk of stroke<br>Has had stroke<br>Recovery from stroke<br>Long-term disability | Responsible for prevention<br>Diagnosis and referral in acute stage<br>Long-term care<br>Pastoral care<br>Purchasing | Acute care of patient<br>Assessment, planning, treatment and evaluation<br>Rehabilitation<br>Co-ordinates care | Health of population<br>Allocation of resources<br>Purchasing<br>Monitoring<br>Evaluation |
| Desired outcomes | Reduced risk of stroke<br>Early diagnosis and treatment<br>No complications<br>Minimal disability and handicap<br>Good quality of life<br>Support at all stages | Low incidence of stroke<br>Accurate diagnosis and quick transfer to appropriate unit<br>Good communication, co-ordination of care<br>Effective rehabilitation<br>Patient returns home<br>Minimal disability<br>Minimal anxiety and stress | Effective assessment procedures acceptable to all professionals<br>No complications<br>Minimal disability<br>Good communications with primary care team<br>Patient and carer satisfied and understand illness<br>Patient returns home | Effective health promotion/ prevention<br>Low incidence and prevalence of stroke<br>Effective treatment<br>Appropriate length of hospital stay<br>Appropriate discharge destination<br>Care co-ordinated<br>Cost-effective care package |
| Possible outcome and measures/ indicators | Disability and handicap measures<br>Quality of life measures<br>Patient satisfaction | Stroke incidence<br>Mortality<br>Time to transfer to hospital<br>Disability and handicap measures<br>Patient satisfaction<br>Co-ordinated care | Mortality<br>Complication rate<br>% assessed at one week<br>Incontinence at one week<br>Discharge destination<br>Disability<br>Handicap<br>Patient satisfaction | % Hypertensives treated<br>Incidence, mortality<br>Length of stay<br>Disability<br>Handicap<br>% Discharged home<br>% Patients on aspirin<br>% With key worker<br>% Attending day centre<br>Stroke register in use |

# Impairment, disability and handicap

*(also see Chapter 1)*

Pathology represents a chain of causal circumstance which gives rise to changes in the structure or functioning of the body. Symptoms and signs are the manifestation of these changes, and as such the components of the medical model of disease. In behavioural terms, an individual becomes aware of his/her unhealthiness.

*Impairment represents disturbance at the organ level:* 'In the context of health experience, an impairment is any loss or abnormality of psychological, physiological, or anatomical structure or function.'

*Disability represents a departure from the norm for an individual:* 'In the context of health experience, a disability is any restriction or lack (resulting from an impairment) of ability to perform an activity in the manner or within the range considered normal for a human being.'

*Handicap is a social consequence of a disease:* 'In the context of health experience, a handicap is a disadvantage for a given individual, resulting from an impairment or a disability, that limits or prevents the fulfilment of a role that is normal (depending on age, sex, social and cultural factors) for that individual.'

This model suggests a hierarchy between impairment, disability and handicap, with handicap being the worst consequence of disease. It also suggests a linear relationship between each dimension. However, this is not always the case. In some circumstances a condition may not cause any disability but is nonetheless handicapping. For example, acne vulgaris does not interfere with the ability to carry out any task but may interfere with carrying out roles in life, such as meeting new people.

It is important, therefore, to understand the relationship between impairments, disabilities and handicaps, to be able to measure more precisely the outcome of health care. This relationship is not always direct, and it is possible to have improvements in impairment, without any in handicap. The target of treatments must not be directed solely at the biological end of disease consequences, and measurements of outcome must include measurements of disability, handicap and impairment.

As mentioned earlier, measurement of outcome of health care is becoming increasingly important. This is especially true for the outcome of care which consumes large amounts of the NHS budget, such as the care of stroke patients. Apart from the cost and cost-effectiveness of stroke care, there are other important applications of stroke outcome measurements. They are useful for clinical purposes (diagnostic and treatment purposes), in research, such as in trials of the effectiveness of new treatments, or in studies of the natural history and prognosis of the disease.

Using WHO's classification of impairments, disabilities and handicaps (WHO 1980), the outcome of stroke can be examined in relation to its consequences. Wade (1986) has identified a wide range of impairments caused by stroke that may lead to different levels of disabilities and handicaps. The main impairments are cognitive loss, communication loss, motor loss and sensory loss. These basic deficits lead to a wide range of disabilities related to self-care, mobility and continence (Chapters 1 and 4).

## Criteria for stroke outcome measures

According to Wade (1986), the ideal stroke outcome measure should be valid (measuring what it is intending to measure), reliable (with as little inter-observer and short-term test/retest variability as possible), sensitive to clinically relevant changes, simple to administer, and communicable to non-specialists. When deciding on which outcome measure to use, the investigator should assess whether to use a disease-specific or broad-ranging instrument; the type of scoring the instrument is based on; the validity, reliability and sensitivity of the scale; the appropriateness of the instrument for the study population; and the acceptability of the instrument to the group under study (Hunt et al. 1986).

From a clinical viewpoint the measures of interest have focused mainly on survival, recurrence of stroke, physical recovery and the occurrence of complications (Chapters 1 & 4). But interest in more general outcomes, eg, the quality of life, is developing. The drawback of general measures is that it may be more difficult to equate a particular finding with either the structure or process involved in the care. A search of the medical literature for quality of life scales reveals a vast array of possible instruments. This area of work suffers from investigators devising new measures rather than using those already available. Many of the instruments have not been adequately assessed for validity and reliability.

# Examples of outcome measures for stroke

Literally dozens of outcome measures have been used for both research and clinical assessment purposes for stroke. This chapter does not intend falling into the trap of listing all the potential measures. Measures that have been used in the assessment of patients in hospital and community studies in south London over the last few years will be discussed. The practical aspects of using such scales will be discussed.

The UK Clearing House for Health Outcomes has produced a table of the range of scales that have been quoted in the extensive literature and discussed at a meeting of outcome measures for stroke (Table 2).

The following discussion gives some examples of the available outcome measures for stroke patients. The scales do not all fit conveniently into the categories of impairment, disability and handicap that have been advocated.

# General health measurements

These attempt to describe several key dimensions of health. They are of limited use as outcome measures, apart from relating the overall scores of the group on the various different dimensions to overall levels of impairment, disability and handicap.

A large number of general health measures exist. Some of the scales are very broad in the range they attempt to cover, and they may overlap with the measures aimed at assessing function. Some are very long and impractical for use in a battery of tests. A small number have been used with stroke patients. Only a small representative sample will be considered here. The first, the Sickness Impact Profile, is considered by many people to be the 'gold standard' (McDowell and Newell 1987).

The Sickness Impact Profile (SIP) was developed in America and measures the impact of sickness on daily activities and behaviour (Bergner et al. 1981). The items on the SIP were developed after interviewing a wide range of subjects. An anglicised version of the SIP, the Functional Limitations Profile (FLP), has been developed (Patrick et al. 1985). It does not differ greatly from the original in design. Both have 136 Yes/No statements, and the scores are summed for 12 different categories. The categories are ambulation, body care and movement, mobility, household management, recreation and pastime,

## Table 2: Available measures (UKCHHO) Leeds)

| Outcome | Classification | Examples |
|---|---|---|
| **Impairment** | Arousal<br>Motor<br><br>Sensory<br>Cranial nerves<br>Cognition<br><br><br><br><br><br><br>Psychological<br><br>Severity | Glasgow Coma Scale<br>Ashworth Scale, MRC grades, Motricity Index, Motor Club Assessment, Fugl-Myer Assessment<br>Clinical<br>Swallowing, visual acuity, hemianopia<br>PASAT (attention and information processing), BIT (neglect), FAST (asphasia), PICA (communication), RPAB, RBMT (new memory), MMSE (orientation language), CAPE (orientation and learning), BDEA (communication), Weschler Adult Intelligence Scale<br>GHQ, HAD, Wakefield Self-assessment Depression Memory, Beck Inventory, Hamilton Inventory<br>NIH, Canadian, Orgogozo, Scandinavian Stroke Scale, Hemispheric Scale |
| **Disability** | Physical interaction (mobility and personal care)<br><br><br><br>Psychological interaction<br>Global disability | ADL Activities of Daily Living (in excess of 40 identified), Barthel ADL, Index, Gait Speed, Functional Ambulation Categories, FAT (proximal control and dexterity), NHPT (manual dexterity)<br>Hodgkinson Mental Test,RBMT, FAST.<br><br>Extended ADL e.g. Nottingham ADL, Rivermead ADL (RMI), Frenchay Activities Index, SIP, OPCS Disability Scale, FIM. |
| **Handicap** | Orientation, mobility, dependence, self sufficiency, occupation, social integration | NHP, Rankin Score, Life Satisfaction Index, FAI, Nottingham EADL, Jeffrey's Measurement, Edinburgh Rehabilitation Status Scale, Functional Autonomy Measurement, London Handicap Scale, Oxford Handicap Scale. |
| **Multi-dimensional** | Global outcome<br>Quality of life | WHO Handicap Scales, NHP, Quality of Life Well-being Scale, SF-36, Life Satisfaction Index, HOI-Type Stroke Scale. |
| **Other** | Prognostic outcomes<br>Negative outcomes<br><br>Patient / carer satisfaction, expectations etc.<br><br>Process (proxy) outcomes | Incontinence, Conscious level, Allen Score<br>Mortality, complications<br><br>Pound Questionnaire, Caregiver strain index, CHIPS, Kellner's Questionnaire<br><br>Key worker, Stroke unit, Readmissions, Discharge destination, Number of patients on aspirin. |

**Key for Table 2**

| | | | | | |
|---|---|---|---|---|---|
| BDEA | Boston Diagnostic Asphasia Examination | FAI | Frenchay Activities Index | NHPT | Nine Hole Peg Test |
| BIT | Behavioural Inattention Test | FAST | Frenchay Asphasia Screening Test | PASAT | Paced Auditory Serial Addition Test |
| CAPE | Clifton Assessment Procedures for the Elderly | FAT | Frenchay Arm Test | PICA | Porch Index or Communicative Ability |
| CHIPS | Cohen, Hoberman Inventory of Physical Symptoms | FIM | Functional Independence Measure | RBMT | Rivermead Behavioural Memory Test |
| | | GHQ | General Health Questionnaire | | |
| | | HAD | Hospital Anxiety and Depression Scale | RPAB | Rivermead Perceptual Assessment Battery |
| EADL | Extended Activities of Daily Living | MMSE | Mini Mental State Examination | | |
| | | NHP | Nottingham Health Profile | SIP | Sickness Impact Profile |

social interaction, emotion, alertness, sleep and rest, eating, communication and work. Some of these categories can be combined to give overall scores for two dimensions, physical and psychosocial. However, the SIP and FLP sum different categories in calculating these dimensions and cannot be compared directly. The SIP and FLP do not have dimensions for pain or an assessment of subjective feelings about health. These instruments define quality of life purely in behavioural terms. The SIP has been used to assess stroke patients (de Haan *et al.* 1993), but it takes up to 30 minutes to complete.

Two of the most widely used general health questionnaires in the UK are the Nottingham Health Profile (Hunt *et al.* 1980) and the anglicised version of the Short Form 36 (Brazier *et al.* 1992).

### *The Nottingham Health Profile*

The Nottingham Health Profile (NHP) was developed in the UK to measure social and personal effects of illness. It is based on lay perceptions of health status, i.e. it measures perceived health problems (Hunt *et al.* 1980). It assesses subjective rather than objective health problems and as such can be a predictor of need for health services. It is short and easy to complete. The NHP has two parts (Hunt *et al.* 1981). The first part consists of 38 statements with weighted scores in the areas of pain, physical mobility, sleep, energy, social isolation, and emotional reaction, to which a respondent is required to answer yes or no. The second part asks about any effects of health problems on seven areas of daily life: paid employment, jobs around the home, social life, sex life, family relationships, hobbies/interests, and holidays. It does not have weights: a count of affirmative responses is used as a summary statistic. It is not possible to calculate an overall health status score, although aggregation within categories is permitted. The NHP has been much assessed for its validity and reliability (Hunt *et al.* 1985; Bowling 1991). The latter assessments have been satisfactory for the first part but there are reservations about the reliability of the second part.

Ranges of 'normal values' are available for different populations. The NHP has been widely used, including with stroke patients (Ebrahim *et al.* 1986). The NHP has been criticised for being too negative and for not being sensitive to low levels of ill health. From a practical viewpoint, however, it is a widely used and simple measure.

### The Short Form 36

The Short Form 36 (SF-36) was developed from the larger Rand Health Insurance Battery. The original instrument is long and unsuitable for use in routine investigations. The SF-36 is straightforward, takes about five minutes to complete, and measures health along the following dimensions: physical functioning, social functioning, role limitations because of physical and emotional problems, mental health, vitality, pain and general health perception. The SF-36 has not been used with stroke patients, but has been used widely for other groups, including the elderly (Lyons *et al.* 1994). In one study (Brazier *et al.* 1992) the SF-36 identified health problems in people who had good health scores on the NHP. Work on the validity and reliability of the SF-36 is ongoing but has been found to be satisfactory (Brazier *et al.* 1992; Lyons *et al.* 1994). There are reservations about the use of certain questions with the elderly and suggestions for improving this have been made (Hayes *et al.* 1995). This involves minor but significant changes to the wording of five parts of three questions.

### EuroQOL

The EuroQOL is a measure which intends to complement other quality of life measures and to facilitate the collection of a common data set for reference purposes. It can be used in economic assessments of interventions (EuroQol Group 1990). McKenna has found it difficult to use with stroke patients, even with the help of an interviewer, and there is a tendency to respond to the visual analogue scale at random (McKenna 1993).

## Measures of impairment

Physical impairments following a stroke can be assessed by questionnaire or clinical examination. Psychological impairments are more complex and require either more specialist clinical examination or the use of specifically developed instruments.

### The Motricity Index

The Motricity Index measures the extent of motor loss after stroke. It gives an overall indication of a patient's limb impairment. It was developed when it became apparent that a single movement at three arm and three leg joints gave as much information as the complete range of movement at all joints (Demeurisse *et al.* 1980). The three movements assessed for the arm are: pinch grip, elbow flexion and shoulder abduction.

The three movements for the leg are: ankle dorsiflexion, knee extension and hip flexion. With the patient seated, each movement is rated on a five-point scale. The points on the scales are given weighted scores to reflect the significance of each point as a proportion of total recovery. The total 'arm score' is the addition of the scores for the three arm movements; the total 'leg score' is the total score for the three leg movements; and the total 'side score' is the addition of the arm and leg scores, divided by two. One point may be added to each limb score so that the top score is 100%.

The Motricity Index has been shown to be sensitive in detecting early recovery (Sunderland *et al.* 1989). The same study examined its validity, by comparing the results of the Motricity Index with the results obtained using a sensitive electronic dynamometer as a 'gold standard'. The study found a high correlation between the two methods. The Motricity Index has been shown to be reliable, but the inter-rater reliability was tested on a small number of patients (Collin and Wade 1990).

### *The Frenchay Aphasia Screening Test*
The Frenchay Aphasia Screening Test (FAST) was developed to diagnose language loss after stroke (Enderby *et al.* 1987). It has been designed to cover the four major aspects of language which may be disturbed in the aphasic patient: comprehension, expression, reading and writing.

Comprehension is tested using two drawings on either side of the test card. Patients are given instruction, of graded length and linguistic difficulty, to point to various objects, etc. One point is scored for each fully correct response.

Expression is tested by asking the patient to describe the picture on the test card. He/she is given points according to the completeness of his/her response. The patient is also asked to name as many animals as he/she can think of in 60 seconds. The score depends on the total number named.

Reading is tested by giving a patient five written instructions in graded difficulty. Writing is tested by asking a patient to write a description of the picture in a maximum time of five minutes. The score depends upon the number of correctly spelled words used, and the level of grammatical construction used.

The sub-scores are summed. The maximum score is 30. The presence of aphasia is indicated by a score of less than 27 for people aged up to 60, or 25 for people aged over

60. The authors tested the validity and reliability of the FAST (Enderby *et al.* 1987). However, only a small number of patients were used and no further tests have been published.

# Psychological impairments

General health questionnaires often include assessments of factors considered to be emotional. This is not comprehensive enough for a quality of life study. Additional psychological assessments aim to assess cognitive function or the patients' feelings of depression and anxiety.

## *The Mini Mental State Test*

The Mini Mental State Examination (Folstein *et al.* 1975) is a simple and widely used measure for assessing cognitive function. It was originally developed for psychiatric patients (Folstein *et al.* 1975), but has been used with neurological patients (Dick *et al.* 1984; De Paulo *et al.* 1980). The authors found it to be a valid and reliable test of cognitive function. The scale is heavily dependent on verbal function and therefore inappropriate in patients with dysphasia.

## *The Hospital Anxiety and Depression Scale*

Several studies have considered depression in stroke patients. These have often used scales intended to assess the depth of depression (Wade et al 1987). Although stroke patients are known to be at increased risk of depression, psychological measures should consider other impairments such as anxiety. The Hospital Anxiety and Depression Scale (HAD) is a short and simple assessment of anxiety and depression (Zigmond and Snaith 1983). The HAD consists of 14 items on two sub-scales (seven for anxiety and seven for depression). The patients are rated on four-point scales, which represent the degree of distress (0-4). Items are summed on each of the two sub-scales, a maximum score for anxiety and depression separately being 21. For both scales 0-7 is normal, 8-10 borderline, and more than 11 disturbed. The anxiety items are part of the Present State Examination, while the depression items included make no reference to physical problems to ensure that scores are independent of physical illness. The HAD was designed for general medical outpatient use, but has been more widely used, including with stroke patients (Gibson *et al.* 1991).

The validity and reliability of the HAD was found to be satisfactory (Zigmond and Snaith 1983). However, these tests were performed on outpatients between the ages of 16 and 65 attending general medical clinics, and therefore the generalisation of these results is questionable. Measurement of depression is difficult in patients with dysphasia.

## Measures of disability

These functional measures are related directly to any outcome as they reflect what individuals are able to do for themselves. The Barthel Index (Mahoney and Barthel 1965) has been widely used in stroke studies. It is a simple rating scale to assess functional independence and disability. The subjects are assessed for their ability to carry out 10 different self-caring tasks such as dressing, feeding, walking and toileting. Ten different activities are assessed, and different values are assigned to them. The total score is then calculated, the maximum being 20 (totally independent) and the minimum 0 (totally dependent).

The Barthel Index has been criticised for being too simplistic and for being used too widely when it was initially intended only for inpatient assessment. Like other rating scales, a change in the total number of points does not reflect equivalent changes in the level of disabilities across different activities, and undetected changes can occur beyond the endpoints of the scales. The scale also lacks any assessment of the ability to carry out tasks in the community or any measures of communication, mental and emotional factors or of family involvement. The Barthel Index is among the most thoroughly studied scales, and numerous groups have shown it to be a valid and reliable measurement (Wade and Langton Hewer 1987; Wolfe *et al.* 1991). The Barthel has its limitations, but it has become an accepted standard outcome instrument in stroke research at the population level.

### The Rivermead ADL

The Rivermead ADL was developed by Whiting and Lincoln (1980) for assessing activities of daily living in patients following a stroke or head injury. The scale is hierarchical, so that the successive items are progressively more difficult. This characteristic gives the Rivermead ADL an advantage in that the total score obtained reflects not only the severity of disability, but also the actual items which are passed or failed. Therefore it makes it possible to describe a patient's ability on the basis of his/her total score.

The Rivermead ADL was reported to be valid and reliable (Whiting and Lincoln 1980). However, this study was performed on 15 patients only, who were below the age of 65. The scale was re-validated in 1990 (Lincoln and Edmans 1990) for older patients, and the same results were achieved.

# Measures of handicap

## *The Rankin Handicap Scale*

The development of the Rankin scale was based on research into the prognosis of patients with a cerebrovascular accident (Rankin 1957). It was developed to measure independence rather than performance of specific tasks, and in this it incorporates mental as well as physical adaptation to the neurological deficits. The Rankin scale has been modified (UK-TIA Study Group 1988). The original scale has five grades of disability, while the modified one has six grades, ranging from no symptoms to severe disability.

The reliability of the Rankin scale has been reported in several studies (Wolfe *et al.* 1991; Tomasello *et al.* 1982; Van Swieten *et al.* 1988) and it has been shown to be high. There are, however, some reservations about inter-observer variation (Wolfe *et al.* 1991). It is a simple measure, but combines impairment, disability and dependency into one score.

## *The Frenchay Activities Index*

There are several scales intended to measure social networks. This is clearly an important area for an individual, particularly the elderly. The general health instruments measure social isolation and social functioning. A widely used measure of social outcome in stroke research is the Frenchay Activities Index (FAI). This is an unusual instrument, in that it was designed specifically for stroke patients (Holbrook and Skilbeck 1983). The scale collects information about changes to a person's lifestyle over time. In general, ADL scales do not assess an individual's ability to carry out more complex activities such as recreation, hobbies, and social interaction. These activities are related to handicap rather than disability. The FAI asks about domestic chores, leisure and work areas as well as outdoor activities. It is short, quick and can be self or interviewer-completed. Assessments of validity and reliability have been found to be sufficient, although there are suggestions for improving reliability (Schuling *et al.* 1993).

## Assessing carers

Apart from the scales discussed above, some instruments are specific to carers. The Caregiver Strain Index (Robinson 1983) is such an instrument. It is short and simple to complete. It was developed from structured interviews with the carers of hip and heart disease patients, but has been used with the carers of stroke patients (Greveson *et al.* 1991). The validity of the index was found to be satisfactory by its designers. More work is needed on reliability.

## Other possible stroke outcome measures

### Simple questions

As a result of the need to follow up a large number of patients in a trial, Lindley *et al.* (1994) found that by asking two simple questions, by phone or by post, they were able to predict the outcome of stroke reasonably well. The two questions were:

*"In the last two weeks, did you require help from another person for everyday activities?"* and *"Do you feel that you have made a complete recovery from your stroke?"*

The authors compared the responses with an assessment made at interview by a nurse who was blind to the answers to the above questions. The authors found that the help question had a 75% accuracy in identifying patients with a Barthel score of less than 20, and the recovery question had a 90% accuracy for identifying someone with no handicap. The authors concluded that such simple questions could be used to assess outcome after stroke.

### Satisfaction questionnaires

There has recently been an increase in the number of studies addressing consumer satisfaction with stroke services. These aspects of outcome are important as they incorporate the patient and family perspective on services into the outcome assessment. The major problem is their interpretation, as with other satisfaction surveys. It is important to determine what determines satisfaction so that services can be altered. Such questions have to be phrased to keep bias to a minimum. Much work in this area has been undertaken by Pandora Pound at the Royal Free Hospital, London. Pound *et al.* (1994a) found a relatively high level of satisfaction with inpatient care, including communication, and the personal social skills of staff. However, a longitudinal survey of patients' and carers' experiences after stroke reported mixed views (Anderson 1992). Pound *et al.* (1994b) highlighted the need to incorporate the patient's satisfaction with therapy services into any satisfaction questionnaire. The impact of physiotherapy is not confined to reducing physical disability, but may also affect well-being.

## Executive summary and priorities for research

The expectation of the health services is that effective services will be provided. To monitor their effectiveness, the components of quality require monitoring. This chapter focuses on the outcome of care, but this is influenced by factors other than just the health services. An important influence on the move to measure outcome is the Department of Health's priority in this area. Although the authors acknowledge the importance of outcome measurements, their use has to be set in a context. The limitations of the scales currently being used in stroke research to measure what they purport to measure is discussed, and there is a need for a national group, such as the Royal College of Physicians Working Party on Stroke Outcome or the United Kingdom Clearing House on Health Outcomes, to undertake evaluations of recommended scales, in both hospital and the community. There is also a need to produce guidelines.

These are major questions that require resolution. What type of outcome is important? Is it a health outcome or a health service outcome? If it is a health service outcome, will a proxy process measure be a valid substitute in areas where the process has been shown to be effective? Whose outcome is important? Is it the patient, carer, family, or a combination? When is the optimal time to assess outcome, and how feasible is it to assess outcome using different methods (e.g. postal questionnaire, telephone)? What are the implications of measuring outcome at a population level?

Measuring the outcome in routine clinical practice is worthless unless there is an effective intervention one can introduce to improve it. There is a requirement to measure the process of care that contributes to that outcome, in order that purchasers and providers can estimate how much extra resources are required to improve the process of care and consequently the outcome. One could argue that until the health services can adequately assess and provide effective care for stroke patients, measuring the outcome is premature. The development of outcome measures should therefore be in tandem with measuring the process of care, and using process measures as proxy measures of outcome. These concepts are discussed further in the models of care chapter.

**The following are considered priorities for research:**

1. The development of national guidelines on outcome measures, for both patients and carers, that fulfil all the criteria of an effective measure.

2. Further development of effective patient and carer measures which more sensitively estimate outcome, and which can be used in routine practice.

3. The determination of the relationship between the process of stroke care and outcome.

4. The development of proxy measures of outcome based on evidence of effectiveness.

5. The evaluation of the effect of incorporation of these measures into stroke service contracts.

# References

Anderson R. The aftermath of stroke. The experience of patients and their families. Cambridge: Cambridge University Press, 1992.

Bergner M, Bobbitt R, Carter W, Gilson B. The Sickness Impact Profile: development and final revisions of a health status measure. Medical Care 1981; 19: 787-805.

Bowling A. Measuring health: A review of quality of life measurement scales. Milton Keynes, Open University Press, 1991.

Brazier J, Harper R, Jones N, O'Cathain A, Thomas K, Usherwood T Westlake L. Validating the SF-36 health survey questionnaire: new outcome measure for primary care. BMJ 1992; 305: 160-4.

Collin C, Wade D. Assessing motor impairment after stroke: a pilot reliability study. J Neurol Neurosurg Psych 1990; 53: 576-9.

De Paulo JR, Folstein MF, Gordon B. Psychiatric screening on a neurological ward. Psychol Med 1980; 10: 125-32.

de Haan R, Horn J, Limburg M, Van der Meulen J, Bossuyt P. A comparison of five stroke scales with measures of disability, handicap and quality of life. Stroke 1993; 24: 1178-81.

Demeurisse G, Demol O, Robaye E. Motor evaluation in vascular haemiplegia. Eur Neurol 1980; 19: 382-9.

Dick JPR, Guiloff RJ, Stewart A *et al.* Mini-mental state examination in neurological patients. J Neurol Neurosurg Psych 1984; 47: 496-9.

Donabedian A. Exploration in quality assessment and monitoring. Volume 1. The definition of quality and approaches to its assessment.

Ann Arbor, Michigan: Health Administration Press. 1980.

Ebrahim S. Clinical epidemiology of stroke. Oxford University Press, 1990.

Ebrahim S, Barer D, Nouri F. Use of the Nottingham Health Profile with patients after a stroke. J Epidemiol Community Health 1986; 40: 166-9.

Enderby P, Wood V, Wade D. Frenchay Aphasia Screening Test. NFER-Nelson 1987.

EuroQOL Group. EuroQOL - a new facility for the measurement of health-related quality of life. Health Policy 1990; 16: 199-28.

Folstein M, Folstein S, McHugh P. 'Mini-Mental State': A practical method for grading the cognitive state of patients for the clinician. J Psychiat Res 1975; 12: 189-98.

Gibson L, MacLennan W, Gray C, Pentland B. Evaluation of a comprehensive assessment battery for stroke patients. Int J Rehab Research 1991; 14: 93-100.

Greveson G, Gray C, French J, James O. Long-term outcome for patients and carers following hospital admission for stroke. Age Ageing 1991; 20: 337-44.

Hayes V, Morris J, Wolfe C, Morgan M. The SF-36 health survey questionnaire: is it suitable for use with older adults? Age and Ageing 1995; 24: 120-125.

Holbrook M, Skilbeck C. An activities index for use with stroke patients. Age Ageing 1983; 12: 166-70.

Hunt SM, McEwen J, McKenna SP. Measuring health status; a new tool for clinicians and epidemiologists. J Roy Coll Gen Pract 1985; 35: 185-8.

Hunt SM, McEwen J, McKenna SP. Measuring health status. Croom Helm, London 1986.

Hunt SM, McKenna SP, McEwen J, Backett EM, Williams J, Papp E. A quantitative approach to perceived health status: a validation study. J Epidemiol Community Health 1980; 34: 281-6.

Hunt SM, McKenna SP, Williams J. Reliability of a population survey tool for measuring perceived health problems: a study of patients with osteo-arthritis. J Epidemiol Community Health 1981; 35: 297-300.

Lincoln NB, Edmans JA. A re-validation of the Rivermead ADL Scale for elderly patients with stroke. Age Ageing 1990; 19: 19-24.

Lindley R, Waddell F, Livingstone M, Sandercock P, Dennis M, Slattery J, Smith B, Warlow C. Can simple questions assess outcome after stroke? Cerebrovascular Disease 1994; 4: 314-24.

Long AF. Clarifying and identifying the desired outcomes of an intervention: the case of stroke. Outcomes Briefing 1995; 5: 10-2.

Lyons R, Perry H, Littlepage B. Evidence for the validity of the Short Form 36 questionnaire in an elderly population. Age Ageing 1994; 23: 182-4.

Mahoney F, Barthel D. Functional evaluation: The Barthel Index. Maryland State Med J 1965; 14: 61-5.

McDowell I, Newell C. Measuring health: A guide to rating scales and questionnaires. New York, Oxford University Press, 1987.

McKenna S. Commonly used measures of health status in European clinical trials. Br J Med Econ 1993; 6C: 3-15.

Patrick D, Sittampalam Y, Somerville S, Carter W, Bergner M. A cross-cultural comparison of health status values. Am J Public Health 1985; 75: 1402-7.

Pound P, Bury M, Gompertz P, Ebrahim S. Views of survivors of stroke on benefits of physiotherapy. Quality in Health Care 1994b; 3: 69-74.

Pound P, Gompertz P, Ebrahim S. Patients' satisfaction with stroke services. Clinic Rehab 1994a; 8: 7-17.

Rankin J. Cerebral vascular accidents in patients over the age of 60: 2. Prognosis. Scott Med J 1957; 2: 200-15.

Robinson B. Validation of a caregiver strain index. Journal of Gerontology 1983; 38: 344-8.

Schuling J, de Haan R, Limburg M, Groenier KH. The Frenchay Activities Index: Assessment of functional status in stroke patients. Stroke 1993; 24: 1173-7.

Seale C, Davies P. Outcome measurement in stroke rehabilitation research. Int Disability Studies 1987; 9: 155-60.

Sunderland A, Tinson D, Bradley L *et al.* Arm function after stroke. An evaluation of grip strength as a measure of recovery and a prognostic indicator. J Neurol Neurosurg Psych 1989; 52: 1267-72.

Tomasello F, Mariani F, Fieschi C, *et al.* Assessment of inter-observer difference in Italian multi-centre study on reversible cerebral ischaemia. Stroke 1982; 13: 32-4.

UK-TIA Study Group: The UK-TIA aspirin trial: Interim results. BMJ 1988; 296: 316-20.

Van Swieten JC, Koudstaal PJ, Visser MC, Schouten H, van Gijn J. Interobserver agreement for the assessment of handicap in stroke patients. Stroke 1988; 19: 604-7.

Pound P, Bury M, Gompertz P, Ebrahim S. Views of survivors of stroke on benefits of physiotherapy. Quality in Health Care 1994b; 3: 69-74.

Wade DT. Assessing disability after acute stroke. In: Stroke: therapeutic and socio-economic aspects. Clifford-Rose F (ed). Royal Society of Medicine Services Ltd, 1986.

Wade D, Legh-Smith J, Hewer R. Depressed mood after stroke: A community study of its frequency. British J Psych 1987; 151: 200-5.

Whiting S, Lincoln N. An ADL assessment for stroke patients. Br J Occup Ther 1980; Feb: 44-6.

WHO. The international classification of impairments, disabilities and handicaps. WHO, Geneva 1980.

Wolfe C, Taub N, Woodrow J, Burney P. Assessment of scales of disability and handicap for stroke patients. Stroke 1991; 22: 1242-4.

Zigmond A, Snaith R. The Hospital Anxiety and Depression Scale. Acta Psychiatr Scand 1983; 67: 361-70.

# CHAPTER 16

## ECONOMIC EVALUATION OF STROKE CARE

*Roger Beech*

**Chapter outline**

# Introduction

This chapter focuses on financial and economic aspects of stroke care. Firstly, available evidence is presented for assessing the overall costs of stroke care from the perspective of the National Health Service (NHS) of the United Kingdom, from that of an individual hospital, and in terms of the burden of care falling on stroke sufferers and their families or other informal carers. Secondly, the results are presented of economic evaluations of stroke care treatments. These are linked to the primary and secondary prevention of stroke and to the organisation and delivery of services for acute stroke care.

Economic evaluations should consider both the cost inputs and outcomes of care. Previous chapters in this review have presented evidence on the efficacy of interventions for stroke care. This chapter only covers studies that have considered both the costs and outcomes of care, that is studies where a formal economic evaluation was conducted.

# The overall costs of stroke care

A recent Effective Health Care Bulletin (1995) stated that stroke care consumes around 4% of NHS expenditure. This is a widely quoted figure and stems from analysis undertaken by the Office of Health Economics (1988).

Their analysis covered the costs of inpatient treatment, outpatient follow up, and general practitioner consultations for stroke. The estimates excluded home nursing costs and costs of prescribed drugs. Based upon 1985 activity data and costs they estimated that the annual cost of inpatient care for stroke was £532 million in England and Wales. This figure was the product of the overall acute bed days consumed by stroke care during 1985 and the average daily cost of care in an acute bed. Activity data for the period also indicated that stroke care accounted for 0.3% of outpatient referrals or around £1 million per annum based upon the average costs of an acute outpatient consultation. A similar method was used to estimate that consultations for stroke care consumed £6.4 million of GP costs per annum or £13 million if the costs of home visits were allowed for. In total, therefore, the overall costs of stroke care were estimated as nearly £550 million at 1985 prices and activity levels or 3.9% of NHS expenditure in England and Wales.

More recently Isard and Forbes (1992) have estimated the costs of stroke care for the NHS in Scotland. The analysis covered inpatient, outpatient and primary care and community home nursing services for the year 1988. Again, activity data and average cost data were combined to derive estimates of total costs.

They estimated that during 1988 there were 17,932 discharges for stroke. These discharges consumed a total of 169,587 bed weeks at an average cost of £489 per bed week. The overall costs of inpatient care were therefore estimated as £82 million or 5.5% of total hospital expenditure. Annual estimated costs rose to £96 million, or 4.3% of NHS expenditure in Scotland, when the costs of outpatient, primary and community care were included.

They contrasted these findings with the results of a previous study by Carstairs (1976) which had used the same methodology. Carstairs' results, based upon 1974 activity and prices, had indicated that stroke care accounted for 4.7% of NHS expenditure and 6% of hospital running costs. The main reason for the decrease in proportionate costs over the period 1974 to 1988 appears to be that the costs of stroke care increased at a lower rate than those of other NHS services: stroke expenditure increased by 34% whereas NHS expenditure increased by 45%. Indeed, there was a 20% increase in admissions for stroke in Scotland over the period 1974 to 1988.

One of the main findings to come from the study by Isard and Forbes probably relates to the 34% rise in stroke expenditure over the period 1974 to 1988. The demographic effects of an ageing population mean that this trend is likely to continue. Malmgren *et al.* (1989) have predicted that first-in-a-lifetime stroke in England and Wales will increase by 30% in real terms during the period 1983 to 2023. A study of the costs of medical care in the Netherlands (Bergman *et al.* 1995) also predicted that the total costs of stroke care would rise in real terms by 30% during the period 1991 to 2010 due to the effects of an ageing population. That study also found that stroke care accounted for around 4% of total health care costs.

Based upon the findings of these studies it can be concluded that stroke care currently consumes between 4-5% of NHS expenditure. Although this proportion may remain around the same during the next 20 years, there is likely to be a dramatic increase in real terms in the total health service costs consumed by stroke care. It is important that research is undertaken to develop methodologies for predicting what this rise in costs might be given different assumptions about demographic changes and the costs and processes of care for stroke.

The study by Isard and Forbes also estimated that the hospital costs of stroke care were £4,626 per discharge. Wolfe *et al.* (1995) also derived estimates of the average costs per stroke case. Their study focused on admissions to hospitals serving two health districts in southern England, one in an urban setting and the other in inner London. They focused on care received by patients during the year following their first ever stroke. Cost data collected related to inpatient and outpatient acute care, rehabilitation services and GP services. Registers were used to record the amount of care patients received from these various sources. Data on the costs of the care these sources provide, for example, the cost of a physiotherapy session, were obtained from local hospital finance departments and from published sources.

Results based upon 98 admissions in the inner London and 108 admissions in the urban setting indicated costs per case of £3808 in the inner London hospitals and £2649 in the urban hospitals. Inpatient care accounted for 93% of total costs in both settings, a finding in line with the 97% found in a study by the Office of Health Economics (1988), and the 87% found by Isard and Forbes (1992). In terms of the amount of care patients received in the two hospitals, there were no significant differences between them in patient stay but patients in the urban hospital received significantly less rehabilitation and CT scan rates were significantly lower in the urban hospitals. However, unit costs were higher in the inner London hospital and this led to its higher costs per case.

Various factors can influence differences in the costs of stroke care between hospitals. These include differences in the quantity and type of care a 'typical' stroke patient can expect to receive, differences in the prices of services within a hospital which in turn will be linked to factors such as staffing levels and skill mix, and differences between hospitals in the accounting methods they use to derive price information. Without a knowledge of the scale of these factors it is impossible to make meaningful comparisons of the costs of care in different hospitals.

With the current purchaser/provider mechanism for funding the NHS, information on the costs of stroke care in different hospitals, and on the reasons for any variations, has potential value for purchasers and providers. As argued by Sandercock (1993), a knowledge of the way care is currently provided is the first step on the road to improvements in care. For key elements of care, standard approaches are therefore needed for collecting data on the amount of services a stroke patient receives. These key elements include length of stay by bed type, use of major diagnostic and therapeutic interventions, and the amount of rehabilitation care provided. Standard approaches are also needed to identify the resources consumed by these elements of care, for example staff, materials and equipment, and the costs of these resources.

All of the studies referred to above have focused on the cost implications of stroke for services provided by health care agencies. Stroke also has cost implications for patients and their informal carers. These implications include expenditure on goods and services, such as adjustments to the home environment or payment for private cleaning or nursing services, and loss of earnings or time away from normal activities. The importance of quantifying these cost areas has been recognised by the Office of Health Economics (1988) amongst others, but this review of the literature was unable to obtain details of any studies which had documented patient and carer costs for stroke in the United Kingdom.

Some information on these effects can, however, be obtained from a study by Anderson (1992) who followed-up a cohort of 173 admissions for stroke in Greenwich Health Authority. Eighteen months after their stroke, half of the cohort reported having made adaptations to their home. For the majority of stroke sufferers, their main source of help was from family members and other informal carers. Amongst informal carers, 25% had had to change jobs or give up work in order to look after the stroke patient, and 25% reported a financial loss due to factors such as travel expenses or loss of earnings.

Stroke has substantial cost implications for patients and their carers. More information is needed therefore to document the scale and the type of these inputs to care.

## Economic evaluations of interventions for stroke

This section reports the results of studies which have assessed the economic impact of interventions for the primary and secondary prevention of stroke, and for the treatment of acute stroke. As previously stated, the review will only cover studies which have considered both the cost inputs and outcomes of care. Selected studies are discussed in detail to expose the methodologies that are currently used to assess the economic implications of interventions for stroke and to allow readers to judge the reliability of their findings. Costs are given in the currency of the host country of the study.

Before discussing specific studies, a definition of cost-effectiveness would be helpful. A treatment is said to be cost-effective if it leads to lower costs per unit of outcome than alternative treatments, for example, a preventive therapy that had lower costs per stroke prevented or life years gained. If a treatment is more effective, but also more expensive than a relevant alternative the costs of securing an improved outcome are usually reported.

## (a) Primary prevention of stroke

The evidence presented in Chapter 2 indicated that treatments considered to be of significant benefit in the primary prevention of stroke included the treatment of hypertension and the treatment of atrial fibrillation.

Gustafsson *et al.* (1992) assessed the cost-effectiveness of treatment with anticoagulants or aspirin as primary preventive measures for stroke in patients with non-valvular atrial fibrillation. The three strategies considered were the sole use of either anticoagulants or aspirin, or the preferred use of anticoagulant treatment with aspirin given to patients not suitable for anticoagulant treatment. The analysis was based on the introduction of these treatment strategies for the population of Sweden (8.5 million people).

Starting with the overall population, the stages in the analysis were: to identify the number of inhabitants with atrial fibrillation; the number eligible for the different treatment options; the number of strokes prevented because of the option; and the increased number of intracranial haemorrhages resulting as an adverse consequence of anticoagulant treatment. Data to furnish the model used for the analysis were obtained from the results of published trials. Key variables included in the analysis were: the prevalence of atrial fibrillation increased from 0.5% in 50-59 year olds to 8.8% in 80 year olds; 50% of at-risk patients in the age band 50-69 would be suitable for anticoagulant treatment, decreasing to 30% in the 70-80 age band; 90% of patients would be suitable for aspirin treatment; the annual incidence of stroke in patients with non-valvular atrial fibrillation is 5%; anticoagulant treatment reduces the rate of stroke by 64% and aspirin treatment by 25%; and finally three different assumptions were made regarding the effect of anticoagulant treatment on the incidence of intracranial haemorrhage: an increase of 0.3, 1.3 and 2.0%.

Data on the costs of treatment were also obtained from published research. The annual costs per patient for anticoagulant treatment were taken as 5,000 Swedish krona (£530) and of aspirin treatment 100 Swedish krona (£10). These costs include costs incurred by health services and costs incurred by patients such as loss of earnings and travel for treatment costs. The lifetime costs of a stroke were estimated as 180,000 Swedish krona when only health service costs were considered or 270,000 Swedish krona when patient costs and costs such as sickness benefit were included.

The results of their analysis indicated that of the overall population of Sweden (8.5 million), 83,000 individuals would have atrial fibrillation, of whom 22,000 would be suitable for anticoagulant treatment, 75,000 for aspirin treatment, and 55,000 suitable for aspirin treatment where anticoagulant treatment was contraindicated. The annual number of strokes prevented by the various treatment strategies ranged from 260 where only anticoagulant treatment was offered and the increased incidence of intracranial haemorrhage set at 2.0%, to 1,300 where anticoagulant and aspirin treatment were used in combination and the increased risk of intracranial haemorrhage was set at 0.3%. This combined treatment option reduced annual strokes by 1,080 when the complication rate was set at 2.0%. Aspirin-only treatment reduced the estimated annual number of strokes by 910.

When the costs of the interventions were balanced against the savings from the strokes prevented, aspirin treatment and anticoagulant treatment were both shown to lead to overall savings and hence be cost-effective, if the risk of haemorrhage was set at 0.3% or 1.3% and both the health service and indirect costs of stroke were considered. For aspirin treatment, the estimated saving per stroke prevented was 262,000 Swedish krona (a saving of 172,000 Swedish krona when only health service costs were considered); for anticoagulant treatment and a complication rate of 0.3% a saving of 99,000 Swedish krona per stroke prevented (a saving of 9,000 Swedish krona when only health service costs were considered), and with a complication rate of 1.3% a saving of 3,000 Swedish krona per stroke prevented (an increased cost of 87,000 Swedish krona when only health service costs were considered). When complication rates were set at 2.0%, anticoagulant treatment caused costs to increase by 147,000 Swedish krona per stroke prevented, or 237,000 Swedish krona when only health service costs were considered.

The author argued that the best treatment option is anticoagulant treatment, with aspirin treatment only being given to those with contraindications. This recommendation appears to stem from this strategy having the most impact in terms of the annual number of strokes prevented. They estimated that it would reduce annual incidence and cost by around 4%. However, in terms of cost-effectiveness, the results of this study suggest that the sole use of aspirin in eligible patients is the best strategy.

Although the costs of prevention strategies and the treatment of stroke are likely to be different in the United Kingdom, the relative costs are likely to be the same. Hence the general conclusions of this study are likely to be applicable to the NHS.

Gage *et al.* (1995) also used modelling techniques to assess the cost-effectiveness of warfarin and aspirin treatment as preventive measures for stroke in patients with atrial fibrillation. The three strategies considered were: warfarin initially, with aspirin substituted if contraindications existed; the reverse strategy, with aspirin as the first choice treatment; and no therapy. As in the study by Gustafsson *et al.* the model was largely furnished by the results of published trials.

Gage *et al.* extended the work of Gustafsson *et al.* by assigning stroke patients to groupings according to their risk status. The risk factor variables considered were a history of stroke or transient ischaemic attacks, diabetes, hypertension and heart disease. Patients with two or more risk factors were regarded as being at high risk for stroke, patients with one risk factor at medium risk, and with no risk factors apart from atrial fibrillation at low risk. Given the nature of the risk factors this study has relevance for both the primary and secondary prevention of stroke.

All patients were aged 65 at baseline and the analysis simulated the outcomes for this cohort over a 10-year time horizon. Patients in the high-risk group were assumed to have an annual rate of stroke of 5.3%, in the medium-risk group between 2.6% and 4.6% depending on which risk factor was present, and in the low-risk group an annual rate of 1.6%. Hence, in comparison to the study by Gustaffson, only the high-risk group of patients had a similar annual rate of stroke. Where strokes were predicted, probability data were used to subdivide them into no residual deficit, mild neurologic residua, moderate to severe neurologic residua, and fatal.

In addition to these clinical outcomes, the quality of life was assessed for time spent by patients in the three categories of non-fatal strokes as well as time spent in the two categories of receiving warfarin or aspirin for stroke prevention. These quality of life estimates compared the utility of a year of life spent in the above five categories relative to a year of life spent in 'perfect' health. These utility data were obtained from interviews with 74 patients with atrial fibrillation. Data were collected by describing life within the various categories then asking respondents to assign a utility value.

As the model was run over the 10-year time horizon, predictions were made of the clinical outcomes and the time periods individuals would spend on preventive treatment and in the period following a stroke. These durations were then combined with the relevant utility estimates to assess the quality adjusted life years generated by the alternative strategies over the 10-year planning period. Durations in these states were also combined with data on the health service costs of prevention and treatment for stroke to assess the total expected cost of a patient by intervention type and risk group over the 10-year period. The average cost estimates were based upon the reimbursement rate for Diagnoses Related Groups 14 and 15 in the Medicare programme of funding and on data of the cost of a year on drug treatment obtained from a survey of eight pharmaceutical laboratories. All future costs and life years were discounted at a 5% rate. Data on indirect costs such as lost wages were not included.

Over the 10-year time horizon the quality adjusted life expectancy of high-risk patients on warfarin as the preferred therapy was 6.51 years, on the aspirin preferred therapy 6.27 years, and on the no therapy strategy 6.01 years. High-risk patients on warfarin also had the lowest projected 10-year costs. Relevant values for warfarin patients were $12,500, for aspirin patients $13,200, and for no therapy patients $15,300. Hence, in high-risk patients warfarin therapy was the most effective and cost-effective strategy. Aspirin therapy was also more effective and cost-effective than no therapy. These findings are in line with the results of the study by Gustafsson *et al.* (1992) although differences in the precise strategies considered and the methods of analysis used make direct comparison difficult.

The quality adjusted life expectancy in medium-risk patients on warfarin treatment was 6.60 years, on aspirin 6.46 years and on no therapy 6.23. However, although warfarin had better outcomes than aspirin therapy, its expected costs over the 10-year time period were greater: $10,900 compared with $9,700. This led to aspirin treatment being more cost-effective than warfarin with the cost of securing the additional outcome from warfarin treatment being $8,000 per life year gained. Both aspirin and warfarin therapy were more cost-effective than no therapy.

The expected quality adjusted life expectancy in low-risk patients was 6.70 years for warfarin treatment (projected cost $9,000), 6.99 years for aspirin treatment (projected cost $5,400), and 6.51 years for no therapy (projected costs $6,300). Here aspirin was found to be the most cost-effective treatment followed by no therapy then warfarin.

These results suggest that in patients with atrial fibrillation aspirin is more effective and cost-effective than no therapy. Warfarin is cost-effective in high-risk patients.

Both of the previous studies reviewed have used modelling techniques using data drawn from a wide variety of routine sources to explore the cost-effectiveness of alternative treatment strategies. Such modelling techniques have an important role in helping to generate broad conclusions about the merits of options. Sensitivity analysis is then used to test the reliability of those conclusions given different working assumptions. Where the conclusions are consistent, the use of models may avoid the need for more detailed studies. Where the conclusions are not consistent, the models help to prioritise future research by identifying the areas of greatest uncertainty.

However, from the perspective of countries other than the host for the research and from that of an individual hospital, although the broad conclusions of such studies are probably generalisable their precise results in terms of outcomes, costs and savings are not. If required, such data would need to be generated via a local audit exercise with the results of the published studies being used to identify the key data to collect.

The final paper reviewed here also used a macro approach and a range of working assumptions to explore the potential economic gains from the control of hypertension and reduced smoking as preventive measures for stroke. Based upon the results of published trials, Gorelick (1994) estimated that in the United States up to 246,500 first-ever strokes could be prevented by hypertension control (49% of the overall number of first-ever strokes in the United States per annum) and 61,500 first-ever strokes prevented by reduced smoking levels in populations (12% of the United States total). He argued that £25 billion per year is currently spent on stroke care when both health service and indirect costs such as insurance benefits are included. Given this, Gorelick states that even if interventions were only 10% successful in reducing the number of preventable strokes, better hypertension control and reduced smoking policies would lead to potential economic savings of $1.23 billion and $310 million respectively.

This analysis is somewhat crude and is being used to make the general points that hypertension control and reduced smoking as primary preventive measures for stroke are likely to be beneficial from an economic perspective. A review by the World Hypertension League (1995) discussed economic issues surrounding hypertension control. This demonstrated the difficulties of undertaking studies to assess the cost-effectiveness of treatment for hypertension. They found that there was considerable variation in the results reported by studies but, as might be expected, the general conclusion was that the cost-effectiveness of treatment increased as the risk of hypertension-related disease, such as stroke, increased. The best cost-effectiveness ratios, in terms of costs per life year gained, were obtained in older subjects with a diastolic blood pressure of 100-110 mmHg. The studies reviewed also indicated that treatment with a diuretic was more cost-effective than treatment with more expensive drugs such as ACE inhibitors.

### (b) Secondary prevention of stroke

The economic impacts of warfarin and aspirin as measures of secondary prevention have already been discussed. Oster *et al.* (1994) considered the cost-effectiveness of ticlopidine in comparison to aspirin as a means of preventing stroke in high risk patients. High-risk patients were defined as having had a recent transient ischaemic attack, reversible ischaemic neurological deficit, amaurosis fugax or minor stroke. Although studies have suggested that ticlopidine is more effective than aspirin in preventing stroke in such patients, it is much more expensive than aspirin and hence there are questions about the relative cost-effectiveness of the two strategies.

Again, modelling techniques were used to compare the costs and outcomes of a hypothetical cohort of 100 patients receiving either 500mg of ticlopidine or 1300mg of aspirin daily. At baseline all patients were aged 65 and, as in the study by Gage *et al.* (1995), the expected medical costs of prevention and treatment for stroke were projected from baseline to the point where any surviving patients were aged 100. Outcomes were in terms of quality adjusted life years of survival. The model was furnished by data from the literature and a series of working assumptions.

In comparison to aspirin therapy, use of the model indicated that ticlopidine therapy led to two fewer strokes amongst the cohort of patients and increased life expectancy by around one half month per patient. However lifetime medical costs per patient were $2341 higher for ticlopidine treatment or between $31,200 to $55,500 per life year gained depending upon the utility values used in the quality of life assessment.

Oster *et al.* (1994) concluded that ticlopidine therapy is 'cost-effective by current standards of medical practice'. This conclusion presumably stems from thinking the higher costs of ticlopidine are justified by the improved outcomes that it is predicted to generate. In the opinion of the author of this chapter, such a conclusion is premature and more work is needed to assess the relative merits of ticlopidine therapy.

Two recent editorials in the British Medical Journal (Baird 1995; Lambert 1995) addressed the issue of whether or not health care purchasers should invest in carotid endarterectomy in people with severe symptomatic carotid artery stenosis. Their conclusions were inconsistent. Baird was in favour of the treatment, arguing that carotid endarterectomy is an effective treatment provided it is undertaken by skilled staff, and that the costs of the operation (£3000) are small when set against the costs of the treatment of a stroke (£45,000). However, he recommended that audit data be routinely used so that surgeons can judge the outcomes of the intervention and that these data be made available to patients, GPs and purchasers.

Lambert was more guarded in his conclusion. He estimated, based upon the population of England, that 1,730 operations would be performed per year leading to a maximum reduction of 154 in the number of first-ever strokes occurring each year. This represents less than 0.2% of the number of first-time strokes that occur in England each year. Given these findings, Lambert argued that carotid endarterectomy should not be a priority for purchasers because, from a population perspective, the potential health gains from the investments are small relative to those for health care interventions for conditions other than stroke.

Using the figures quoted by Baird, a crude comparison of the costs of prevention and treatment for stroke also leads to an inconclusive finding regarding the merits of carotid endarterectomy. The extra 1,730 surgical procedures would cost an additional £5.2 million per annum. Savings in the treatment costs of the 154 strokes prevented per annum would be £6.9 million. However, Lambert argued that the potential for annual reductions in the number of strokes was unlikely to be achieved. More research is needed to assess the cost-effectiveness of carotid endarterectomy in the secondary prevention of stroke.

### (c) The treatment of acute stroke

Current evidence indicates that stroke care in stroke units reduces mortality and leads to speedier recovery in those patients who survive (Garraway *et al.* 1980; Langhorne *et al.* 1993; Jorgensen *et al.* 1995). Stroke unit care implies care given in a systematic manner by an organised multidisciplinary team usually operating from a designated hospital ward or wards. Comparative data on inpatient acute stay were the only information found to judge the relative cost-effectiveness of stroke unit and conventional care.

In the study by Garraway *et al.* (1980) patients were randomised to either stroke unit care or care on general medical wards. Mean patient stay on the stroke unit was 55 days and on the general medical wards 75 days. In spite of this reduction in stay, clinical outcomes were better for stroke unit patients.

More recently, Jorgensen *et al.* (1995) compared the care received by stroke patients in two adjacent communities in Greater Copenhagen. Patients from one community were admitted to a hospital providing general care on medical and neurological wards and from the other to a hospital with a stroke unit. Patient characteristics were similar for the two groups but stroke unit care reduced mean patient stay by 30%, 39 days compared with 55 days on general wards.

Jorgensen *et al.* chose their study design because it avoided the potential effects of bias that could exist in a randomised controlled trial based on one hospital. The difficulty with their chosen design, however, is the assumption that their 'control' hospital is representative of conventional care in Denmark. As the results in Chapter 3 indicated, there are large differences in stroke care provided by hospitals both within and across countries. Hence Jorgensen *et al.* might have reached a different conclusion if they had chosen a different 'control' hospital even though its mix of admissions might have been similar to the study hospital.

Intuitively, it might be expected that organised and systematic care provided in stroke units would lead to reduced hospital stay. Available evidence tends to support this impression and, given that inpatient care is expensive, leads to a preliminary conclusion that stroke units are both effective and cost-effective. However, more research is needed to clarify this issue and in particular to check that costs are not merely being shifted to agencies beyond the inpatient setting.

A key component of this research should be a detailed description of the precise nature of care given in both control and test situations. This description should include data such as the nature, quantity and timing of key interventions received by patients and the numbers and qualifications of staff involved in stroke care. Such data will help others judge how applicable the studies' results are to their own localities as well as judging how care packages can be recreated locally. In their study, Jorgensen *et al.* (1995) did provide some description of stroke unit care but care in the control hospital was described as 'traditional treatment offered to patients at Danish hospitals without a stroke unit'. The need to disentangle precisely what is meant by stroke unit care, given that it is not a standardised concept, is a fact that has been acknowledged by others (Langhorne *et al.* 1993; Jorgensen *et al.* 1995).

With patients discharged from acute inpatient care at the University Hospital Nottingham, Gladman *et al.* (1994) compared the costs of hospital-based and domicillary-based physiotherapy and occupational therapy. Three patient groupings were considered: patients discharged from an elderly care ward; patients discharged from a stroke unit, which tended to be a younger group of patients; and patients discharged from general medical wards, an intermediate grouping of patients in terms of age. For the first grouping, hospital-based therapy was in a geriatric day hospital and for the latter two groupings in an acute hospital outpatient department. Patients had been randomly assigned to either the hospital-based or domiciliary-based therapy option as part of the DOMINO study (DOMiciliary rehabilitation In NOttingham). The results of the study suggested that, for care of the elderly patients, day hospital therapy may lead to lower mortality, and for stroke unit patients, home therapy may lead to improved household and leisure abilities at six months amongst patients. For the third group of patients, no differences in outcome were detected.

The health service costs of the different therapy options were assessed. These costs included staff costs, either ambulance costs or travel costs incurred by therapists, and hospital overheads. The average cost of a domiciliary therapy session was estimated as £36.80 (£34 staff costs), a day hospital session £52.40 (£46.90 staff costs) and an outpatient session £17.80 (£12.50 staff costs). When these costs were combined with data on the average number of sessions received by patients, for elderly care patients domiciliary care was the less expensive option (mean cost per patient £485.50 compared with £964.60 for hospital-based care). For stroke unit patients, hospital care was cheaper (£467.90 compared with £925.20 for domiciliary care), the same being true for general ward patients (£265.50 for hospital care and £367.90 for domiciliary care).

The main reason why hospital care was more expensive than domiciliary care for elderly care patients appears to be that patients attending the day hospital received twice as much therapy: mean visits per patient were 10 for domiciliary and 20 for hospital care. For the other patient groups, the lower costs of a therapy session in hospital was the main reason why hospital care was less expensive than domiciliary care.

Again, the results of this study would have benefited from more details being provided on the way care was organised and delivered for the various options. For example, there are big differences between the staff costs of a therapy session in outpatients, a session in a day hospital, and a domiciliary session. Without details of skill mix and numbers it is difficult to understand the reasons for cost differences or for readers to judge how representative the results are of care in their locality. Indeed, although this study is focusing on the location of care, perhaps this is a secondary issue, the primary issue being the most appropriate staffing for a session in terms of skill mix, therapist-to-patient ratio and duration.

Young and Forster (1993) also compared the cost-effectiveness of day hospital and domiciliary physiotherapy for elderly stroke patients. They extended the work of the Bradford community stroke trial, a randomised trial which had indicated that home therapy was slightly more efficacious than hospital therapy (Young and Forster 1992). Health care inputs received by patients during the eight-week period following discharge from inpatient care and entering the trial were recorded prospectively. The key cost areas considered were home and hospital physiotherapy, district nursing services, and home care services such as meals on wheels.

Median costs per case were significantly lower for patients in the domiciliary group (p<0.001), cost values being £385 per domiciliary patient and £620 per hospital-based patient. The main cost elements were those of physiotherapy, median costs per case being £205 for the domiciliary arm and £530 for the hospital based arm. Two main factors caused home physiotherapy to be cheaper. Unit staff costs per therapy session were lower for home therapy: £20 per session compared with £49 per session for care in a 15-place day hospital and £35 per session in a 30-place unit. Home unit patients also received a median of 11 visits over the eight weeks compared with 15 attendances for the day hospital group.

Both the studies by Gladman *et al.* (1994) and by Young and Forster (1993) indicate that, for elderly patients, domiciliary care is less expensive than hospital care because the unit costs of a therapy session are lower and because patients need fewer therapy sessions to achieve the same or improved outcomes. Young and Forster argued that it would not be possible to reduce the unit costs of a hospital session to that of a home session because fixed overhead costs are higher for a hospital session. This difference might be maintained in the short term but, if home care becomes more widely practiced, its overhead costs might rise because of the need to develop an infrastructure to co-ordinate and manage the service. In addition, the proportionate size of hospital overheads will vary from locality to locality, a fact that will affect the relative costliness of hospital and home therapy. This is important for potential adopters of a home therapy service. Young and Forster did not address the issue of whether the nature of the home physiotherapy session could be recreated in the hospital environment such that fewer sessions are needed. This is probably the more interesting issue.

The studies reviewed in this section about interventions for the acute management of stroke are to a large extent concerned with changes in the way care is organised. More studies are needed which broadly consider the way care is organised in different hospitals. The European Biomed study of stroke that is being undertaken by staff within the Department of Public Health Medicine, UMDS, is an example of such a study. Preliminary results which showed large variations in practice between hospitals, and in particular in lengths of stay, were presented in Chapter 3. Such variations have large potential financial and economic consequences. By studying care in different settings, elements of the service which improve the efficient delivery of care can be highlighted. These might be clinical or managerial. The potential link between variations in practice and variations in outcomes between hospitals can also be explored so as to generate information about which patterns of care appear to be the most effective.

## Executive summary and priorities for research

This chapter has focused on the overall costs of stroke and on the economic benefits of key interventions for the prevention and treatment of stroke. The review of the literature is not exhaustive. The aim has been to generate relevant information for guiding practice in the United Kingdom.

In terms of overall cost, stroke care consumes between 4-5% of health service expenditure. Although this proportion may remain the same, actual expenditure on stroke care is likely to rise in real terms over the next 20 years because of the effects of an ageing population. Stroke also has major cost implications for patients and their carers in terms of financial expenditure, lost income and time away from normal activities but limited information is available on the precise scale of these effects in the United Kingdom. Finally, information on the costs of stroke care and the way it is delivered in different hospitals has potential value for purchasers and providers by helping to highlight areas where services could be improved. In the light of these findings research is needed:

1. To develop methodologies for predicting the potential rise in the overall costs of stroke care over coming years. These approaches should then be used to assess the future costs of care given different assumptions about demographic changes and changes in the costs and processes of care for individual patients.

2. To assess the cost implications of stroke for patients and their carers.

3. To highlight key elements of care where standard approaches are needed for collecting data on the quantity of services a stroke patient receives and on the costs of those services. These data should then be used to generate information about care in different hospitals.

The methodologies for assessing the economic impact of alternative treatment and organisational policies for stroke care currently range from macro-economic modelling techniques, which draw on the findings of a range of published studies, to specific studies alongside individual clinical trials. Both have an important role in stroke research. Macro techniques generate broad conclusions about the merits of interventions whereas individual trials allow specific issues and areas of uncertainty to be explored in greater detail. There is also a place for studies which describe care in different settings as these can be used to generate information about the merits of alternative treatment patterns and to highlight issues which require more detailed research.

When conducting economic appraisals it is important that details of the delivery and organisation of care are collected and reported for both test and control situations. These details will help readers judge how applicable the findings are to their locality and how they could implement the innovation locally. Such details were often lacking from the studies reviewed in this chapter. The potential impacts of innovations on patients and carers should also be considered. Such impacts can affect issues such as patient compliance which in turn will affect the likely success of the treatment in question. Again, patient and carer effects were often ignored in the studies reviewed here. Finally, economic analysis can be a complex task. Methodological errors and errors in interpreting study results can be avoided by including a health economist, or a scientist from a related discipline, as a member of any research team. This does not seem to have been done in some of the studies reviewed here.

In general there is a shortage of research on the economic implications of treatments for stroke. Consequently more research is needed:

1. On the economic implications of treatments for the prevention and acute management of stroke.

2. On alternative arrangements for the overall delivery and organisation of stroke care.

# References

Anderson R. The aftermath of stroke: the experience of patients and their families. Cambridge: Cambridge University Press, 1992.

Baird RN. Should carotid endarterectomy be purchased? Treatment avoids much morbidity. BMJ 1995; 310: 316-7.

Bergman L, van der Meulen JHP, Limburg M, Halbema TDF. Costs of medical care after first-ever stroke in the Netherlands. Stroke 1995; 26: 1830-6.

Carstairs V. Stroke: Resource consumption and the cost to the community. In: Gillingham FJ, Maudsley C, Williams E (eds) Stroke. London: Churchill Livingstone 1976, 516-28.

Effective Health Care Bulletin. Stroke rehabilitation. Leeds: University of Leeds, School of Public Health, 1992.

Gage BF, Cardinalli AB, Albers GW, Owens DK. Cost-effectiveness of warfarin and aspirin for prophylaxis of stroke in patients with nonvalvular atrial fibrillation. JAMA 1995; 274: 1839-45.

Garraway WM, Akhtar AJ, Prescott RJ, Hockey L. Management of acute stroke in the elderly: preliminary results of an acute trial. BMJ 1980; 280: 1040-3.

Gladman JRF, Lincoln NB, Barer DH. Outcomes in a randomised controlled trial of domiciliary and hospital-based rehabilitation for stroke patients after discharge from hospital. J Neurol Neurosurg Psychiatry 1993; 56: 960-6.

Gladman J, Whynes D, Lincoln N. Cost comparison of domiciliary and hospital-based stroke rehabilitation. DOMINO Study Group. Age Ageing 1994; 23: 241-5.

Gorelick PB. Stroke Prevention: an opportunity for efficient utilisation of health care resources during the coming decade. Stroke 1994; 25: 220-4.

Gustafsson C, Asplund K, Britton M, Norrving B, Olsson B, Marke LA. Cost-effectiveness of primary stroke prevention in atrial fibrillation: Swedish national perspective. BMJ 1992; 305: 1457-60.

Isard PA, Forbes JF. The cost of stroke to the National Health Service in Scotland. Cerebrovasc Dis 1992; 2: 47-50.

Jorgensen HS, Nakayama H, Raaschou HO, Larsen K, Hubbe P, Olsen TS. The effect of a stroke unit: reductions in mortality, discharge rate to nursing home, length of hospital stay, and cost. A community-based study. Stroke 1995; 26: 1178-82.

Lambert M. Should carotid endarterectomy be purchased? Purchasers need a broader perspective. BMJ 1995; 310: 317-8.

Langhorne P, Williams BO, Gilchrist W, Howie K. Do stroke units save lives? Lancet 1993; 342: 395-8.

Malmgren R, Bamford J, Warlow C, Sandercock P, Slattery J. Projecting the number of patients with first-ever strokes and patients newly handicapped by stroke in England and Wales. BMJ 1989; 289: 656-60.

Office of Health Economics. Stroke 1988.

Oster G, Huse DM, Lacey MJ, Epstein AM. Cost-effectiveness of ticlopidine in preventing stroke in high-risk patients. Stroke 1994; 25: 1149-56.

Sandercock P. Managing stroke: the way forward. Organised care saves lives. BMJ 1993; 307: 1297-8.

Wolfe CDA, Taub N, Bryan S, Beech R, Warburton F, Burney PGJ. Variations in the incidence, management and outcome of stroke in residents under the age of 75 in two health districts of southern England. J Pub Health Med 1995; 17(4): 411-8.

World Hypertension League. Economics of hypertension control. Bulletin of the WHO 1995; 73: 417-24.

Young JB, Forster A. The Bradford community stroke trial: results at six months. BMJ 1992; 304: 1085-9.

Young J, Forster A. Day hospital and home physiotherapy for stroke patients: a comparative cost-effectiveness study. Roy Coll Physicians of London 1993; 27: 252-8.

# CHAPTER 17

# DEVELOPING A DISTRICT STROKE SERVICE

*Tony Rudd, Charles Wolfe*

*This chapter is based on an article published in Cerebrovascular Disease (Rudd & Wolfe 1996).*

**Chapter outline**

# Summary of the evidence on the prevention and management of stroke in the United Kingdom

A summary of the evidence presented in the previous chapters is outlined to consolidate the evidence on our current knowledge on stroke, its prevention and management. Where the studies have previously been discussed the references are not quoted in the text. Building on this model, stroke services can be suggested that then require formal evaluation in districts around the country.

Death from cerebrovascular disease ranks third in men and women, accounting for 10-12% of deaths in industrialised countries and stroke is the most common cause of adult disability. For every 100,000 population there will be 200 new strokes a year, 40 recurrent strokes and 600 stroke survivors, of whom one-third will be severely disabled. There are significant variations in the SMRs for stroke around the UK that would suggest that certain districts will have to provide considerably more services than others, be they preventive, or services for people who have had strokes. Determining the balance between prevention and cure will be difficult and the following points should be considered.

The United Kingdom government has set a target in *The Health of the Nation* to reduce the death rate for stroke by at least 40% by the year 2000 in those aged under 75 years. Further targets have also been set to reduce risk factors considered to increase the risk of stroke such as smoking, saturated fatty acid intake, obesity, hypertension and alcohol consumption. How realistic these targets are is open to debate because the potential benefits of health promotion and other preventive strategies are disputed both at an individual and population level. Risk factors for stroke have not been as clearly identified as for coronary heart disease, and this is even more evident when considering the various subtypes of stroke. At an individual patient level, primary prevention of stroke by general practitioners, particularly the recognition and treatment of hypertension and atrial fibrillation, may be effective. Secondary prevention with aspirin for ischaemic stroke and previous TIAs, warfarin for patients with atrial fibrillation, and carotid endarterectomy for those with severe carotid stenosis is likewise now supported by a substantial body of research evidence. However those risk factors classified as inherited, social and environmental are not considered in *The Health of the Nation* strategy.

The mortality targets are based on trends over the past 20 years and assume a similar decline to the year 2000. It is not clear in the UK what proportion of the decline, if any, has been and will continue to be due to risk factor reduction strategies. The current rapid decline in stroke mortality predates the widespread use of antihypertensive regimens and there is debate, not about the effectiveness of antihypertensive therapy in the trial setting, but about the efficaciousness at the population level, especially in ethnic minorities. Studies of the effectiveness of population interventions to reduce the risk of stroke have been conducted mainly in men in the United States and their extrapolation to the whole United Kingdom population should be treated with caution. After 10.5 years in the MRFIT study a 13% reduction in stroke mortality was observed in an intervention group where hypertension was controlled, and smoking and dietary habits modified by a range of interventions. In the north Karelia study it has been estimated that 66% of the fall in stroke mortality in men, and 50% of the fall in stroke mortality in women over the last 20 years could have been due to the reduction in risk factor prevalence. In the United Kingdom preliminary data from the OXCHECK study, however, fail to show any conclusive benefit from health promotion in primary care.

The evidence does not exist for effective models of service for prevention in the UK, largely because stroke has not been considered separately from cardiovascular disease and the risk factors are not well defined.

The dilemma facing policy makers and health service planners, therefore, is that risk factor reduction on its own is not going to solve the problem of stroke and the management of stroke remains the focus of any stroke service. Tertiary prevention, or the effective treatment of established disease, is also contentious but there is now evidence to suggest that a properly co-ordinated package of care is more effective than ad hoc treatment provided in non-specialist settings. No drug treatment for stroke has yet been shown to have more than a marginal impact on stroke mortality and morbidity and the effectiveness of various components of rehabilitation is in question.

## Current service provision

It has been estimated that around 4-5% of the NHS budget is spent on stroke care, but this is an underestimate of the overall cost of stroke, as social services, voluntary organisations, the private sector (including nursing homes) and carer costs are not included. The cost to the NHS in a district will be around £2.1 million per year at an estimated cost of £3555 per case, with 93% being spent on providing hospital accommodation and nursing care to the admitted patient (Wolfe *et al.* 1995). The King's Fund Consensus Conference in 1988 described stroke services as being haphazard, fragmented and poorly tailored to patients' needs. A recent survey of hospital consultants by The Stroke Association indicated that management of acute stroke was still in many units suboptimal, when compared to the King's Fund statement and the Royal College of Physicians' guidelines (Lindley *et al.* 1995).

Information on the services received in the community by stroke patients is virtually non-existent but the little that there is would suggest that there is a considerable amount of unmet need both in terms of secondary prevention, and management of stroke patients and their carers, although there are pockets of good practice on which models could be based.

How then should resources be distributed between primary, secondary and tertiary prevention and what models of care should be adopted? The following sections outline those aspects of a service that should be considered when developing an effective co-ordinated model service.

## A conductive health service

The recognition by the Department of Health in the document *The Health of the Nation*, and increasingly by local purchasing authorities, that stroke is a major public health issue and responsible for the use of a considerable proportion of resources is to be welcomed. Close examination of the organisation of care and of the efficacy of the various components of care is overdue and the emphasis that the Research and Development initiatives of the National Health Service as well as the European Community Biomed programme are now placing on stroke should begin to provide answers to some of the current issues surrounding the development of a high-quality stroke service. Stroke may in addition provide a model which may be applicable to other chronic diseases which have until recently similarly attracted little research attention, but nevertheless have been responsible for the consumption of large proportions of health and social service resources.

## Existing models of good practice

Theoretical discussion documents have been produced to describe stroke service requirements and these have been drawn on when building up a model service. They give little practical advice on how to actually set about designing a clinical service, particularly in a multicultural inner-city district for example. Of more importance is to draw on the experiences of those who have made significant changes to the stroke services. This paper describes how stroke services could be developed in a district, based upon published evidence of good practice and the personal experiences of the authors involved in such an exercise over the last five years.

As long ago as 1989, the Royal College of Physicians recommended that each health district establish specific services for patients with stroke (Royal College of Physicians 1989). Traditionally the management of stroke patients is viewed as part of the work of every physician involved in admitting acutely ill patients. Elderly care physicians in some districts have developed specialist stroke services, although these tend to be available only to patients over a specific age. Neurologists in the UK, particularly compared to those in Europe, have a poor record for showing interest in the commonest of all neurological diseases, with some notable exceptions and there are fewer neurologists per head of population than in most other countries. Few districts have a physician whose responsibility it is to co-ordinate services for stroke patients although The Stroke Association has piloted four such posts and some districts are appointing stroke co-ordinators, often with nursing backgrounds, although neither of these models has been evaluated. The Stroke Association convened a meeting in 1995 to discuss district stroke service developments (Stroke Association 1995). Although the Association quite rightly says that terms such as seamless and multidisciplinary are used without thought and no one knows how to achieve them, it did not come up with any suggestions as to how to develop these themes. The four district services were set up five years ago but no formal evaluations have been published to guide the development of services in districts not as fortunate as these few.

The World Health Organisation has produced a report on multidisciplinary quality development in stroke care (WHO 1995). A multidisciplinary group discussed the professional functions and responsibilities of the nurse, the physiotherapist and the occupational therapist in the process of stroke management. Unfortunately the role of the primary health care team, doctors and other agencies is not considered. It highlighted the need to set goals, develop a team structure and monitor quality but in a theoretical fashion that is not helpful to those setting up services. Of more concern is that the group appeared not to draw on the evidence of effectiveness for its suggestions, relying instead on intuition. For stroke teams in the acute phase of care, the group recommended there be a co-ordinator but not a leader; there should be input from therapists, doctors, nurses and social workers; early rehabilitation should be considered to last up to three months; and the care manager should take an important role in improving communication between patients and the team. For stroke teams in the later stages, the group envisaged a different team structure, increasing therapy input and reducing medical input. This report was to be used as a basis for discussion at the Pan-European Consensus meeting on Stroke in Helsinborg, November 1995.

At the WHO Pan-European Consensus meeting (1995), essential principles for good practice were drafted and targets set for the year 2005. Such consensus statements cannot reflect the needs in particular countries, or indeed districts within a country. They again reiterate previous statements of good practice that should be considered: the need for organisation with an individual responsible for co-ordination; the need to treat stroke as a medical emergency with immediate access to hospital; all patients should have access to a specialised stroke unit or stroke team; the interests and needs of patients and their families should remain the principal concern of all professionals; support by self-help groups and voluntary patients' associations should be encouraged and should include information provision; rehabilitation should be planned in close collaboration with patients and their families and continue for as long as is required. In some instances the group made specific recommendations on how to achieve these aims using evidence from the literature but in others, such as the objective to reduce case-fatality from stroke by 20% by the year 2005, there is no clear guidance given to indicate which route is considered effective in achieving the target.

A Scottish Intercollegiate group is developing guidelines along a familiar path for services in Scotland. At present these appear to be very medically led with little discussion of multidisciplinary teamwork (Scottish Intercollegiate guidelines network. The management of patients with stroke 1995).

Wade and The Rivermead Specialty Team (1993) outlined their objectives of a stroke service, which are similar to those of the WHO Consensus statement but produced several years earlier in the UK. They usefully described audit measures that have been developed by Dennis that could be used to assess the quality of the service but there are no reports to suggest such data can be collected in a routine fashion in all districts. These issues are discussed further in the section on audit.

A recently convened workshop on contracting for stroke services was held in London (Royal College of Physicians/NAHAT meeting, 1995). Although the wording of a stroke service contract could not be defined, the essential components of such a service were discussed and are currently being written up. The views of the workshop are reflected in the ensuing model of service and displayed in Table 1. There is a considerable way to go to achieve such contracts for the best models of service. A survey of purchasers undertaken by Juliet Solomon for the workshop had a "lacklustre response". Of the responses, 75% stated that their contracts for stroke services were subsumed within their acute medical or care of the elderly contracts. Only two formal contracts detailing costs and activity levels were sent. The respondents had in the main signed up to co-ordinated, multidisciplinary care but there was little agreement on what a stroke unit constituted. Most mentioned prevention as part of 'The Health of the Nation' strategy, acknowledged the need for CT scanning facilities, the importance of early assessment for rehabilitation and the need to consider carers.

The resource and cost consequences of introduction and the type of recommendations suggested by the previously quoted groups have been ignored and will require evaluation in future service developments.

**TABLE 1: Essential components for stroke care**

- Lead named clinician responsible for stroke services

- Primary prevention strategy linked to *Health of the Nation* Targets

- Access to    -      hospital beds including intensive care

              -      investigatory facilities: outpatient and inpatient

              -      rapid processing of TIA referrals

              -      vascular, neurosurgery and neurology

- Specialist multidisciplinary co-ordinated rehabilitation services both in hospitals and in the community e.g. stroke unit, day hospitals, domiciliary therapy.

- Discharge planning and collaboration with social services

- Secondary prevention strategy

- Development of guidelines for the prevention and management of stroke both in primary and secondary care and audit.

- Carer support, including information provision

- A programme of in-service training for staff

- Continuing care in NHS facilities

# Service developments

## 1. Primary prevention

It is the responsibility of health authorities to achieve *The Health of the Nation* targets but this requires close collaboration with physicians, general practitioners and health promotion departments. As indicated, there is questionable evidence as to the effectiveness of population-based intervention programmes. Strategies should be through medical efforts to deal with high-risk individuals (e.g. hypertension, atrial fibrillation) and through public initiatives involving multisectoral collaboration to encourage healthier lifestyles for the whole population. Locally produced protocols and standards implemented with widespread local agreement may prove effective. The structures to promote improved care also need developing. Anticoagulation, for example, if it is to become more widely prescribed, will need to be done in primary care rather than as is usually still the case, in hospital-based clinics. There needs to be further research at a local level on how to target different groups of the population (e.g. different ethnic groups or localities) and close co-operation with Family Health Service Authorities (FHSAs) on these issues is necessary, such that locality-based purchasing of specific preventive packages is developed.

## 2. Stroke register

Maintaining a community stroke register is time consuming and costly. Its value lies principally as an epidemiological and health services research tool. The Oxfordshire Community Stroke Study (1988) was a model for how such a database can inform service providers but the results are now 10 years old and there is doubt as to how applicable some of the results might be to urban areas with high proportions of ethnic minorities. Locally, the data produced from the West Lambeth register (Wolfe *et al.* 1993), which was the first United Kingdom register based in an inner-city district, provided clear evidence of anomalies in service provision. Some 78% of stroke patients were admitted to hospital for a median of 21 days. The overall level of rehabilitation received was low, especially for patients not admitted. Follow-up after discharge appeared haphazard with 31% of patients not seeing their GP within three months of returning home. The high admission rates with little continuity of rehabilitation, poor rates of follow up after discharge and resultant gaps in secondary prevention all showed the need for service developments. Identical problems were demonstrated simultaneously in three districts in the South East Thames Region. These findings are likely to be widely applicable in other cities around the country.

While it may not be feasible to develop a community-based register, having an individual responsible for collecting the names and basic data of all patients admitted to the hospital each week ensures that patients are not 'missed' by therapists and forms the basic data set upon which the design of a service and audit of the service can be developed. The hospital-based register is of particular value in identifying those patients who develop their stroke while in hospital, most notably while on surgical wards, where notification of therapists is most often overlooked. Maintenance of effective computerised hospital records may avoid the need for an individual physically walking around each ward in the future, but at least locally this is not yet sufficiently reliable to act as a substitute. The type of data collected by the register needs to be determined locally, but should be sufficient to enable recognition of the major areas where treatment deviates from previously determined standards of care such as those set nationally (Royal College of Physicians 1994) or locally (West Lambeth Health Authority 1992), and includes demographic data to enable future patient contact where necessary.

Dennis (personal communication) has suggested the types of data that could be incorporated into a minimum data set for comparing case-mix and these include: demography, age, living conditions, premorbid function, risk factors for stroke; clinical state on admission to include date of onset, date of admission, incontinence, ability to walk without aid of another person, whether patient can lift both arms against gravity, blood pressure, orientation, and speech assessment using a component of the Glasgow Coma Scale. Components of this minimum data set could be incorporated into the register. Most other data sets that have been developed are primarily for research purposes and are impractical for day-to-day use.

### 3. District stroke working party

The information from local hospital and community registers painted a picture of haphazard services. The West Lambeth District Stroke Working Party has previously reported its role in developing a locally agreed protocol for the management and audit of stroke in the light of these levels of service provision (West Lambeth Health Authority Stroke Steering Group 1992). The working party brought together senior individuals from all the relevant disciplines both from within the hospital, from the

West Lambeth Community Care Trust and social services who had or should have had a particular interest or expertise in stroke. It performed two major functions. Firstly it produced a local document acceptable to the clinicians working with stroke patients, outlining appropriate management guidelines from admission through to discharge to the community. Secondly it brought together, for the first time, the relevant professionals and identified stroke as being a disease for which there was a coherent specialised team available. With relatively little effort, the profile of stroke was raised within the district and stroke service development was put onto the agenda in both purchaser and provider settings.

### 4. Stroke clerking sheet

One of the problems the working party highlighted was the poor quality of data collection by admitting physicians. For patients staying in hospital, often for long periods, and being treated by a large number of different individuals from a range of departments, good quality data are essential. In addition, the educational opportunities for junior doctors were possibly also being missed. A formatted clerking sheet was therefore prepared, to be used whenever a patient presented in the emergency department. Specific sections on stroke risk factors, premorbid functional ability, cognitive function, swallowing assessment and neurological tests particularly relevant to stroke were included. Lists of important investigations and contact phone numbers for referring to therapy departments were provided to act as an aide memoir for the doctor. Other pro formas have been developed subsequently such as the one produced by the Royal College of Physicians (Royal College of Physicians Stroke Audit Package 1994).

### 5. Multidisciplinary education and working

Evidence to support the value of the use of individual therapies after stroke is not as strong as would be liked. What is, however, clear is that professionals working as part of a team do so more effectively than when operating separately. Effective rehabilitation has also been shown to be cost-effective, even for the most disabled and aged patients. Avoiding the need for institutionalisation in nursing homes, which is one of the most costly decisions a physician is ever likely to make, is worthwhile even when achieved in only a small percentage of patients treated.

Until about five years ago, in the West Lambeth district patients with stroke were admitted to many different wards under the care of a large number of different physicians. Except for those patients admitted to wards for the care of the elderly, rehabilitation was provided by specialist neurophysiotherapy, occupational therapy and speech therapy each based in separate departments in different parts of the hospital without organised multidisciplinary working. The average number of patients in the hospital at any one time with stroke was between 30 and 40. Agreement from all the physicians was obtained to convene weekly meetings of the therapists together with one of the elderly care physicians and any interested junior medical staff, nurses or social workers. The meetings ensured that all relevant therapy referrals had occurred and that all team members were working to a common agenda. The role of the physician is to identify those patients not progressing as expected, to review them and to offer appropriate advice to the responsible physician. This model is one way of introducing multidisciplinary working in a large district general hospital without necessarily having to develop a stroke unit capable of providing for all stroke patients within the hospital. It can only work where physicians are not excessively territorial about their patients. With increasing specialism being demanded by patients and purchasers alike, the model has the advantage of allowing all junior doctors to continue with the management of stroke patients while at the same time not compromising quality of care.

One key component to effective teamwork is that the various health care professionals involved have the same goals and objectives. Educating these groups together as part of the team will hopefully achieve this but requires further evaluation. The use of such a group as a district stroke steering group could provide the forum for developing an educational programme involving primary and secondary care sectors. The development of guidelines and minimum data set pro formas can potentially act as a prompt to health care professionals.

### 6. Stroke units

Meta-analysis of 10 trials of stroke units against alternative models of care has demonstrated that they are effective in reducing mortality. Taken individually, the trials are inconclusive; each is of different design with varying outcome measures but mortality is a measure unlikely to be interpreted differently between centres. How much the analysis is affected by publication bias is of course impossible to assess. Even without hard research evidence to support their development, there are clearly arguments that can be used to justify their existence. Concentration of expertise in one area of a hospital reduces time wasted on administration. Development and implementation of management protocols is likely to be more effective. Involvement of the nursing staff in the rehabilitation process becomes easier and research, teaching and training are all facilitated. Expected developments in the acute management of stroke such as thrombolysis and administration of NMDA receptor antagonists will require a much improved system than exists in many hospitals at present to effectively administer such treatments. Stroke units admitting directly from home may provide such a structure. Whether stroke units are effective at reducing long-term complications such as post-stroke depression, pain due to shoulder subluxation, urinary incontinence or catheterisation, contractures, pressure sores and inappropriate institutionalisation still needs to be assessed.

Organising a stroke unit to combine the specialist skills of the neurophysiotherapists with the specialist skills of the elderly care therapists provides a flexibility that gives considerable advantages. At some stage in rehabilitation the stroke patient will need advice from a physiotherapist with neurology expertise; all stroke patients with significant residual disability, regardless of age, will benefit from the experience that elderly care physiotherapists have in solving problems of long-term impairments. Sharing care medically between a general physician with an interest in stroke, a geriatrician or a rehabilitation specialist and a neurologist has proved beneficial for the St. Thomas' unit in providing a breadth of understanding that would otherwise have been difficult of the individual patient's problems ranging from the pathology to the handicap. Inclusion of a clinical neuropsychologist in the rehabilitation team to evaluate difficult perceptual and cognitive problems and to work with the other therapists in overcoming barriers to rehabilitation, is in our experience valuable but needs formal evaluation to determine the clinical and financial consequences of such a service.

## 7. Stroke clinic

There is a need to follow up patients after stroke, to ensure compliance with therapy for secondary prevention and to provide a structure by which early detection of complications and the need for re-evaluation by therapists can be identified. Local audit has shown that even with a relatively well-organised stroke service, simple secondary prevention measures such as prescription of aspirin following cerebral infarction are not always achieved. Only 30% of patients discharged from our unit had had their blood pressure checked during the first three months after discharge. Basic investigations such as blood sugar or serum lipids are not always done during a hospital admission. A stroke clinic where formalised re-evaluation is performed according to a set pro forma is one way that quality of care after discharge might be improved.

Better communication between primary and secondary health care is also necessary and joint clinics between general practitioners and stroke specialists may be an alternative to the separate services that exist at present. Again, formal evaluation of running stroke clinics has not been reported in the literature and so purchasing authorities will need to consider empirically whether they should be commissioned. The precise function of such clinics will need to be determined locally and organised appropriately. A clinic primarily aimed at secondary prevention will need to be close to investigation facilities, anticoagulant clinics and other specialist clinics such as vascular surgery, neurology and cardiology. Whether in the future such clinics could effectively be run by the majority of GPs in their surgeries remains to be seen. The organisation needed, for example to take blood for anticoagulant monitoring and arrange transportation to the laboratory, and the expertise needed to adjust the dosage appropriately are as yet difficult to achieve in the community. Clinics primarily aimed at reviewing disability and deciding on further rehabilitation intervention may well, however, be better situated in GP-run health centres or day hospitals.

### 8. Community rehabilitation

Organisation of care after discharge from hospital has been reported in two major studies, one comparing domiciliary therapy with day hospital treatment and the other comparing hospital outpatient therapy with domiciliary therapy. Most districts offer a combination of services, although these are often better organised for elderly patients than younger people. Domiciliary therapy appears to offer slight advantages over the other methods, including financial ones, but differences are small and there is some variation according to the client group. Whether it is possible to effectively substitute inpatient hospital rehabilitation therapy with domiciliary care is currently under evaluation at our hospital in a randomised controlled trial of early discharge from hospital, with rehabilitation by a specialist team of stroke therapists at home compared with conventional services. A previous study looked at provision of a stroke rehabilitation team in the community to assess whether it had an impact on rates of hospital admission and outcome and found little benefit. For how long it is justifiable to continue with rehabilitation is also debatable. Evidence suggests that providing physiotherapy a year or more after stroke may improve function while the therapy continues, but the patient quickly relapses once it is withdrawn. Whether it is possible to maintain improvement by continuing with some level of support needs evaluation. Patients not admitted to hospital, according to the evidence from Wolfe *et al.* (1993), receive virtually no medical or rehabilitation support. Little data exists on this subset of stroke patients to indicate what their needs really are and this is again in the process of being studied with a randomised controlled trial of specialist rehabilitation from a dedicated team of stroke therapists compared with conventional services. In Holland, Schuling *et al.* (1992) found non-admitted patients to be generally older, with milder strokes and more likely to be in nursing homes than the admitted patients. While this may hold true elsewhere, perhaps indicating less of a need for effective community rehabilitation, the structures still need to be in place to deal with those with more severe strokes who wish to remain at home and advice on secondary prevention needs to be easily accessible.

Handicap and quality of life are issues that often seem to be neglected in stroke rehabilitation and may be easier to address in the patient's own home rather than in an institutional setting. Development of tools for measurement of these parameters may also encourage advances in their treatment.

### 9. Carers' group

Perhaps the most important members of the rehabilitation team are the principal carers. It is they who will continue with the management treatment in the months and years following the stroke. Education and support for carers should therefore be one of the top priorities for any stroke rehabilitation service (Kernich *et al.* 1988). Running a carers' group to which all relatives and friends are invited, and providing guidance on how to survive as a carer, is popular and possibly helpful. Sessions range from practical advice on how to lift a disabled person or assist in his or her walking, to benefit entitlements and risk taking. Maintaining a resource centre on the stroke unit containing useful literature provides further help for carers but is again a resource that needs to be funded if it is to remain effective. In the UK The Stroke Association has considerable expertise in providing carer support but it is entirely dependent upon voluntary contributions and much of its work, particularly when demonstrated to be effective, could be taken over by the statutory bodies.

## 10. Regional stroke special interest group

Collaboration with colleagues in neighbouring districts in developing regional strategies for care, in applying for funds to provide services for patients across the region, and for providing mutual support, has worked well locally. Development of a minimum data set for use in five districts in the South East Thames area will also facilitate collaborative research. Similar collaboration between a number of centres in the European Community and affiliated states is also underway, comparing different models of health care for stroke both in terms of clinical effectiveness and cost. There is still little guidance in the literature about how to measure an input into stroke treatment and what process measures to record, and even less relating how inputs relate to outcomes. Evaluating the relationship between outcome and resource data, collected in a standardised way from a large number of services providing care in different ways, should provide useful information to purchasers and providers to guide service developments in the future.

## Audit

### Guideline production and audit

Clinical audit is now an integral part of the NHS but its uptake and effectiveness has not been evaluated. The NHS spends in the region of £48 million a year on audit with the aim to improve the quality of care for patients. This review is mainly concerned with research evidence. Audit is not research and results from audit studies are not generalisable. The conclusions drawn from audit have to be considered alongside research evidence and both have a contribution to shaping health service provision at a local level (Smith 1992). Health care purchasers contract for specific audits in their contracts with provider units and it has been argued that healthcare commissioners should purchase guidelines or protocols rather than simple procedures.

Clinical audit is the review of patient care and has been defined in many ways, including "systematic, critical analysis of the quality of medical care, including procedures used for the diagnosis and treatment, the use of resources and resulting outcome and quality of life for patients" (Department of Health 1989). Its main purpose is to identify opportunities and implement improvements in the quality of care, medical training and continuing health care professional education and the effective use of resources.

**The main steps in undertaking an audit include (the audit cycle):**

*Setting the standards for care*

*Collecting data on the quality of care*

*Comparing practice with standards*

*Changing practice and/or altering the standards*

*Setting standards of care for stroke*

The King's Fund Consensus Statement (1988) and the Royal College of Physicians (1989) both produced standards of care for stroke in the late 1980s which formed a national basis for guidelines. These guidelines were developed by consensus and incorporated the feelings of experts at the time. Since that time there have been advances in the rigour with which guidelines are developed and in assessing their effect on medical practice (Grimshaw and Russell 1993; Thompson *et al.* 1995). Guidelines are systematically developed statements to assist practitioner and patient decisions about appropriate health care for specific clinical circumstances. Grimshaw and Russell (1993) evaluated 59 published guidelines (none on stroke care) and concluded that explicit guidelines do improve clinical practice when introduced in the context of rigorous evaluations. However, the size of the improvements in performance varied considerably. There is a growing literature on the factors that influence the effectiveness of guidelines (Thompson *et al.* 1995).

In the field of stroke care, the Department of Health has produced guidelines on the effectiveness of rehabilitation (Effective Health Care 1992). Although many provider units and purchasers have produced reviews of the evidence to support or refute various interventions or services (e.g. Northamptonshire Health Authority 1994), few have disseminated these as guidelines. The Northamptonshire review was subsequently produced as guidelines under a project aimed at 'Getting Research into Practice and Purchasing' (GRIPP). Many health authorities are developing overviews of the evidence for effective stroke care, which would appear to be a duplication of effort.

In England the West Lambeth Health Authority published district guidelines for stroke services , adapting the Royal College guidelines for local use (West Lambeth Health Authority Stroke Steering Group 1992). Based on these guidelines, standards were set in the main domains of care for stroke patients. In addition, earlier sections of this chapter could form the basis of local guideline development.

*Collecting data on the quality of care and comparing practice with standards*

The quality of care can be assessed by describing the structure, process and outcome of care. Although the outcome of care is the most appropriate measure, it is the most difficult to collect and there is reliance in many audits on the processes involved in care. These processes are those determined by the guidelines. There is a need to link process to outcome particularly from a purchasing perspective, as the resource required to improve outcome has to be estimated. There has been no work in this area for stroke. Wade (1994) outlines some process and outcome measures that can be used to assess the quality of care. He highlights the current problems of using routine NHS data for audit and the reliance on information from specific evaluations, particularly stroke registry data. Wolfe *et al.* (1993) were able to compare the processes of care in three districts using stroke registers as outlined above. The use of outcome measures is discussed in a previous chapter.

There are many case series reports describing the natural history of stroke care and outcome in different units. There are only a few published audits of stroke care. Stone and Whincup (1994) described only the process of care in relation to the Royal College of Physicians' guidelines. Stojcevic *et al.* (1995) audited the process and outcome of care in Tunbridge Wells Health Authority and demonstrated that the appropriate use of investigations increased over the study period of 18 months, that the use of rehabilitation was low and that the type of bed (medical or care of the elderly), age and sex of the stroke patient were significant predictors of receiving the appropriate service. It is assumed that the majority of audits are undertaken locally and not disseminated through the academic press.

The Royal College of Physicians of England has produced a computerised audit package (1994), developed by experts in the field but without primary care or rehabilitation input. The aim of the package is to develop methods for auditing hospital care and to enhance the quality of patient care, although only process of care is assessed.

Such groups as the WHO Pan-European Consensus Group (1995) made recommendations on measures of the quality of stroke care that could be considered. These included access to a stroke unit, access to CT facilities, case-fatality rates at 28 days, mortality and morbidity at one year, the keeping of records of pressure sores and urinary incontinence, destination on discharge, access to long-term follow up, use of secondary preventive interventions e.g. aspirin, access to aids and appliances, availability of home support, and appropriate information provision for carers. Many of these are structure or process variables which would have to be interpreted in the light of local circumstances and their relationship with outcome determined.

### Changing practice and/or altering the standards

There are no papers which demonstrate the effect of guidelines on a change in outcome for stroke patients or their carers.

### Health economics

Although guidelines have been advocated and incorporated into contracts, the financial implications of developing a service to the desired standards have not been well researched. Bowen *et al.* (1994) studied the financial implications of implementing a stroke protocol on hospital costs of stroke care in an urban community hospital in America. There were no differences in outcome between the patients treated with the protocol and those who were not (non-random allocation of patients). There were significant savings in hospitalisation costs for patients with acute stroke after the introduction of a treatment protocol. These savings were almost entirely related to decreased length of stay. The protocol led to modest differences in tests ordered and treatment provided.

### Further research

There is a need to develop national multidisciplinary guidelines for the whole of stroke care, including primary care, which can then be adapted over time and at a local level. These guidelines require evaluation.

The use of a national audit package using standardised terminology is to be encouraged. The Royal College of Physicians' audit package is a start but requires development, incorporating a multidisciplinary approach to audit and the inclusion of outcome measures at fixed assessment points. The feasibility of developing the data sets needs to be assessed and the software required for such a national audit requires development.

Audits should include process, proxy outcome and outcome measures. Although previous chapters and sections above have outlined some proposed process and outcome measures for use to monitor the quality of stroke services, there is no national agreement on which measures are suitable. Measures should have the correct properties (valid, reliable, sensitive to change in clinical condition, easy to use, administration by postal questionnaire would be an advantage) and be evaluated in several districts.

The financial implications of implementing effective guidelines and undertaking ongoing audits require evaluation.

### Information requirements

The current routinely available data in the NHS are of poor quality and are not adequate for assessing the needs for stroke services and for monitoring service developments. In primary care computerisation of records should enable GPs to record the prevalence of risk factors and the interventions undertaken to reduce identified risk, be this as a primary or secondary preventive measure. Important measures to consider include the following for monitoring prevention:  proportion of patients with atrial fibrillation or ischaemic heart disease who are on aspirin or anticoagulants; proportion of patients who have a duplex scan after stroke; and stroke recurrence rates. We have indicated the need to develop an appropriate classification of stroke and a measure of case mix. Ideally these should substitute the current ICD classifications used in the NHS, or be completed at the same time. For acute treatment,  30-day mortality rates, proportion of patients treated by a stroke team/unit, and measures of impairment, disability and handicap as outlined in the chapter on outcome measures could be used. It is vital that the outcome assessments are undertaken at fixed time-points after stroke, such as six months, and that as much of the assessment as possible can be undertaken by postal questionnaire.

# Executive summary and priorities for research

High-quality services for stroke patients can often be developed without major investment in extra resources. The majority of patients are already admitted to hospital, stay a long time and are therefore costing the NHS large sums of money. Some research has already been done which has indicated how the organisation of care can improve outcome. More is currently being undertaken, looking particularly at the interface between hospital and community care. Thus re-allocation of resources may be all that is needed to improve care, and purchasers have a responsibility to carefully analyse the evidence and commission appropriately i.e. not according to what has traditionally been the way that care has been provided, but according to what is most likely to improve outcome. More studies are needed to explore the 'black box' of rehabilitation to define which components of care are appropriate for which particular patients. The European Community is funding studies which are comparing the way that different health systems treat stroke patients and how these alternatives vary in cost and efficacy. It may be that collaborative studies between different countries will be one way of indicating which components of care are effective. Italy, for example, has very rudimentary occupational and speech therapy; while it would probably be considered unethical now to conduct a randomised controlled trial of speech therapy versus no speech therapy after stroke in this country, it may be possible to design a study which answers the same question using national differences.

For a disease as common as stroke there is a good case to be made for each district appointing an individual with special responsibility for developing and co-ordinating stroke services. In our case, public health and clinical research provided the purchasers with clear evidence of the problem; they then responded by making stroke a priority area and collaboratively funded the development of further research into the provision of community care for stroke. Close collaboration now exists between purchasers and providers in attempting to implement substitution in the community of hospital services in a planned way following evaluation.

Changes in the NHS over recent years have led to a greater need to evaluate the quality and quantity of services provided and in many instances to define specific services for specific diseases to satisfy the needs of purchasing authorities. For stroke, some aspects of care are based upon flimsy evidence of benefit and these now should be subjected to formal evaluation. Other aspects of management have been shown to be of benefit and there is no longer any excuse to delay the implementation of the changes necessary to introduce them.

From these conclusions, there are specific areas that require development of methodologies and evaluation.

The priorities for research are therefore:

1. The formal evaluation of a district stroke service, including an economic evaluation.

2. Evaluation of the benefits of clinical co-ordination of stroke services, which should include the benefits of a clinical nurse specialist.

3. Estimation of the components of an effective team and the measurement of the 'chemistry' of a team.

4. The development of locally-based preventive strategies for stroke.

5. The evaluation of different ways of providing support and information to carers.

6. The evaluation of the effect of introducing a contract for model stroke services.

7. The refining of the definition of a stroke unit.

8. The development of a national minimum data set for stroke both in primary and secondary care which should be piloted and validated. The software required to maintain such information requires development.

9. Revision of the routine NHS sources of data to incorporate minimum data set items.

# References

Bowen J, Yaste C. Effect of a stroke protocol on hospital costs of stroke patients. Neurol 1994; 44: 1961-4.

Department of Health. National Health Services review working paper 6. Medical audit. London: DOH, 1989: 3.

Effective Health Care Bulletin 2. Stroke rehabilitation. University of Leeds School of Public Health, 1992.

Grimshaw J, Russell IT. Effect of clinical guidelines on medical practice: a systematic review of rigorous evaluations. Lancet 1993: 342: 1317-22.

Kernich CA, Robb G. Development of a stroke family support and education program. J Neurosci Nurs 1988; 20: 193-7.

King's Fund Consensus Conference. Treatment of stroke. BMJ 1988: 297: 126-8.

Lindley RI, Erastus OM, Marshall J *et al.* Hospital services for patients with acute stroke in the United Kingdom: The Stroke Association survey of consultant opinion. Age Ageing 1995; 24: 525-32.

Oxfordshire Community Stroke Project. Incidence of stroke in Oxfordshire: first yearÕs experience of a community stroke register. BMJ 1983; 287: 713-7

Royal College of Physicians. Stroke Audit package. RCP, 1994.

Royal College of Physicians. Stroke: towards better management. London: RCP, 1989.

Rudd A, Wolfe CDA. Developing a district stroke service. Cerebrovascular Disease 1996; 6: 89-96.

Scottish Intercollegiate Guidelines Network. The management of patients with stroke. Discussion document 1995.

Shuling J, Groenier KH, Meyboom-de Jong B. Home treatment of patients with cerebrovascular accidents (in Dutch). Ned Tijdschr Geneesud 1993; 137: 1918-22.

Smith R. Audit and research. BMJ 1992; 305: 905-6.

Stojcevic N, Richardson E, Warburton F, Wolfe C. Audit of stroke services in a district health authority. Faculty of Public Health Medicine Conference, Spring 1995, Cardiff.

Stone SP. Whincup P. Standards of the hospital management of stroke patients. J R Coll Physician Lond 1994; 28: 52-8.

Stroke Association. Positive Steps. A progress report on district stroke services. 1995.

Thompson R, Lavender M, Madhok R. How to ensure that guidelines are effective. BMJ 1995: 311: 237-42.

Wade DT. Stroke (acute cerebrovascular disease). In: Health care needs assessment. Volume 1. (eds) Stevens A, Raftery J. Radcliffe Medical Press, Oxford. 1994: 111-255.

Wade DT, Rivermead Speciality Team. Services for people with stroke. Quality Health Care 1993; 2: 263-6.

West Lambeth Health Authority Stroke Steering Group. Setting district stroke standards and objectives. J Roy Coll Physicians of London 1992; 26: 172-6.

Wolfe CDA, Taub NA, Bryan S, Beech R, Warburton F, Burney PGJ. Variations in the incidence, management and outcome of stroke in younger residents of two health districts in southern England. J Pub Health Medicine 1995; 17: 411-8.

Wolfe CDA, Taub NA, Woodrow E, Richardson E, Warburton FG, Burney PGJ. Patterns of acute stroke care in three districts of southern England. J Epidemiol Community Health 1993; 47: 144-8.

World Health Organisation. Multidisciplinary quality development in stroke care. Report of a WHO consultation. Reykjavik, Iceland, April 1995.

World Health Organisation. Pan-European Consensus Meeting on Stroke Management. Helsingbord, Sweden, November 1995.